Victor Horsley

Victor Horsley

The World's First Neurosurgeon and His Conscience

Michael J. Aminoff
University of California, San Francisco

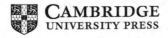
CAMBRIDGE
UNIVERSITY PRESS

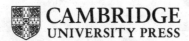

CAMBRIDGE
UNIVERSITY PRESS

Shaftesbury Road, Cambridge CB2 8EA, United Kingdom

One Liberty Plaza, 20th Floor, New York, NY 10006, USA

477 Williamstown Road, Port Melbourne, VIC 3207, Australia

314–321, 3rd Floor, Plot 3, Splendor Forum, Jasola District Centre, New Delhi – 110025, India

103 Penang Road, #05–06/07, Visioncrest Commercial, Singapore 238467

Cambridge University Press is part of Cambridge University Press & Assessment, a department of the University of Cambridge.

We share the University's mission to contribute to society through the pursuit of education, learning and research at the highest international levels of excellence.

www.cambridge.org
Information on this title: www.cambridge.org/9781009069991

DOI : 10.1017/9781009071734

First published 2022
First paperback edition 2023

A catalogue record for this publication is available from the British Library

ISBN   978-1-316-51308-8   Hardback
ISBN   978-1-009-06999-1   Paperback

Neurosurgery saved the life but sadly
not the person of Monique Aminoff.
She therefore died not once but twice.
This book is dedicated to her memory.

It is also dedicated to my father,
Abraham S. Aminoff,
whose love and support of her never faltered.

Contents

Preface   ix
Acknowledgments   xii

1. **Early Days**   1

2. **The Other Side of Gower Street**   10

3. **At the Brown**   22

4. **Dividing the Indivisible: The Localization of Cortical Functions**   38

5. **The Making of a Specialty**   52

6. **The Grammar of Neurosurgery: Technical Underpinnings**   61

7. **The Neurosurgery of Specific Disorders**   70

8. **Measures of the Man**   89

9. **The Politics of Protection**   105

10. **Not So Trivial Pursuits: The Slide into Politics**   117

11. **Antivivisectionist Claims and Clamor**   128

12. **Bitter Tears: Horsley and the Suffragist Movement**   137

13. **Last Orders: The Temperance Movement**   143

14. **Syphilis and the Public Health**   151

15. **A Surgeon Goes to War**   156

16. **Aftermaths and Appraisals**   170

Appendix 1: Horsley's Procedure for Cranial Surgery   177
Appendix 2: Appointments, Honors, and Awards   179
Appendix 3: Victor Horsley's Professional Publications   182
Appendix 4: Sir Victor Horsley's Correspondence with The Times *of London*   198
Index   200

Preface

Historians encounter Horsley's name in many different contexts, but he is now largely forgotten by a public that owes him a great deal. His life was one of paradoxes, shaded by nuances and crises that varied with the circumstances. He was born in England in 1857 and, as a young surgeon-scientist, became the superintendent of the premier institution for advanced medical research in Britain. In this capacity, he helped to define the then-unknown function of the thyroid gland, examined the cause of rabies and the means to eliminate it from Britain, and studied the localization of function in the brain. The experience gained in the laboratory enabled him to construct a new clinical specialty, that of neurosurgery. He showed that operations on the brain could be accomplished safely and effectively, and was the first surgeon to devote most of his time to the nervous system, an area of the body then largely unexplored. He thus became a celebrity, a famous doctor with the only major established and successful neurosurgical practice in the world. It seemed he could do no wrong until he fell out of favor with his colleagues who felt threatened by his social activism and began a professional boycott that caused his clinical practice to wither. What manner of man, widely admired by so many, aroused such passion among his colleagues?

In his later years, he turned increasingly from clinical work, using his fame and influence to promote social causes and devoting more time to medical and national politics. A brilliant healer of physical illness, he felt the need to improve the circumstances and context in which people lived, and used all his energy to influence social policy. It was as if he needed something new with which to challenge himself, something for which to fight, something that complemented his medical work.

The causes that he embraced to right injustices or social inequities kept him in the public eye. His combative manner sometimes offended those who opposed him, however, and the non-smoking teetotaler must have seemed insufferably righteous to those who did not share his views. No cause was too small for him if he judged it worthwhile. In addition to reforming the autocratic institutions of the medical profession to make them more responsive to their members, he advocated in support of the temperance movement and for equal opportunities for women, for the education and welfare of children, and for health insurance and paid sick leave for wage-earners (through Lloyd George's national insurance bill). He fought to protect the public from unqualified doctors or nurses, and doctors from frivolous or malicious lawsuits. At the same time, he battled the antivivisectionists, opposed the use of alcohol and tobacco, and led the medical opposition to the forcible feeding of the suffragists. He called for the government to establish a ministry of health and for an independent office of national statistics, for improved certification of disease, and for the provision of sex education for children and the improved treatment of sexually transmitted disease. Almost all of his suggestions were adopted eventually, although he did not live to see them all come to fruition. At the outbreak of World War I, while in his fifties, he volunteered for military service and died on active duty in Mesopotamia in 1916, fighting the establishment to improve the medical care of the troops. His death, tragic as it was, had an air of inevitability about it, for it would be difficult to imagine an elderly Victor Horsley, increasingly infirm, dependent on others, dying in his own bed.

Horsley was a man full of contradictions. He resented both opposing views and those who held them but was an academic, a famous professor at a university where discourse and disagreement were encouraged and not to be taken personally. He was clear-headed and thoughtful but capable of the most injudicious acts to further his own sense of social justice. He could, it seems, behave badly without any hesitation if the cause was good.

How was it that he was able to operate on the brain successfully when others failed? What led to his increasing involvement in medical and then national politics? What caused this man of position and substance to advocate so ardently for the poor, the sick, and the needy, and to attempt to right injustice and inequity wherever he encountered it. Why did this brilliant surgeon-scientist resign before the age of fifty from a leading teaching hospital in the capital of the British Empire, then at its grandest? What made him, in his sixth decade, volunteer for active military service during World War I in one of the most inhospitable regions of the world, where he died from heatstroke? Questions of this sort attracted me to study his life.

I was a student and then a junior doctor at the very hospital in London where Victor Horsley trained and subsequently was on staff, and although he had died fifty years earlier, his spirit was still very much alive at University College Hospital during the 1960s, as well as at the National Hospital. Fascinated by his achievements and reversals of fortune, I resolved to write a biography of the man who was a neurosurgical pioneer and the public conscience. Alas, within a year of my commencing the necessary research, a monograph by another was published on the same topic, and so I laid aside my own project, feeling its redundancy.

More than half a century has passed since that time. I became a neurologist and clinical neurophysiologist, and – despite moving from London to San Francisco – developed an increasing interest in the history of the neurosciences. It was thus that I came back to the life and achievements of Victor Horsley, which had so fascinated me as a young man, particularly because I believe that no published biography has yet done him justice. It remains difficult to grasp the reach of Horsley's career and interests. Stephen Paget's biography of him was a labor of love that came out in 1919, shortly after Horsley's death, and is more than one hundred years old; that by J. B. Lyons was published in 1966, fifty years after Horsley's death. Both books provide only a limited analysis of Horsley's laboratory and clinical studies and his social activism, and do not place them in the context of more recent work, leaving many questions unasked or unanswered. Moreover, they provide scholars with little in the way of

systematic documentation of source material or of Horsley's writings, despite their importance. Nevertheless, both biographies were valuable in helping me to find my way when sometimes I got lost as I delved into Horsley's life, with its twists and turns, and I remain indebted to their authors.

It is time for a reappraisal of the life of a pioneer who helped to shape not only the development of neurosurgery as a specialty but also the context and circumstances surrounding the very practice of clinical medicine, and who worked to promote legislation advancing the welfare of society. Many of the issues with which he struggled still resonate today. His achievements have not received the wide appreciation that they deserve, and he is unknown by many people. Others simply associate his name variously with a hemostatic bone wax, with a complicated apparatus for locating targets within the brain, and with outbursts of righteous indignation. One of my goals in writing this book was to set the record straight, to make the man and his achievements known to a new generation and to bring them back to the collective consciousness. There are many underlying themes to the book, however, including the interplay of science and politics, medicine and human rights, and the responsibility of physicians to themselves and for the welfare of society. The book includes discussions of social policy and their evolution, and Horsley's influence on them.

The broad range of Horsley's activities has made it difficult to capture the essence of the man. His frequent letters to the editors of *The Times* and other newspapers, however, provide some insight to his views, as does the enormous amount of non-digitized archival material that exists at University College London and in the National Archives at Kew. I was fortunate to be able to examine these archives on visits to England. Happily, I also kept the notes I had made when, in 1966, I interviewed the eighty-year-old Sir Francis Walshe, a formidable neurologist who had acted as Horsley's house surgeon in London and later spent time with him while on military service in Egypt during World War I. Today, no-one who worked with Horsley is alive to share their personal recollections of him.

It has been difficult to follow a strictly chronological course in this account without confusing the reader, because it would have meant breaking off one narrative to catch up with others.

Accordingly, I have taken the main events chronologically, but have then followed them through to the end so that each topic is discussed coherently and comprehensively in one place. I hope this will make it easier for readers to follow the twists and turns in a remarkable life.

I like to think that if Victor Horsley were alive today, he would be delighted at the manner in which scientific advances are underwriting new developments in neurosurgery and clinical medicine. He would certainly smile also at the general acceptance of the numerous causes and beliefs for which he once advocated so tirelessly, even as he would direct his efforts at righting other inequities.

Acknowledgments

Many people in the United States and Britain generously assisted me while I was preparing this book. At the University of California in San Francisco, Aaron Daley helped by tracking down reference material for me, often from obscure sources, with tremendous energy and initiative and assisted me in compiling the bibliography of Horsley's published writings. In the process he has become quite a Horsley fan himself. Theresa Devine helped by preparing some of the illustrative material. The library staff at the university – especially Andres Panado, Evans Whitaker, Bazil Menezes, and Ryan White – went to a great deal of trouble in obtaining reference material for me from many other institutions. I thank them all.

It is a pleasure to acknowledge also the assistance I received also from Jane Kirby, librarian and archivist at Bedales School; Peter Allen, archivist at Cranbrook School; Dawn Boyall, media relations manager of the Medical Defence Union; Lori Podolsky, archivist at McGill University; Richard Temple, archivist at the Senate House Library of the University of London; and Sarah Lawson, librarian at the Queen Square Library of the UCL Institute of Neurology. I am especially grateful to Steven Wright of the UCL Library Services for his help in accessing the Horsley Papers held at University College London and in the National Archives at Kew. In 1966 the late Sir Francis Walshe graciously shared with me his personal recollections of Horsley, whose house surgeon he had been and with whom he later served in the Middle East during World War I, and I greatly appreciated his insights.

The source of the various illustrations in the book is indicated in the figure legends. Many illustrations came from the Wellcome Collection in London, where William Schupbach helped me to find my way and Holly Peel provided me with certain improved high-resolution images. Other figures were from the Queen Square Archives in London, and I thank Sarah Lawson for her help in providing these. Mrs. Corinna Rock, the last surviving grandchild of Victor Horsley, graciously allowed me to include certain family photographs, for which I am grateful.

Professor emeritus Robert B. Layzer of the University of California in San Francisco read a penultimate version of the entire manuscript and Anne M. Sydor, PhD, read three of the chapters. I thank them both for their comments and suggestions. Various chapters were read by my wife, Jan, who has been a wonderful support and companion for more than forty-five years, and my gratitude to her is boundless. Our three children also looked over parts of the book. Alexandra is a pediatric rheumatologist working with the Kaiser Permanente Medical Group in Oakland, California; Jonathan is a federal defence attorney in Los Angeles; and Anthony is a federal prosecutor in Alexandria, Virginia. Their advice and comments were helpful as the book developed and I am grateful for their insights. Penny, Doushie, and Mollie provided loyal companionship and unconditional trust – as only a cat and dogs can do – while I worked on numerous drafts of this book and are remembered with great affection.

Anna Whiting at Cambridge University Press was always helpful and I am grateful for her support and encouragement. I am grateful also to Katy Nardoni for seeing the book through the production process and to Bethan Lee for her careful copyediting of the manuscript.

I am sure that there are many others who deserve my thanks, and I hope they will forgive me if I have not mentioned them by name.

Michael J. Aminoff,
San Francisco, California

Early Days

Chapter 1

It was a year of contrasts, culture, and crises. In 1857, James Buchanan presided over a United States in which African Americans were not regarded as citizens and slaves could not sue for their freedom. Queen Victoria sat comfortably on the British throne with Palmerston as her prime minister, while India mutinied. Charlotte Brontë, Charles Baudelaire, Charles Dickens, Gustave Flaubert, William Makepeace Thackeray, and Anthony Trollope were among the many writers with new books published during the year, and new musical offerings by Franz Liszt and Giuseppe Verdi were to be heard in the concert halls. In America an economic crisis led to recession, the collapse of a New York financial institution, and a run on the banks.

William Howard Taft – a future president of the United States and, later, chief justice of the supreme court – was born in 1857, as was Robert Baden-Powell, founder of the Boy Scout movement, Edward Elgar the composer, Joseph Conrad the writer, and two future Nobel laureates in medicine or physiology. Ronald Ross was honored in 1902 for his work on the transmission of malaria, and Charles Sherrington in 1932 for his studies characterizing the operation of the nervous system.

In that same year, on 14 April, a son was born in Kensington, London, to the artist John Callcott Horsley (1817–1903) and his second wife, Rosamund Haden (1820–1912), who had married in 1854. The boy had a remarkable pedigree. John Callcott Horsley was a painter, a member of the Royal Academy, and the designer of the first commercial Christmas card. His *Rent Day at Haddon Hall* received much acclaim, as also did *The Pride of the Village* and a number of his other paintings, many still on display in museums and galleries. He was known to Queen Victoria's husband, the Prince Consort, through his paintings and through his selection by a commission overseen by the prince to paint some of the frescoes for the

Houses of Parliament.[1] In his later years he had a major role in organizing the winter exhibitions of Old Masters at Burlington House, persuading private owners to lend their treasures for public display.[2]

John's father – William – was an organist and composer, especially of glees. A friend of Felix Mendelssohn, he is said to have been the first to hear Mendelssohn's music for *A Midsummer Night's Dream*, played for him at the family home in Kensington, London (at what is now 128 Church Street). William married Elizabeth Hutchins Callcott, the daughter of another composer and the niece of the well-known landscape painter, Augustus Wall Callcott (1779–1844), who was knighted by Queen Victoria in 1837 and appointed Surveyor of the Queen's Pictures in 1843.

John's wife Rosamund, known in the family as Rose, was from a distinguished medical family. Her father Charles Thomas Haden had a practice in London's smart Sloane Street, was an early enthusiast of the stethoscope, and was a medical author and editor. In 1815, he became a close friend of Jane Austen and looked after her father, who had a lung complaint. Rose's brother, Francis Seymour Haden, was a surgeon and etcher who founded the Royal Society of Painter-Etchers and Engravers in 1880 to promote original etching as an art. He presided over the society for its first thirty years; it was renamed the Royal Society of Painter-Printmakers in 1991.

Victor – the third child of John Callcott Horsley and Rosamund Haden – was named after Queen Victoria,* whose youngest child (Princess Beatrice) was born on that same day in April 1857, and he was also given his mother's maiden name of Haden. The boy's father provides an account of the circumstances in his

---

* The queen's full name was Alexandrina Victoria Guelph.

Recollections of a Royal Academician. Marianne Skerrett, head dresser to Queen Victoria and a friend of the Horsleys, was required to read to the queen. Two days after the birth of Princess Beatrice, "when she was reading the announcements of births, marriages, etc., the arrival . . . [of our son] . . . was noted . . . and there was quite a lively discussion between Her Majesty and the Prince Consort as to whether there was any good masculine version of the name Beatrice, on which they had already agreed for the Princess, which could be bestowed upon my son. The Prince said he could think of none . . . Her Majesty laughingly agreed with him" and then sent her request that the boy be named Victor Alexander after her.[3] Just over a year later, John Horsley was to paint the Princess Beatrice for the queen. The portrait shows Osborne House, the royal family's private residence on the Isle of Wight, with the sea in the background, although the sittings were all at Buckingham Palace. The painting remains in the royal art collection.

Victor had two elder brothers, Walter Charles born in 1855 and Hugh John in the following year, and a younger brother – Gerald Callcott – born in 1862. He also had three younger sisters: Emma Mary born in 1858, Fanny Marian a year later, and Rosamund Brunel in 1864. Walter became an artist and Gerald an architect; both Hugh and Emma died of scarlet fever at the age of 10 and are buried in the churchyard at St. Dunstan's, Cranbrook, Kent. Fanny married Benjamin Arthur Whitelegge, a physician and civil servant (chief inspector of factories at the Home Office) and lived to be almost ninety. Rosamund became a talented artist and costume designer for the Royal College of Music and published two works relating to her family: in 1934 *Mendelssohn and His Friends in Kensington,* based on the letters of her paternal aunts between 1833 and 1836, and in 1937 a biography of *Maria, Lady Callcott,* the writer. She married Francis Gotch, a classmate of Victor at University College, who was to become professor of physiology at Oxford. She died in 1949.

Cranbrook Days

Soon after Victor's birth, his father bought an old country house at Willesley, near Cranbrook in Kent. The countryside was pretty, access to the metropolis was easy by rail, and the area was becoming increasingly popular with a group of artists (the "Cranbrook colony") who settled there in the latter half of the nineteenth century, painting scenes of everyday rural life. In fact, it was because he was tempted by the painter Thomas Webster's account of Cranbrook that Horsley went there in the first place.[4] He commissioned the young, relatively unknown architect Richard Norman Shaw (1831–1912) to restore and enlarge the house, which had been built in the early eighteenth century. He chose well, for Shaw went on to achieve great eminence in his field, designing many country homes and commercial buildings as well as New Scotland Yard, for many years the headquarters of London's Metropolitan Police but now government offices.

The rooms in the house were well proportioned, and a grand oak-paneled drawing room with leaded windows overlooked the handsome lawns. There was a separate lodge and stable block. The house still stands, but much of it is hidden from public view by tall hedges and trees, and new housing developments have reduced the beauty of its setting. In any event, Victor spent much of his childhood there. The family moved back to London when he was sixteen, and Willesley was kept as a holiday home.

Victor's mother, a strong-minded and practical woman, was short, shy, and somewhat stern, and could be quite intimidating when she chose. She had been brought up in France, and so Victor learned French and about French culture at an early age. Victor's father was fussy about even little details and worried constantly about his family, but for good reason. His first wife, Elvira Walter, had succumbed to tuberculosis, and all three of their children had died of scarlet fever. He could be irritable and impatient over the petty frustrations of daily life, but he loved to gossip, liked company, and enjoyed a good joke. He was old-fashioned in his loyalty to queen and country, and campaigned energetically during the 1880s against the study of nudes by students at the Royal Academy, for which he was nicknamed "Clothes Horsley." He himself certainly used models, but never required them to disrobe.

Willesley was a happy place for the Horsley children. Their parents were fair and well meaning, and the household was untroubled. A skittle alley (somewhat similar to a bowling alley) was built by their father behind the house, and the children spent hours there.

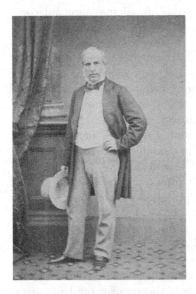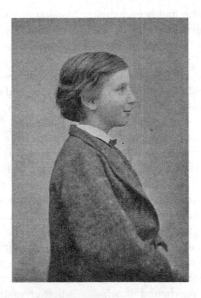

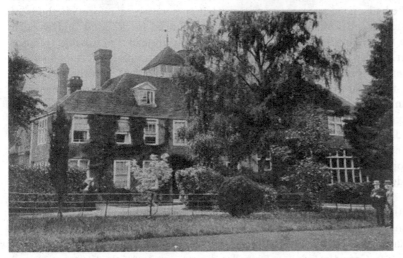

Figure 1.1 *Top left*, John Callcott Horsley, father of Victor, was a painter, Royal Academician, and designer of the first commercial Christmas card. (Photograph by Maull & Polyblank; from the Wellcome Collection, London.) *Top right*, Victor Horsley, aged 11. (From Paget S: *Sir Victor Horsley: A Study of His Life and Work*. Constable: London, 1919.) *Bottom*, the Horsley family home in Willesley, near Cranbrook, Kent. (Image courtesy of the Queen Square Archives and Sir Victor Horsley's family.)

Victor was a free-spirited, good-looking little boy, rather reckless and clumsy in his way, impetuous and often up to mischief. He spent much of his time playing at soldiers or games such as hide-and-seek; riding horses or ponies; playing tennis or skittles; collecting wild birds' eggs and nests; roaming the countryside while avoiding the gamekeepers; and getting into fights. As he got older, he also loved target practice with a pistol, walking for miles in the countryside, or just keeping fit with various exercises. Dances were always fun.

Their house was only about half a mile from the old grammar school at Cranbrook, and that is where Victor went as a day boy from 1866, when he was nine, until the family moved back to London in 1873. The Horsley boys would walk along the road to and from school except when it rained, when they traveled in a covered donkey-cart. Cranbrook school had a long history.[5] In

1518, a wealthy local man who had been yeoman of the King's Armory under King Henry VIII bequeathed the property for "a frescole house for all the poure children of Cranbroke" after his daughter failed to produce a son. Over the following three centuries, the school went through good times and bad, but in the latter half of the nineteenth century – when Victor was a pupil there – it began to grow in size, reputation, and importance. Victor started at the school in the same year that the ambitious and driven cleric, Charles Crowden, became its headmaster with the avowed aim to "make his pupils Christian Gentlemen."[6]

Victor was one of about twenty foundationers (local boys receiving a free classics education) at the school, where there were also about fifty boarders. He showed little interest in much of his studies but did well in subjects he enjoyed, winning prizes in the classics, French, and drawing.[7] He also did well in science: he had a good science teacher, and the school had recently founded a Natural Science Society at which Horsley gave a talk on the subject of water.[8] Indeed, Horsley – praised for his abilities in science – was for several years probably the only boy to be named individually by the headmaster in his annual Speech Day report.[9] He played soccer and field hockey but was not particularly good at sports. Given the many distractions of the Kentish countryside, he was often in trouble at school, but he advanced from class to class on schedule, and his days at Cranbrook were happy.

Some years later (in 1888), he gave the principal speech at the first London dinner of the fledgling Old Cranbrookian organization, expressing his gratitude to the school and to Crowden (who moved on from Cranbrook that year).[9] And when – shortly after the end of the Great War – the school adopted the house system, widely used in British fee-charging public schools, two houses for boarders were created and named for Crowden and another former headmaster, and a single day-boy house was established and named after Victor Horsley, who had died during the war.[10]

As a boy, Victor wanted to be a soldier – a cavalry officer or an officer in the artillery – an exciting prospect for a young lad brought up in a prosperous well-ordered household in the hub of the empire. The teenager frequently played at soldiers and created a Willesley army in which both he and his brother Gerald were lieutenant-

colonels, each signing himself the commander-in-chief.[11] His father, however, was against a military career, if only because of the cost involved. Although the purchase of commissions would soon be abolished, it was common for officers to live beyond their means, and a private income was a necessity, especially in the more fashionable regiments.[12] Instead, John Horsley suggested that Victor become a doctor, a suggestion that he repeated when the subject came up again, and Victor agreed – provided he could become a surgeon, not a physician. The deal was sealed, and Victor was promised a set of scalpels for his next birthday.

The choice was not very surprising for Victor's maternal grandfather and uncle were both distinguished surgeons. Uncle Francis was a particularly colorful character who believed that cremation was a waste of natural resources and found it imperative to reform methods of burial. He denounced brick vaults and wooden coffins, promoting instead a perishable coffin of papier-mâché that was designed to allow the corpse to come into contact with the soil as fast as possible.[13] Another connection to medicine was that Victor's Aunt Fanny (his father's sister) had married Seth Thompson, physician to the Middlesex Hospital in London.

Moreover, there was an entrancing medical anecdote concerning yet another member of the family. His aunt Mary Elizabeth Horsley was married to Isambard Kingdom Brunel (1806–1859), or IKB as he was known to his friends. Brunel was a civil engineer who built dockyards, bridges, tunnels, viaducts, steamships (including the first propeller-driven, iron transatlantic steamer), and the Great Western Railway. London's Paddington station was designed by him. There are numerous memorials to him in Britain, where a university is named after him. In the family, he was better known among the children for his playfulness. While pretending to swallow a gold half-sovereign to amuse them, he accidentally inhaled the coin, which became stuck in his windpipe. After a few days he developed an irritating cough and consulted the famous surgeon, Sir Benjamin Brodie, who attempted unsuccessfully to remove it with forceps through a tracheotomy. It was eventually expelled after six weeks when the poor man was attached to a tilt-table that he himself had designed, turned upside down, and gently struck on the back. After a few coughs, he felt the coin move in his chest and, a few seconds later, fall from his mouth. Thereafter, he always said that the most exquisite moment in his life was when – heels over head – he heard the gold piece strike against his upper front teeth.[14]

Victor could not have been older than fifteen when he began to direct his interests and energy toward a medical career, dissecting birds and other small animals, studying the plates in an atlas of anatomy that was among his father's books, and beginning to use a microscope. In a letter to his mother in June 1873, he lists the material he needed for the preparation of slides for the microscope.[7] He was left-handed but became ambidextrous at a young age, being required to use his right hand to write and for other activities. He also had a common form of red-green color-blindness, but this did not limit him.

At the end of 1873, Victor left Cranbrook School when the family returned to the house in Kensington. Victor spent the next several years living at home there, studying for his chosen profession, serious and focused. Holidays were spent at Willesley, where he started working with a local general practitioner, Dr. Thomas Joyce, using the microscope, studying the local natural history, and even helping with some medical cases. He was prepared for the examination to matriculate at the University of London by Philip Magnus, who at the time held a rabbinical appointment at the West London Synagogue but was supplementing his income by tutoring. Magnus (1842–1933) later became well known as an educator, mathematician, administrator, and a member of parliament. In 1880 he became director of the City and Guilds of London Institute, which eventually came to form part of the Imperial College of Science and Technology. He was knighted for his services to education in 1896 and created a baronet in 1917.

Horsley went on to University College, on London's Gower Street, to study the sciences that he would need for medical school. He was easy-going and cheery, but also confident, assertive, and always sure that his views were correct. Everything seemed to come easily and effortlessly to him. In July 1875 he not only passed the preliminary examinations in science necessary to enter medical school but gained the gold medal of the college in anatomy and two sovereigns from his proud father.

The Medical Student

Horsley was a preclinical medical student from 1875 to 1878. It was an exciting time to study medicine and the biological sciences. The concept of evolution, which had simmered in the background for some years, had received a strong push by the publication in 1859 of Charles Darwin's *The Origin of Species*. Darwin's work was popularized by the zealous Thomas Huxley (1825–1895), while Francis Galton (1822–1911) added a level of precision to studies of heredity by his contributions to statistics. Medical practice itself was changing, as was hospital care following the pioneering nursing reforms of Florence Nightingale (1820–1910) and acceptance of the antiseptic approach of Joseph Lister (1827–1912). The mysterious operations of the nervous system in health and disease were under study, and four new hospitals had opened in the metropolis for patients with neurological diseases, as discussed in Chapter 5. The nervous system was becoming the new focus of academic medicine and – not surprisingly – Horsley was soon attracted to it.

University College had been established as the original University of London in 1826 and took in its first students in October 1828. The medical department was a very active part of the institution from the beginning, and the anatomy department was especially renowned, based on the excellence of its staff. Nevertheless, there were some staffing problems and some of the original professors soon resigned, died, or were driven from office. Thus, Charles Bell (who held chairs of surgery, clinical surgery, and physiology, under the general heading of anatomy), the most famous of the professors, resigned because of mismanagement of the college and disillusionment about his own role; Granville Sharp Pattison (anatomy) was dismissed; James Richard Bennett (anatomy) died; and Robert Carswell (morbid anatomy) resigned to work in private practice and closely with European royalty. In the early 1830s the Quain brothers came to teach anatomy. Richard Quain, demonstrator and then professor of practical anatomy, went on to become professor of clinical surgery. A jealous and difficult man, he readily "imputed improper motives to all who differed from him"[15]; he died in 1887, leaving a fortune to the college. His brother Jones Quain became professor of anatomy and his well-known textbook, *Elements of Anatomy*, became the standard work in the field. He retired in 1835 and a year later William Sharpey, who had trained in Edinburgh, was appointed joint professor of anatomy and physiology. Sharpey was an outstanding teacher but not much of an experimentalist, although he encouraged his students to undertake original studies and always took an interest in their work. He retired in 1874 and died six years later.

Over the following years, the fortunes of the college fluctuated, but its emphasis on scientific enquiry from its inception established a reputation that in the last half of the nineteenth century attracted the best students and faculty in the country. In 1873, T. J. Phillips Jodrell endowed a permanent full-time professorship in physiology, with time being devoted largely to research. Jodrell himself was a somewhat colorful alumnus of the college whose eccentricity led eventually to insanity, but his endowment permitted a major step forward. The Jodrell chair in physiology became one of the most sought-after appointments in academic physiology, enabling its occupant to have a full-time research career without the need to earn a living by other means.

While Horsley was a student, the Jodrell professor of physiology was John Burdon Sanderson (1828–1905), also the first superintendent of the Brown Institution (Ch. 3). Burdon Sanderson had joined the physiology laboratory at University College in 1864, when William Sharpey was its director, and he took it over ten years later. His striking appearance – tall, thin, with piercing blue eyes – and his personality and eccentricities charmed his students, as did his approach in making the subject as experimental as possible. In the 1870s, then, British physiology was coming into its own, largely thanks to groups of researchers who had come together in Cambridge under Michael Foster (who had trained in London at University College) and at University College itself under Sharpey and then Burdon Sanderson.

Burdon Sanderson moved to Oxford as the first Waynflete professor of physiology in 1882, to be succeeded in London by his assistant, Edward Schäfer (1850–1935), who not only taught Horsley but became his first major scientific collaborator. Schäfer, whose father was of German origin, added the name of his teacher, Sharpey, to his own surname in 1918 to avoid contemporary

anti-German sentiment, commemorate his elder son (whose middle name it was), and honor his former teacher. He is best known for his work with George Oliver demonstrating the effects on the blood pressure of adrenal extracts and his discovery thereby of adrenaline. Schäfer proposed the generic term "endocrine" for the secretions of the ductless glands and predicted the existence of a pancreatic secretion regulating glucose metabolism, which he referred to as "insuline". He is also renowned for his description of a widely adopted method of artificial respiration in the prone position.

With regard to anatomy, G. Viner Ellis (1812–1900) succeeded Jones Quain, in 1850, and in 1877 was succeeded in turn by George Dancer Thane (1850–1930). Ellis, austere and seemingly remote, with an intolerance especially of smoking, required an exact observation of fact and unadorned expression of the findings of dissection. He refused to clothe "the dry bones of anatomy with any flesh of human interest" but he took his students' success or failure very personally. His grief when University College men failed badly in the Royal College of Surgeons examinations was such "that on one occasion ... he appealed to his class, with tears rolling down his face, to remove this disgrace from him."[16] He was secretive about his private life but was popularly held to keep two *ménages*. Horsley was one of a small deputation of students that went to Sharpey to enlist his support for a memorial being raised by the students to Ellis, who was about to retire.[17] Thane, professor of anatomy between 1877 and 1919, inherited a somewhat diminished department, segments of which had been lost to the physiology department, but he succeeded in restoring interest in anatomy. He had an encyclopedic knowledge of the subject and took a personal interest in his students, keeping a written record of their subsequent careers.[18]

The three years from 1875 to 1878 were spent by Horsley in hard study at University College, working late into the night to capture the essence of anatomy under Ellis and Thane, and physiology under Burdon Sanderson and Schäfer. But his efforts paid off. He was able to report on two studies of his own to the Students' Medical Society in the winter of 1875 and 1876, winning a prize of five pounds

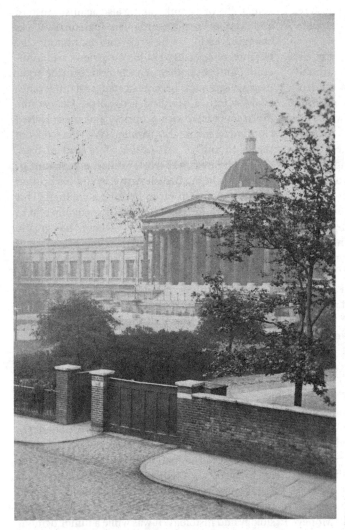

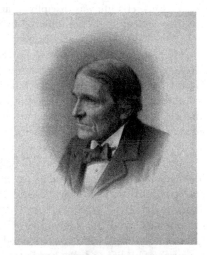

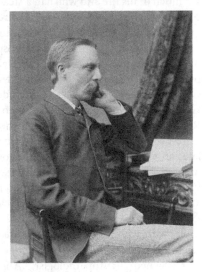

Figure 1.2 *Left*, Photograph of University College London, Gower Street, in 1871. (Photograph by Sawyer & Bird.) *Top right*, John Burdon Sanderson, Jodrell professor of physiology at the college and first superintendent of the Brown Institution. (Lithograph by G. B. Black.) *Bottom right*, Edward Schäfer (later Sharpey-Schafer), who succeeded Sanderson in the Jodrell chair and became a pioneer of hormone research. (Photograph by Elliott & Fry.) Horsley studied physiology under both men and later collaborated with Schäfer in studies of cerebral (cortical) function. (Images from the Wellcome Collection, London.)

for the second, on the microscopic structure of intervertebral discs.[17] He shared the second-prize silver medal in physiology with Francis Gotch (his future brother-in-law) in 1877, and won the silver also for practical physiology in that same year. At the time "the traditional views of physiology were essentially anatomical in character, and one of the most impressive features of Burdon Sanderson's lectures was the vivid interest of his teaching that physiology was the philosophy of function and the study of active life and living things."[19] Horsley was deeply impressed by this approach.

The tedium of study was relieved by occasional outings on the river or with his little sister Rosamund, who seemed to worship him and to whom he was particularly close. During their Sunday afternoon walks together in Kensington Gardens, Horsley would amuse her with little factoids of anatomy or biology that he had picked up from his studies. But these were minor distractions. His life was disciplined and austere, and he was seemingly uninterested in the frivolities of the dance floor or the theater.

After completing his preclinical studies, Horsley spent a month rambling around Germany with his friend John Silk, a student from King's College, admiring the countryside and culture, and learning German, of which he already had a passing knowledge through a German governess who lived with the family. He went with Burdon Sanderson's visiting card in his diary, and the card served as an introduction and "passport" to the universities and laboratories along their way.[20] Another friend dating from those early days at University College was Charles Bond, with whom he remained in contact for much of his life and who had a steadying effect on his sometimes hot-tempered nature.[17]

There were many others with whom Horsley interacted in the classroom, on the hospital wards, or in student societies: several especially talented persons were medical students at University College in the 1870s. They included Francis Gotch, mentioned earlier, who married Rosamund; Bilton Pollard, who became a respected London surgeon; Sidney Martin, later an experimental pathologist whose appointment to a professorial chair Horsley was to oppose (p. 18); Charles Beevor, who became a neurologist and worked with Horsley on the localization of function in the cerebral cortex (p. 42); Frederick Mott, with whom Horsley wrote one of his first scientific papers and who subsequently became a renowned neuropathologist; Angel Money who, despite his improbable name, became a respected pediatrician and medical author; Dawson Williams, who would serve as editor of the *British Medical Journal* for some thirty years; Dudley Buxton, who became an influential anesthesiologist; and J. E. Hine, afterwards a missionary in Africa and bishop of Northern Rhodesia, who had the remarkable distinction of possessing three doctorates – in medicine, divinity, and law.

As a student, Horsley distanced himself from alcohol once he realized that even a small amount made him sleepy and affected his concentration. It was during his student years, also, that he developed a dislike for tobacco, and he would engage in long, somewhat tedious, debates – often over Sunday dinners at home – about the evils of tobacco or alcohol. Indeed, he was becoming

something of a crank, railing also against mustard and similar condiments. His personality was changing and – as he grew into manhood – he became more assured of his own views and intolerant of those of others. Discussions became arguments, arguments became heated, and intolerance evolved into a youthful arrogance. He became more concerned with propriety and even devised clothing to ensure that women were covered from throat to ankle.[21] Also during his student days, Horsley joined the Artists' Rifles, a regiment of volunteers in the British Army, as did his brother Walter (who went on to become a colonel). This enabled him to keep up his marksmanship and to go on annual maneuvers, which he greatly enjoyed; he only stopped when the pressures of forthcoming examinations in surgery became too difficult to ignore.

There can be no doubt that the scientific approach favored at University College and by his teachers profoundly influenced the young Horsley and also stimulated his interest in hormone-related diseases, a field in which he subsequently played a decisive role. Meanwhile, more academic honors followed the student when, in the winter of 1877, he acted as one of the junior anatomy demonstrators[17] and, in 1878, he was awarded the Filliter exhibition (a cash prize of thirty pounds) in pathological anatomy. He also passed the first of the series of examinations required for the degree of bachelor of medicine of the University of London, gaining first class honors and the gold medal in anatomy, and first class honors in physiology and histology. It was while a junior demonstrator in anatomy that he examined the relationship between the vertebrae and the segmental levels of the spinal cord. His anatomical dissection clarifying this relationship formed the basis of the drawing by William Gowers (p. 57) – then on the staff of University College Hospital – in his book on the spinal cord.[22]

Horsley had already developed considerable intellectual curiosity about fundamental issues such as the brain–mind relationship. He was one of a small group of students who joined together (as the "Philomathic Society") to put down on paper their original thoughts on philosophical topics, such as the nature of the soul or whether absolute right or wrong can exist independently of "a theistic existence."[17,23] In fact, he was finding certain Christian concepts difficult to reconcile with the scientific knowledge he was acquiring from his studies and was becoming more agnostic in his beliefs.

Having completed his preclinical studies, Horsley now moved on to the wards at University College Hospital, just across Gower Street from the college. But his performance as a student had a major impact on his subsequent career. Burdon Sanderson would later help to secure for him an appointment as professor-superintendent of the Brown Institution (see Chapter 3), then a leading research institution, and Schäfer would invite his collaboration in studies of the localization of function in the cerebral cortex of animals, as discussed in Chapter 4. These studies established his reputation as a researcher and gained him the technical expertise to develop neurosurgery as a clinical specialty.

Notes

1. Boase TSR: The decoration of the new Palace of Westminster, 1841–1863. *J Warburg Courtauld Inst* 1954; **17**: 319–358.

2. Horsley JC: *Recollections of a Royal Academician. Edited by Mrs. Edmund Helps.* p. 279. Dutton: New York, 1903.

3. Horsley JC: *Recollections of a Royal Academician. Edited by Mrs. Edmund Helps.* pp. 129–130. Dutton: New York, 1903.

4. Horsley JC: *Recollections of a Royal Academician. Edited by Mrs. Edmund Helps.* p. 339. Dutton: New York, 1903.

5. Allen P: *Cranbrook School. The First Five Centuries.* Gresham: Isle of Wight, 2015.

6. Anon: Cranbrook School history. Available at: www.cranbrookschool.co.uk [last accessed June 10, 2021].

7. Paget S: *Sir Victor Horsley: A Study of His Life and Work.* pp. 12–14. Constable: London, 1919.

8. Allen P: *Cranbrook School. The First Five Centuries.* p. 88. Gresham: Isle of Wight, 2015.

9. Allen P: Personal communication, January 2016.

10. Allen P: *Cranbrook School. The First Five Centuries.* p. 136. Gresham: Isle of Wight, 2015.

11. Horsley V: *The Willesley Army.* Section D9, Horsley Papers, Special Collections, UCL Library Services (London, UK).

12. Badsey S: *Doctrine and Reform in the British Cavalry 1880–1918.* pp. 67–69. Ashgate: Aldershot (UK), 2008.

13. Anon: Obituary. Sir Francis Seymour Haden, F.R.C.S. *Lancet* 1910; **175**: 1653–1654.

14. Thiselton-Dyer TF: *Strange Pages from Family Papers.* pp. 272–283. Sampson Low, Marston: London, 1895.

15. Power D'A: Quain, Richard. p. 90. In: Lee S (ed): *Dictionary of National Biography, 1885–1900, Vol 47.* Smith, Elder: London, 1896.

16. Anon: Ellis, George Viner (1812–1900). *Plarr's Lives of the Fellows: Online.* Available at: http://livesonline.rcseng.ac.uk/biogs/E001608b.htm [last accessed June 10, 2021].

17. Bond CJ: *Recollections of Student Life and Later Days.* Lewis: London, 1939.

18. Anon: Thane, Sir George Dancer (1850–1930). *Plarr's Lives of the Fellows: Online.* Available at: http://livesonline.rcseng.ac.uk/biogs/E003228b.htm [last accessed June 10, 2021].

19. Horsley V: Obituary. Sir John Burdon-Sanderson, M.D., F.R.S. Late Regius Professor of Medicine in the University of Oxford. Some personal tributes. III. *Br Med J* 1905; **2**: 1490.

20. Horsley V: Personal papers. Section D1, Horsley Papers, Special Collections, UCL Library Services (London, UK).

21. Paget S: *Sir Victor Horsley: A Study of His Life and Work.* p. 24. Constable: London, 1919.

22. Gowers WR: *The Diagnosis of Diseases of the Spinal Cord.* Churchill: London, 1880.

23. Walker JB: Charles John Bond of Leicester (1856–1939). *J R Soc Med* 1984; **77**: 316–324.

Chapter 2

The Other Side of Gower Street

When University College, with its medical department, was built on Gower Street as the original University of London, a small dispensary was opened close by as a teaching facility. It soon became evident, however, that the medical school would need an affiliated hospital to provide clinical training. The college opened a public fund and provided a site on the other side of Gower Street to erect its own hospital, and in 1834 the hospital (originally the North London Hospital but later renamed University College Hospital) was opened. It contained one hundred and thirty beds, but when completed was intended to house another one hundred patients. Over the following years, the hospital was enlarged until it became evident that complete rebuilding was necessary. Between 1897 and 1906 a new hospital was built, largely with funds donated by Sir John Blundell Maple, the owner of a large furniture and furnishings store close to the college. The *fin-de-siècle* red-brick structure had an unusual design, with four diagonal wings, in the form of St. Andrew's cross, radiating from a central block. In 1907 a new medical school, designed by Paul Waterhouse, was erected close to it, the gift of Sir Donald Currie, a shipping magnate.

Clinical Training and Teachers

Horsley was to study and work in both the original and the new hospitals, and this chapter focuses on his time in Gower Street. He obtained his clinical training, from 1878 to 1880, at the old hospital. Training was in the form of an apprenticeship, with students attached for a set period to different senior clinicians, from whom they learned by example. They acted as clinical clerk to a physician or as dresser to a surgeon, writing the case notes of patients to whom they were assigned, following their progress, assisting in their care, and observing any surgical or other procedures that they underwent. Horsley was

attached to various senior physicians, notably Charlton Bastian (1837–1915) and Wilson Fox (1831–1887), for whom he acted as a clinical clerk, and to certain established surgeons, and in particular to John Marshall (1818–1891), whom he served as a dresser. The seniors often developed a personal interest in the students under their charge.

Bastian worked for most of his life at University College, where he had been a student, and he was one of the first neurologists appointed to the National Hospital for the Paralysed and Epileptic at Queen Square (see Chapter 5). His private consulting room was divided by a screen so that – between patients – he could undertake experiments to substantiate his somewhat exotic biological beliefs on the origin of life.[1] As an advocate of "spontaneous generation," he held that life could develop from non-living matter and that one kind of organism could appear as the offspring of another, quite different form.[2] Despite these eccentric views, he was professor of pathology at University College and a fellow of the Royal Society, in large measure because of his studies in parasitology and his work on free nematodes, of which he had described many new species. Among his published works, *The Brain as an Organ of Mind* was particularly well known, having gone into several editions and been translated into French and German. Horsley made two of the drawings in the book.

Wilson Fox was physician-extraordinary to Queen Victoria and the Holme professor of clinical medicine, one of two professorships established especially for providing clinical instruction, the other being in surgery. He had a particular interest in diseases of the lungs, especially tuberculosis, which he believed was a distinct disease rather than a nonspecific chronic inflammation as was then widely believed. A careful clinician with a large practice, he was an enthusiastic teacher, popular with the students.

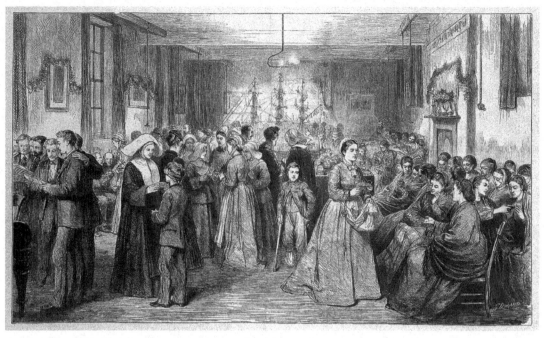

Figure 2.1 Christmas benefit at University College Hospital. (Wood engraving by G. Durand, 1874; image from the Wellcome Collection, London.)

As for the surgeon-anatomist John Marshall, a man of great charm and a friend of Horsley's painter-father, he became president of the Royal College of Surgeons and eventually of the General Medical Council. He was widely regarded as a critical and adventurous surgeon, always ready to explore new approaches.[3] Perhaps because he was already on the hospital staff, he was appointed in 1866 to the chair of surgery at University College in preference to Joseph Lister, who went on to pioneer the development of antiseptic techniques in Glasgow and then Edinburgh, before moving back to London (King's College) in 1877. Horsley, in addition to acting as Marshall's dresser while a student, served as his house surgeon in 1881.

Other contemporary members of the staff with whom the young Horsley would have interacted included the physician Sydney Ringer (1835–1910), who eventually became the Holme professor of clinical medicine. Ringer studied the actions of various inorganic salts on the heart and other tissues, showing that a solution with certain ions in specific concentrations provides a medium in which the tissues can function

normally, thus allowing their study. Ringer's solution is still widely used in clinical contexts and physiological laboratories worldwide. There was also the much-liked surgeon and venereologist, Berkeley Hill (1834–1892), whose uncle Rowland had invented the modern postal system and pre-paid postage stamps. Rickman Godlee (1849–1925) was an assistant surgeon, an exacting and sometimes harsh teacher who in 1884 was to perform the first operative removal of a brain tumor (see Chapter 5). He later became professor of clinical surgery, surgeon to the royal household of Queen Victoria, and surgeon-in-ordinary to King Edward VII and King George V. He and Horsley were to disagree on a variety of issues, discussed in later chapters. Christopher Heath (1835–1905), the fussy Holme professor of clinical surgery, had an unwavering belief in his own views and briskly rejected Lister's antiseptic techniques. He found Horsley difficult, and the two of them clashed in later years when Horsley was appointed to the staff.

In contrast to Heath, Marcus Beck (1843–1893) was a skilled surgeon, inspiring teacher, and a champion of antisepsis who eventually

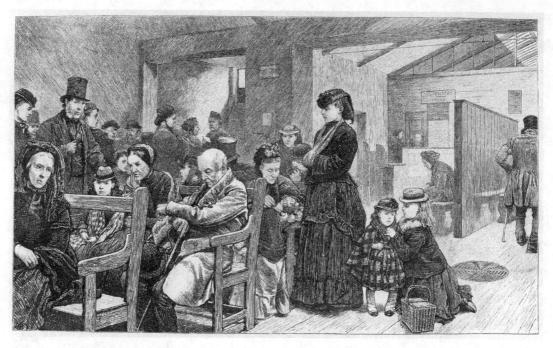

Figure 2.2 The outpatients waiting room and dispensary at University College Hospital. (Wood engraving, 1872; image from the Wellcome Collection, London.)

succeeded Marshall in the chair of surgery. Beck loved his students, just as they worshipped him. He stressed to them his belief that surgical practice required a solid grounding in pathology, a belief that clearly influenced the young Horsley, who held him in the highest regard. Beck – in turn – had no doubt that Horsley was brilliant and would go far.

William Gowers (1845–1915), assistant physician to the hospital when Horsley was a student, went on to become one of the greatest neurologists of the period and collaborated with Horsley in managing many clinical cases. Sir Russell Reynolds (1828–1896), physician to Queen Victoria's household and another distinguished neurologist, was also on staff. He was articulate, popular, but grave. In 1870 he had given a series of lectures on the clinical uses of electricity that Gowers, then his student, transcribed verbatim, so that it could be published in book form.[4] Sir William Jenner (1815–1898), on the consulting staff, was plainspoken and an excellent teacher, and became president of the Royal College of Physicians. He had shown the separate identity of typhus

and typhoid fever, was physician to Queen Victoria, and attended Albert, the Prince Consort, during his fatal attack of typhoid fever. The staff at the hospital thus consisted of outstanding clinicians, teachers, and investigators, who were nationally prominent and acted as wonderful role models for the students in their charge. They served Horsley well.

It was with Bastian that Horsley wrote his first medical paper, which was published in 1880 in one of the earliest volumes of the neurological journal *Brain*. It recounted the autopsy findings after the sudden cardiac death of a twenty-six-year-old clerk, whose small, underdeveloped left upper limb was associated with an extremely small ascending parietal convolution in the right cerebral hemisphere.[5] The case was somewhat similar to another described previously by Gowers, and provided support for the belief that there was a functional relationship between the affected brain region and movement of the opposite hand and fingers, in agreement with the experimental evidence of David Ferrier obtained just a few years earlier

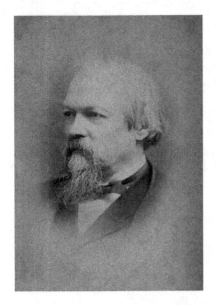
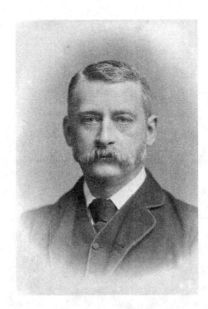

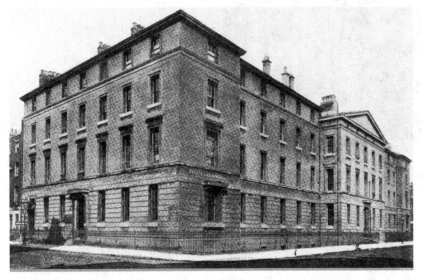

Figure 2.3 *Top left*, John Marshall, surgeon-anatomist and later president of the Royal College of Surgeons. Horsley served as his surgical dresser and then his house surgeon. *Top right*, Marcus Beck, Marshall's beloved successor to the chair of surgery at University College and a great admirer of Horsley. *Bottom*, The original North London Hospital, renamed University College Hospital, where Horsley was a medical student and then worked. (Images from the Wellcome Collection, London.)

and published in his 1876 classic, *Functions of the Brain*.[6]

In November 1880, Horsley passed the examination for membership of the Royal College of Surgeons and thus was able to enter clinical practice. His student days were ending. He had been one of a remarkably talented class, and the nicknames given to him by his peers are revealing: "the professor" because of his broad knowledge and opinionated manner, "Archibald Allright" for his cheery optimism, "the germ" for his interest in bacteriology, and "the vulture" because of his enthusiasm for postmortem examinations.

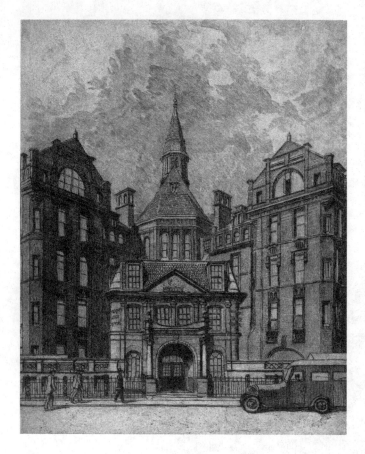

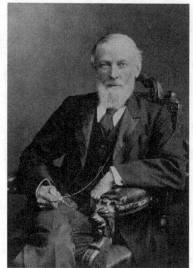

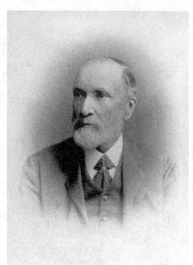

Figure 2.4 *Left panel,* The new University College Hospital was completed in 1906. The building is now a research center. *Top right,* William Gowers was renowned as a master clinician at the hospital. One of Horsley's teachers, he later became his collaborator and colleague. (Images from the Wellcome Collection, London.) *Bottom right,* Charlton Bastian, the physician-neurologist for whom Horsley worked as a clinical clerk, was also professor of pathology at University College. It was with Bastian that Horsley wrote his first medical paper. (Image from the Queen Square Archives.)

Life as a Junior Doctor

After a brief sea voyage to Gibraltar, he became house surgeon for six months to Marshall, who encouraged him to study the structure of nerves. During 1881, he graduated from the university with the degrees of bachelor of medicine and bachelor of surgery (MB, BS). (In Britain and certain Commonwealth countries, medicine was and remains an undergraduate course leading to bachelor degrees; a doctorate in medicine is an advanced degree awarded for original research.) Horsley gained first class honors and a medal in surgery,[7] second class honors in obstetrical medicine and forensic medicine (pathology), and third class honors in medicine (internal medicine).

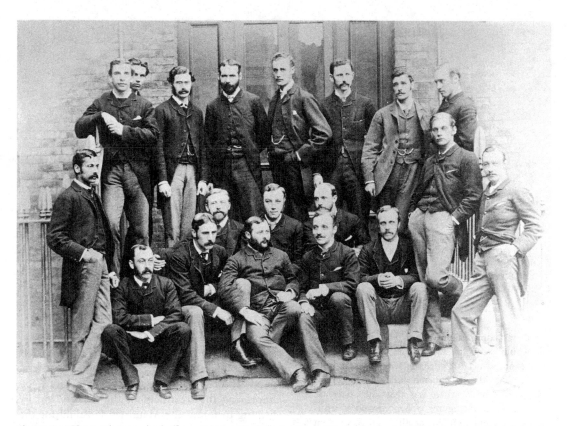

Figure 2.5 The resident medical officers at University College Hospital. Victor Horsley is in the back row, on the left, leaning against the railings. Photograph circa 1880. (Image from the Wellcome Collection, London.)

His co-medalist in surgery was Charles Ballance, who later became an illustrious neuro-otological surgeon. Within a few years of their graduation, Ballance was to assist Horsley in his pioneering removal of a tumor compressing the spinal cord (see Chapter 5).

Horsley became surgical registrar at the hospital and – in 1882 – shared lodgings in Charlotte Street with his friend and former classmate, Charles Bond. He was appointed assistant professor of pathology at University College in that same year, and shortly afterwards moved to new accommodation at 129 Gower Street, which he shared with Arthur Whitelegge, who later married his sister Fanny. An English Heritage blue plaque now marks the house.

Somewhat recklessly, in 1881 and 1882 Horsley studied the effects of anesthetics on himself regardless of the fears of friends and colleagues. He inhaled chloroform, ether, or nitrous oxide and dictated to the other house staff the progressive loss of his abilities, such as when he became unable

to move his limbs, while they recorded the character and content of his speech, his tendon and superficial reflexes, and his level of consciousness. The anesthesia was pushed until he was unconscious and sometimes cyanosed; recovery was often accompanied by muscle spasms, convulsive struggles, and agitation. He published his findings in the journal *Brain*, showing that different anesthetics affected the reflexes differently: during nitrous oxide anesthesia the knee jerk – a stretch reflex – persisted while the superficial reflexes disappeared, in contrast to the findings during asphyxial states or with chloroform.[8] He referred to these experiments in his 1900 Lees and Raper Memorial Lecture but from a different perspective, using them to support his views on the adverse effects of alcohol:

I arranged a table by my side with writing paper on it, held a pencil while the [laughing]

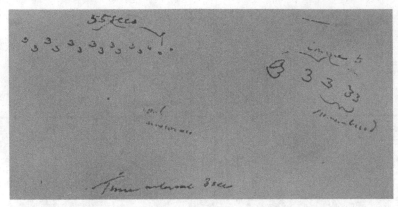

Figure 2.6 Photograph of the paper on which Horsley began writing the number three in alternating rows while inhaling nitrous oxide. There is a gradual decrease in the size of the numeral as consciousness becomes depressed (*left side of figure*), but the arrangement in rows is not disturbed until he becomes unconscious (after fifty-five seconds). As he recovers, he begins writing threes again, but in one line rather than in alternating rows (*right side of figure*). See text for further details. (From Horsley V: *The Effect of Alcohol upon the Human Brain: A Lecture. The Second Lees and Raper Memorial Lecture.* Lees and Raper Memorial Trustees: London, 1900.)

gas was administered to me, and resolved that I would write the figure 3, as being a simple mechanical act, in alternate rows. ... In fifty-five seconds I became unconscious, and concurrently ... [there was a] gradual decrease in the size of the figures, a phenomenon which is the representation in another form of that observed by patients when gradually becoming unconscious from fainting or from an epileptic attack – namely, the apparent diminution of size of objects they are looking at. ... [Although] the figures are written smaller, the more complicated thought is preserved and the writing of the threes in rows has not been disturbed.

As I began to recover consciousness I recommenced writing. I remembered ... that I was to write threes, but although they are written correctly enough, they are no longer in alternate order – that is to say, the idea had been entirely blotted out of my mind by the very slight and fleeting poisoning of the cortical centres by the laughing gas. It is remarkable how easily the cortex of the brain can by a little chemical intervention have blotted out from it the highest impressions ... and hence it is not surprising ... that alcohol in those very small quantities which come within the so-called limit of the dietetic use of the drug first causes an apparent stimulation of the cortex, which is really loss of balance, and then very quickly paralyses its activity.[9]

As a student and then assistant professor of pathology, Horsley collaborated on a bacteriological project with Frederick Mott (1853–1926), his former classmate at University College, who also held junior appointments at its hospital. Mott was to achieve fame by establishing that general paralysis of the insane is due to syphilis, by improving the treatment of the insane, and by helping to found the Maudsley Hospital for the mentally ill in London.

In October 1882, Horsley and Bond holidayed together in Italy, traveling via Gibraltar. They stopped at Pisa, Naples, Pompeii, and Paestum (where Horsley armed himself with a revolver as a defense against roaming bandits), and then in Rome, where they visited the monuments and medieval churches but were shocked by the maggot-infested wounds of surgical patients at one of the hospitals. The antiseptic approach in use at University College Hospital was apparently not yet favored in the eternal city.[10,11] They toured the art galleries of Florence in the company of an artist friend of Horsley's father, Sir Frederic (later Lord) Leighton, painter, sculptor, and then president of the Royal Academy. Leighton was the first painter to receive a peerage, becoming Baron Leighton in the New Year's Honours List of 1896. He died the next day of heart disease. Finally, Horsley and Bond went on to Venice by train but, because local flooding submerged the track in places, the journey from one station to another sometimes had to be made by boat.[10]

The year 1883 was a momentous one for Horsley both professionally and domestically. In June he passed the required examinations to become a fellow of the Royal College of Surgeons of England, the passport to success as a surgeon in Britain and the empire. The examinations were daunting: The first part consisted of a six-hour written examination in anatomy and physiology followed by practical examinations on anatomical specimens and histological slides. The second part involved a four-hour written examination in pathology, surgery, and therapeutics, and then a clinical section that required two patients to be examined for thirty minutes each, followed by an oral examination in front of the entire court of examiners. Candidates also performed mock operations on at least two dead subjects while observed by a pair of examiners, and were examined orally in surgical anatomy and in pathology and surgery.[12] About half the candidates generally passed, the others being referred to repeat the examination in six or twelve months.

Then, in October, he became engaged to be married. As a young man, Horsley had shown little interest in women outside his own family circle, and his intolerance of tobacco and alcohol and rigid views about how women should dress – covering virtually everything – did not help to attract romantic partners. Although he was focused on his work, he found time for travels, social gatherings, fencing, tennis, and other recreational activities, but he did not seek out female companions. His engagement, to Eldred Bramwell, therefore came as something of a surprise to those who knew him.

The Bramwells were a distinguished family: Eldred's father was an engineer, legal consultant, and the younger son of a banker, while her uncle was an influential barrister and judge. Eldred was born in October 1855, the second of three sisters. The family lived at 1A Hyde Park Gate, in Kensington, London, and had friends in common with the Horsleys. The three Bramwell sisters became friends with the Horsley girls, whom they often met when walking in Kensington Gardens, and the Bramwell family even rented Willesley for a summer. Eldred was reserved, somewhat shy, considerate, and highly intelligent. When Horsley hesitated between pure pathology and surgery, it was she who urged him "to go in for surgery."[13] She was practical, sensible, and took herself seriously, but in appearance was rather ordinary. She was to become a wonderful support for Horsley in all his endeavors.

In 1883, Marshall gave the Bradshaw lecture at the Royal College of Surgeons in London, speaking on the relief of pain by nerve stretching, and this was subsequently published in book form together with twelve anatomical illustrations contributed by Horsley.[14] Horsley had been working on the structure of nerves at Marshall's suggestion, but he never published his findings in humans in any detail. He did present them at professional meetings in early 1884, however, reporting that nerves have within their sheaths their own sensory nerves, the so-called *nervi nervorum*, that are distinct from nerves to the blood vessels of the nerves (*nervi vasorum*), and are associated with specialized mechanoreceptors of two kinds, namely Pacinian corpuscles and Krause end-bulbs. These might account for the occurrence and localization of certain nerve pains and – he suggested – perhaps also provide information about the position of the limbs and contribute to the so-called muscle sense (supplementing the information obtained from receptors in the muscles and tendons).[15,16] His findings concerning the presence of *nervi nervorum* and their sensory receptors were confirmed by others more than seventy years later[17] and are now widely accepted.[18,19] There is support for his suggestion that they contribute to nerve trunk pain,[20] but any contribution to the muscle sense is unlikely.

As surgical registrar, Horsley was responsible for overseeing the preparation of annual reports summarizing the cases seen at the hospital, and these were published in the *North London or University College Hospital Report of the Surgical Register*, with a preface by him. Charts detailed every surgical procedure performed over the year. Horsley improved the practical value of the reports by deleting unnecessary material, adding new tables to facilitate analysis of the causes of various disorders, and providing his own conclusions.[21] He also devoted much time to teaching students and house staff not just the theoretical basis of surgery but also how to keep good clinical records of their patients.

In 1883, Edward Schäfer succeeded Burdon Sanderson in the Jodrell chair of physiology at University College, and decided to extend the innovative work of Ferrier and Yeo (see Chapter 5) on cortical localization. He asked

Horsley to collaborate with him, but with time and changing circumstances, Horsley later continued the experiments independently or in collaboration with others.[3] They were important and – in addition – gave Horsley a particular expertise in operating on the brain that helped him as he began to treat certain neurological disorders by surgery (discussed in Chapter 5).

Steps up the Professional Ladder

Horsley resigned his position as surgical registrar in 1884 on his appointment as professor-superintendent of the Brown Institution (see Chapter 3). Nevertheless, he continued to give the series of systematic lectures to the nursing staff that he had begun while registrar, helping to usher in a new approach to the training of nurses.[22] He was appointed assistant surgeon at University College Hospital in 1885, and with this surgical promotion moved from Gower Street to smarter rental premises at 80 Park Street (near Grosvenor Square, Mayfair). He worked hard both clinically in general surgical practice and on his research projects, devoting his Thursday afternoons and Saturdays mornings to research work and the rest of Saturday to pathology. He accordingly tried to avoid seeing patients then except when they had urgent surgical problems. His laboratory work gave him particular satisfaction that he shared with close friends.

In February 1886, Horsley was appointed surgeon to the National Hospital at Queen Square in Bloomsbury. His work there – the foundation of modern neurosurgery – is discussed in later chapters. In the following year he succeeded Bastian as professor of pathology at University College, a position that he held until 1896, during which time he introduced the methods of experimental research into pathology.[23] Contemporary pathologists had focused primarily on morbid anatomy – the anatomical alterations that occur in diseased tissues and organs – and showed little interest in understanding the basis or pathophysiology of such changes.[24] In consequence, Horsley chose not contribute to meetings of the Pathological Society.[25] His own teaching about disease processes was based particularly on experiments that allowed these processes to be studied in detail, and he prepared for class experiments with great care. His enthusiasm inspired many of his students with the intellectual curiosity

necessary for research. He also developed a division of pathological chemistry headed by Vaughan Harley, an Edinburgh graduate. The division became a research center in its own right and Horsley used it as his formal affiliation in various publications. Among his other assistants was Rubert Boyce (1863–1911), later professor of pathology at Liverpool and inaugural dean of the now-famous Liverpool School of Tropical Medicine.

When eventually he stepped down from the chair, Horsley's students and colleagues presented him with some silver and an album of photographs of fifty-one of those who had worked with him or under his direction, listing their achievements. His enemies – the antivivisectionists (see Chapter 11) – proposed that the album's cover should consist of an arrangement of figures of animals in various stages of mutilation.[26] Horsley's resignation from the chair should have been a happy occasion, but his unsuccessful attempts to influence the choice of his successor led to a bitter quarrel with Schäfer, his former collaborator, who had written a strongly supportive letter to secure Horsley the appointment to the National Hospital. Angry words were exchanged both in private and in public, in writing and in person. Despite Schäfer's plea not to take the matter personally, Horsley did exactly that.[27] Time healed the breach, but things were never quite the same again. As for the chair of pathology, Sidney Martin – whose main contributions related to infectious diseases, particularly tuberculosis – was appointed, rather than Vaughan Harley, the chemical pathologist whom Horsley would have preferred. Harley was thereupon appointed professor of pathological chemistry at the college and held the chair until 1919.

As assistant surgeon to University College Hospital, Horsley had several run-ins with the imperious Christopher Heath, his senior on the surgical staff. There is a story that on one occasion, the prickly Heath gave Horsley a dressing down for neglecting his hospital work when it seemed that he was thirty minutes late for an outpatient clinic. Horsley remained untroubled by the outburst and – when asked why he was not with his patients – responded languidly "I've seen them already."[28] Heath's frequent complaints about and to Horsley,[29] and the differences that existed between them – both clinically and in daily life – reflected in part the disparity in their ages but also a certain antipathy between them.

Horsley was appointed full surgeon to outpatients at the hospital in 1893, and surgeon with charge of beds and professor of clinical surgery from 1900 until his retirement from the active staff in 1906 at the age of forty-nine; he then joined the consulting staff. Despite his professional success, he remained prickly and sensitive to gossip or criticism, regardless of its source. In 1894, for example, he wrote accusingly to Sydney Ringer, one of his former teachers, whom he believed had commented adversely on his surgical expertise and reputation to a colleague, an aspersion that Ringer flatly denied.[30]

Horsley retained his interest in general surgery until the turn of the century, but focused his work increasingly toward neurosurgery. On one occasion, he performed an appendectomy on the son of Sir Luke Fildes, the Victorian painter whose *The Doctor* remains on display in London's Tate Gallery and in 1949 was reproduced in posters and on brochures by the American Medical Association as part of a campaign against a proposal by President Harry Truman for nationalized medical care. Fildes was a great friend of Sir Frederick Treves, the abdominal surgeon who had performed one of the first appendectomies in England some years earlier, but Treves was in South Africa – a volunteer at a field hospital during the second Boer War – at the time. Unfortunately, Horsley only removed part of the appendix, leaving its stump behind, and the boy's symptoms later recurred. Treves, by this time back home, was consulted: "I do wish Horsley would stick to his bloody skulls and leave bellies to me."[31] Not surprisingly, Horsley passed a lot of general surgery to his clinical assistant, Wilfred Trotter (1872–1939), who succeeded him. Trotter was an unassuming and meticulous general surgeon with, like Horsley, a special interest in the thyroid gland and nervous system. Among his important contributions was his publication on subdural hematomas, in which he emphasized that early operation may be life-saving. He also authored the well-known *Instincts of the Herd in Peace and War* (first published in 1916), a sociological and psychological classic that analyzes the behavior of individuals when part of a group, the relationship of the group to the individual, and the organization of different (British and German) social orders. In 1928, Trotter was summoned to Buckingham Palace to treat King George V for pleural empyema (which he drained successfully) and was informed that a car would be sent for him; he supposedly responded, "That's alright. I can take the No.14 bus, which goes right by it."

Horsley also held administrative posts at University College, becoming vice dean of the medical faculty in 1891, and dean and chairman of the medical committee of the hospital from 1893 to 1895. In August 1897 he was elected a member of the senate of the University of London,[32] and served on it for three years. The university, established in 1836 with University College as one of its two founding colleges, was then reconstituted as a federal collection of colleges and medical schools, and the composition of its senate was changed. Horsley was also a member of the university's committees on examinations in science and medicine.[33] Meanwhile, he maintained an active laboratory at the college,[13] and he continued his work on the nervous system there and his pioneering approach to clinical neurosurgery at the National Hospital (see Chapters 5, 6, and 7). As if he were not busy enough, Horsley was appointed a special constable in November 1887,[34] just five days after the events of "Bloody Sunday" in which the police and army clashed in London with socialists, the unemployed, and demonstrators against British actions in Ireland. Further unrest and demonstrations followed, but it is not known whether he actually became involved in peace-keeping activities.

Although there were many competing demands on his time, Horsley never seemed in a hurry but always focused intently on the task in hand, giving it his full attention, carrying it out efficiently and with startling speed. Even after he had retired from the active staff because of the pressure of his private practice, his other professional activities, and his increasing public work as a medical and social reformer, he made himself freely available to consult on clinical cases, and his wide-ranging experience always brought fresh insight to bear. Infection was a feared complication of any surgical intervention and Horsley was a firm believer in antisepsis, following the lead of Marcus Beck and John Marshall, who had so influenced him earlier. Indeed, in a photograph taken the day before he was to have his own appendix removed, Horsley appears somewhat bulky due to an antiseptic dressing wrapped around him.[35] His ward teaching was limited – it seemed as if he were too busy – but took the form more of a consultation and discussion between colleagues than the rigid exposition of personal views that characterized his public life.

Horsley's day was a long one. He had developed the trick of taking a brief nap for about fifteen minutes whenever he was exhausted, falling asleep immediately and awakening refreshed and re-energized to take on further tasks. He typically breakfasted at around 7:30 A.M. and was usually in the operating room by 8 o'clock. He would then work almost continuously until 11 o'clock at night. He had large clinical practices at University College Hospital and the National Hospital, as well as a substantial private practice in which his patients were placed in a plush nursing home at No. 9, Mandeville Place. He cared intensely for the welfare of his patients regardless of their social standing, and was kind and considerate of them. He always did their first dressings himself, later ones being entrusted at University College Hospital to his assistants, Wilfred Trotter and Rupert Bucknall. Bucknall was a brilliant young surgeon who unhappily failed to live up to his early promise. He had minor epileptic seizures (transient blank spells) that fascinated the medical students working with him, and unpredictable bursts of rage that frightened them.[36] He eventually was found to have tertiary neurosyphilis,[37] had to resign all his appointments in 1910, and died two years later.

Notes

1. Holmes G: *The National Hospital Queen Square, 1860–1948.* pp. 38–39. Livingstone: Edinburgh, 1954.

2. Anon: Obituary. Henry Charlton Bastian, M.A., M.D. Lond., F.R.C.P., F.R.S. *Br Med J* 1915; **2**: 795–796.

3. Tweedy J: Victor Horsley Lecture: The late Prof. John Marshall, F.R.S. *Lancet* 1923; **202**: 1007–1008.

4. Reynolds JR: *Lectures on the Clinical Uses of Electricity Delivered in University College Hospital.* Churchill: London, 1871.

5. Bastian HC, Horsley V: Arrest of development in the left upper limb, in association with an extremely small right ascending parietal convolution. *Brain* 1880; **3**: 113–116.

6. Ferrier D: *The Functions of the Brain.* Smith, Elder: London, 1876.

7. Anon: *University of London. The Historical Record (1836–1912). Being a Supplement to the Calendar.* University of London Press: London, 1912.

8. Horsley V: Note on the patellar knee-jerk. *Brain* 1883; **6**: 369–371.

9. Horsley V: *The Effect of Alcohol upon the Human Brain: A Lecture. The Second Lees and Raper Memorial Lecture.* p. 10. Lees and Raper Memorial Trustees: London, 1900.

10. Bond CJ: *Recollections of Student Life and Later Days.* Lewis: London, 1939.

11. Walker JB: Charles John Bond of Leicester (1856–1939). *J R Soc Med* 1984; **77**: 316–324.

12. Gant FJ: *A Guide to the Examinations at the Royal College of Surgeons of England for the Diplomas of Member and Fellow.* pp. 22–36. Baillière, Tindall, Cox: London, 1881.

13. MacNalty A: Reminiscences of Sir Victor Horsley. *Ann R Coll Surg Engl* 1962; **31**: 120–126.

14. Marshall J: *Neurectasy or Nerve-Stretching for the Relief or Cure of Pain, Being the Bradshaw Lecture delivered at the Royal College of Surgeons of England on the 6th December, 1883.* Smith, Elder: London, 1887.

15. Horsley V: Preliminary communication on the existence of sensory nerves in nerve-trunks, true "nervi nervorum." *Br Med J* 1884; **1**: 166.

16. Horsley V: Preliminary communication on the existence of sensory nerves and nerve endings in nerve trunks, true "nervi nervorum." *Proc R Med Chir Soc Lond* 1885; **1**: 196–198; Proceedings of the Physiological Society, 1884. *J Physiol* 1885; **5**: xvii–xviii.

17. Hromada J: On the nerve supply of the connective tissue of some peripheral nervous system components. *Acta Anat (Basel)* 1963; **55**: 343–351.

18. Sugar O: Victor Horsley, John Marshall, nerve stretching, and the *nervi nervorum. Surg Neurol* 1990; **34**: 184–187.

19. Vilensky JA, Gilman S, Casey K: Sir Victor Horsley, Mr John Marshall, the *nervi nervorum*, and pain. *Arch Neurol* 2005; **62**: 499–501.

20. Asbury AK, Fields HL: Pain due to peripheral nerve damage: An hypothesis. *Neurology* 1984; **34**: 1587–1590.

21. Merrington WR: *University College Hospital and its Medical School: A History.* pp. 104–105. Heinemann: London, 1976.

22. Merrington WR: *University College Hospital and its Medical School: A History.* p. 254. Heinemann: London, 1976.

23. Merrington WR: *University College Hospital and its Medical School: A History.* p. 219. Heinemann: London, 1976.

24. Horsley V: Introductory remarks delivered in the section of pathology. *Br Med J* 1892; **2**: 248–249.

25. Horsley V: The study of pathology. [Letter to the editor.] *Br Med J* 1892; **2**: 435.

26. Anon: Notes and notices. *Zoophilist* 1896; **16**: 82.

27. Schäfer EA: Letters to Victor Horsley dated March 21, 25, and 31, and April 8, 1896, and Horsley's response dated April 8, 1896. Section A50, Horsley Papers, Special Collections, UCL Library Services (London, UK).

28. Jones E: Sir Victor Horsley. [Letter to the editor.] *Br Med J* 1957; **1**: 1065.

29. Heath C: Letters to Victor Horsley between 1892 and 1899. Section E4/8, Horsley Papers, Special Collections, UCL Library Services (London, UK).

30. Horsley V: Letter to Sydney Ringer dated June 1894. Section E3/12, Horsley Papers, Special Collections, UCL Library Services (London, UK).

31. Abraham JJ: *Surgeon's Journey.* p. 389. Heinemann: London, 1957.

32. Letter from MW Ridley to Lord Herschell, Chancellor of the University of London, dated August 31, 1897 concerning the appointment of Horsley to the Senate. *Senate Minutes, 1897–1898.* pp. 158–159, minute 334. UoL/ST/2/2/14, Archives and Manuscripts, Senate House Libraries, University of London, London, UK.

33. Anon: *University of London Calendar 1898–1899.* pp. 20–21. UoL/UP/1/17/55, Archives and Manuscripts, Senate House Libraries, University of London, London, UK.

34. Certificate no. 299, dated November 18, 1887, appointing Victor Horsley a special constable. Section D9, Horsley Papers, Special Collections, UCL Library Services (London, UK).

35. Merrington WR: *University College Hospital and its Medical School: A History.* p. 46. Heinemann: London, 1976.

36. Walshe FMR: Personal communication, July 15, 1966.

37. Jones E: *Free Associations: Memories of a Psycho-Analyst.* pp. 126–127. Basic Books: New York, 1959.

3

At the Brown

Founded in 1871, the Brown Animal Sanatory Institution of the University of London survived legal challenges to its birth and spawned legal proceedings at its closure. It thrived initially despite chronic underfunding, but it was shut down in 1939 at the onset of war, was damaged by bombs during the hostilities, and was subject to a compulsory purchase order by the local authorities once peace was declared. Nevertheless, it was for a time the premier research institution for the medical sciences in Britain, and to work there was in itself both an achievement and a privilege. Its staff was among the most distinguished in the land.

Thomas Brown and His Institution

The institution was established under the terms of a trust set up by one Thomas Brown of Dublin and the isle of Anglesey, who died in 1852. Brown seems to have had a law degree, probably from Dublin, but there is no record that he ever practiced as a lawyer. In his will, he left to the University of London about twenty thousand pounds to set up an Animal Sanatory Institution within a mile of Westminster or Southwark in the capital, or in Dublin "for investigating, studying, and without charge beyond immediate expenses, endeavouring to cure, maladies, distempers, and injuries, any Quadrupeds or Birds useful to man may be found subject to."[1,2] The interest on the capital sum was to be allowed to accumulate for up to fifteen years, but if the institution had not been established within nineteen years of Brown's death, the trust was to pass to the University of Dublin [Trinity College] to establish professorships in three or more languages, namely in "Welsh, Sclavonic, Russian, Persian, Chinese, Coptic, and Sanscrit."[1]

It was a strange legacy, not least because of the exotic languages selected for study in Ireland, and it has never been clear why Brown wished to support research on animal diseases, even if for the ultimate benefit of humankind.[3] Despite assertions of insanity by the family[1] and legal challenges by the University of Dublin based in part on the ancient Statute of Mortmain (which did not allow the gift of land to the church or corporate bodies), the will was upheld. There were certain restrictions; for example, the money could not be used to buy or rent land or cover building costs on a leased site, although it could be used to rent already-existing buildings. Because the accumulated income was insufficient to cover rental costs plus the salary of staff and any general expenses, the university attempted unsuccessfully to alter the terms of the will through an act of parliament. It was faced with losing the entire bequest to Dublin until Burdon Sanderson – the experimentalist from University College – induced a wealthy merchant to donate two thousand pounds and then a further seven hundred pounds so that property could be bought. This enabled a suitable site to be purchased for the institution at 149 Wandsworth Road, Vauxhall, south of the Thames in an unfashionable suburb of London (but not far from The Oval, the famous cricket ground).

Thus the Brown Institution was established and placed under the charge of a committee, of which Professor William Sharpey (p. 6) was the first chairman. Burdon Sanderson was elected professor-superintendent, with Dr. Edward Emanuel Klein – who was to become an eminent bacteriologist – as his assistant. There was accommodation for the professor-superintendent, and for a veterinary assistant, stableman, and housekeeper. The superintendent was required to give at least five free public lectures a year.

As required by the trust, the institution had a clinical side: its hospital provided mainly out-patient veterinary services to several thousand animals every year, the majority initially being horses but, in later years, smaller animals such as

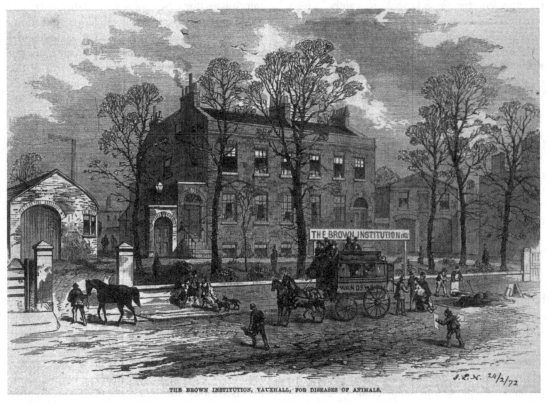

THE BROWN INSTITUTION, VAUXHALL, FOR DISEASES OF ANIMALS.

Figure 3.1 The Brown Animal Sanatory Institution of the University of London, for some years the premier research institution for the medical sciences in Britain. Horsley was professor-superintendent from 1884 to 1890. (Wood engraving made shortly after the institution was founded in 1871; courtesy of the U.S. National Library of Medicine.)

cats and dogs. Experimental work was performed not on these patients but on animals specially obtained for research purposes, and the facilities were so good that for many years they were unequalled in the capital, even though the superintendent had to provide his own equipment. Indeed, the new research center rapidly gained in stature and authority as its staff undertook work for local and national government bodies and various professional societies. Nevertheless, it failed to grow and was eventually sidelined by larger, more central, and financially more robust establishments. It is now all but forgotten, and few appreciate its importance in Victorian Britain when the focus of science departments at medical schools was generally on teaching rather than research.

Almost from its creation, its research staff became a target for the antivivisectionist movement, discussed in Chapter 11. In 1876, after the passage of the Cruelty to Animals Act, which was the first national legislation of its kind in the world and remained in force until 1986, the use of live animals in scientific research was regulated by the Home Office. Licenses were required to perform experiments on living vertebrates, were valid for one year, and required the support of a president of one of eleven named medical or scientific bodies and a professor of medicine or medical science. Experiments had to be performed in registered premises that were inspected periodically. The Brown Institution was so registered.

Its superintendents were widely recognized experimentalists. Burdon Sanderson – professor-superintendent until 1878 – had studied the natural history of cow plague and observed that blood of an affected animal contains an infective agent that can produce the disease in another animal. At the Brown Institution, he also studied pleuropneumonia and anthrax, suggesting the possibility of protective vaccination. His

Handbook for the Physiological Laboratory,[4] which he edited and co-authored, was an important aid to the study of physiology in Britain, but also became grist to the mill for the antivivisectionists. His electrophysiological studies at University College of the leaf of *Dionaea muscipula* (the so-called Venus flytrap, a carnivorous plant that traps insects and spiders if the tiny hairs on the inner surface of its leaves are touched) and then of the frog's heart were important. Many, including the young Horsley, studied under this inspirational but rigorous man. He subsequently became Wayneflete professor of physiology at Oxford, the chair having been endowed by Magdalen College in honor of its fifteenth-century founder.* On his arrival, however he found that no provision had been made for laboratories and equipment. Requests for funding led to spirited objections by non-scientists and anti-vivisectionists. There was an acrimonious debate before funding was agreed by a majority vote of less than five at Convocation, the main governing body of the university.[5,6]

Burdon Sanderson's department became active in research into nerve and muscle, and as its reputation grew it became increasingly popular with students of physiology and related sciences,[5] although it failed to match the success of the Cambridge school.[6] Burdon Sanderson served on many national committees including in 1886–1887 on the Commission on Hydrophobia, with Horsley as its secretary. In 1895, he succeeded the courtly Sir Henry Acland as regius professor of medicine, one of five professorships established at Oxford by King Henry VIII in 1546. He was succeeded ten years later by his former student, the iconic William Osler (1849–1919), a noted bibliophile, historian, and author, who was one of the founders of the American Association of Physicians and a member of the founding staff of the Johns Hopkins Hospital and its school of medicine.

Victor Horsley became the fourth professor-superintendent of the Brown Institution, probably due to the influence of Burdon Sanderson, and he served from 1884 to 1890. He followed William Greenfield and Charles Smart (C. S.) Roy. Greenfield prepared an effective vaccine against anthrax by repeated subculture in vitro and described his results some months before the experiments of Pasteur, but he has never received the credit he deserves.[7] The

unfortunate Roy – he died at 43 – studied the circulation and cardiac physiology, devising various instruments for this purpose, such as the cardiometer to record changes in heart volume and the myocardiograph to obtain graphic records of the contraction of part of the heart's wall.[8] Horsley's predecessors all eventually left London and moved on to chairs at famed universities – Burdon Sanderson, as mentioned, to Oxford, Greenfield to Edinburgh, and Roy to Cambridge. They had been responsible for remarkable scientific advances despite the lack of adequate financial support. Funding of the institute was meager, and there were always unanticipated expenses. For example, on one occasion compensation of 132 pounds had to be paid "to the father of a child who was frightened, fell, and cut its face when a chimpanzee from the Institution jumped over the wall, and to the landlady who had a nervous attack."[1]

Horsley, following in the tradition of his predecessors, was also responsible for important scientific advances. His work on the thyroid gland and on rabies was performed mainly at the Brown Institution, as were some of his studies on the localization of motor centers in the brain and on the involuntary movements (canine chorea) that may occur after distemper in dogs. His work on rabies led to the muzzling orders and related safeguards that resulted eventually in the eradication of the disease in Britain. Indeed, the decade that began with Horsley's stewardship was probably the most fruitful in the entire history of the institution.[1]

After the end of World War II, the capital of the Brown bequest grew because – with the closure of the institution – there were no expenses to charge against it. It was only when the University of Dublin (Trinity College), recognizing that the original conditions of the trust were being met no longer, made claim on the money that the University of London was obliged to act. An application was made to set aside the original conditions of the will, with the two universities sharing the capital sum and this was eventually agreed in 1971. It was a sorry end to the first medical and veterinary research institute to be founded in England.

Horsley's Work on the Thyroid Gland

Horsley's work on the thyroid gland is best appreciated in the context of the state of contemporary endocrinology.

---

* William Waynflete (?1398–1486) was also bishop of Winchester and lord chancellor of England.

Background

The court physician to King Louis XV of France, Théophile de Bordeu (1722–1776), first formulated in 1775 the concept that individual organs – particularly the testicles and ovaries – release substances that influence the body as a whole.[9] In 1849, Arnold Adolph Berthold (1803–1861), a German physiologist, showed the effect of the testicles on distant parts of the body, especially on secondary sexual characteristics.[10] Castrated young cockerels developed into docile capons without any interest in hens, and they lacked the combs, wattles, and spurs of normal roosters. Castrated cockerels that underwent implantation of a testicle in the abdominal cavity, however, developed into normal combative animals with a lusty interest in hens. Autopsy showed that the grafted testicle had gained a blood supply but had no nerve connections. Berthold thus concluded that the testicles had acted through the blood to influence the physical and behavioral characteristics of the animals. Contemporary scientists did not follow up this experimental work,[11] however, and no significant further developments occurred until the work of Claude Bernard (1813–1878) and Charles Édouard Brown-Séquard (1817–1894).

They were an interesting pair. As young men, both had briefly nurtured literary aspirations that they discarded soon after their arrival in Paris, Claude Bernard from provincial France, and Brown-Séquard from Mauritius in the Indian Ocean. Both studied at the Paris faculty of medicine and became noted animal experimentalists, and each sought the chair of medicine at the Collège de France when vacated by the death of François Magendie (1783–1855). Bernard – Magendie's former laboratory assistant – was successful and thus remained in Paris during his long career. Brown-Séquard, by contrast, became a peripatetic physician-scientist, traveling between Europe, North America, and Mauritius, holding important positions in both the old world and the new but unable to settle down for long until, with the death of Bernard, he in turn succeeded to the prestigious chair. Bernard was calm, deliberate, and disciplined in his work; Brown-Séquard was impulsive, intuitive, and erratic.[12]

These two men, so different from each other, founded the concept of internal secretions.[13] Bernard believed that such secretions served to maintain the composition of the blood – he showed, for example, that the liver manufactures sugar from stored glycogen and releases it directly into the circulation. He concluded that the internal environment is kept constant by the interaction of different processes in the body. Brown-Séquard reported that various tissues influence distant parts of the body by secreting chemicals into the blood, thereby maintaining the normal state of the organism. His belief in humoral integrative mechanisms was a logical extension of his earlier views concerning the integrative action of the nervous system and the functional processes subserving this role.[12] His work led directly to the development of modern endocrinology and hormone replacement therapy.

In lectures that he gave in Paris in 1869, Brown-Séquard first suggested that "all glands, with or without excretory ducts, give to the blood, by an internal secretion, principles which are of great importance if not necessary."[14] He came to believe that the internal secretion from the testicles energized the nervous system and muscles in some manner – castration during childhood was known to affect the development of men, and he thought that weakness in the elderly may relate at least in part to a decline in testicular function. On June 1, 1889, he reported to the Société de Biologie in Paris that – after preliminary studies in animals – he had injected himself subcutaneously on several occasions over a two-week period with a small quantity (1 cc) of an aqueous solution of the mashed-up testicles of dogs and guinea pigs. There was, he found, a marked increase in his strength and stamina, improved mental energy and concentration, a more powerful urinary stream, and greater regularity in his bowel movements. These changes persisted for about a month after the last injection before waning.[15,16]

Brown-Séquard's report stunned some, embarrassed others, and led to his ridicule by many. The aging professor was well aware that the changes described may have been spurious, due to suggestion, and so he did not try his injections on patients, preferring to wait for more evidence to accumulate. As others reported similar anecdotal findings, however, reputable physicians and researchers began to show more interest in his work. Brown-Séquard came to believe that if a certain condition responded to treatment with an extract of a specific organ, it was likely that the individual disorder was caused by impaired production of the relevant internal secretion.[17] Over time, he expanded this concept to suggest that not merely the glands but many other tissues contributed internal secretions to the blood supply, thereby influencing the activity of other parts of the body.[18,19] His laboratory was soon approached with requests to prepare extracts of different organs for therapeutic trials.[20]

In 1895, Edward Schäfer (see p. 6), then of University College and subsequently at the University of Edinburgh, spoke about the internal secretions – material secreted into the blood – in an address to the British Medical Association, pointing out that it was not only the ductless glands but any organ of the body that could furnish these secretions.[21] This is precisely the sense in which Brown-Séquard and his assistant d'Arsonval generalized the concept in 1891,[17] although they did so without the experimental evidence that subsequently accumulated and justified Schäfer's views.

Horsley and the Thyroid Gland

Brown-Séquard's approach must have influenced work proceeding in England by Horsley and others on the treatment of myxedema, a disorder attributed in 1873 to atrophy of the thyroid gland by Sir William Gull (1816–1890), a physician of some eminence at Guy's Hospital in London. Gull had treated the Prince of Wales for typhoid fever in 1871, and subsequently was created a baronet and physician-in-ordinary to Queen Victoria. Myxedema was so named because symptoms were thought to arise from mucous swelling of connective tissues. The function of the thyroid gland was then unknown, but an enlarged gland (goiter), thyroid atrophy, congenital absence of the gland, or its total surgical removal was associated with a distinctive clinical disorder. Patients gained weight, tired easily, and developed dry and roughened skin, hair loss, a hoarse voice, constipation, weakness, muscle and joint pains, cold intolerance, depression, irritability, memory changes, slowed thinking, reduced libido, menstrual changes, and a slowed heart-rate. Untreated, coma and even death could occur.

The work in England must have been influenced also by the early studies of Moritz Schiff (1823–1896), a German physiologist who, after having studied under François Magendie in Paris and served as a military surgeon in Germany, worked as an experimental scientist first in Bern and then in Florence. He finally settled in Geneva as professor of physiology, a chair originally offered to Brown-Séquard, who first accepted and then declined it. Schiff, a somewhat exotic character with a wild beard, reported in 1859 that dogs and guinea pigs died after total removal of the thyroid gland and later that death was prevented by injection of thyroid extracts or transplantation of the thyroid into the abdominal cavity.[22] Correspondingly, the Swiss surgeons Emil Theodor Kocher (1841–1917) and Jacques-Louis Reverdin (1842–1929), together with Reverdin's cousin Auguste Reverdin, separately noted in the 1880s that humans who underwent thyroidectomy for goiter sometimes developed hypothyroidism ("cachexia strumipriva"). Convulsions and a fatal outcome could occur soon after surgery, presumably because the neighboring parathyroid glands – then unknown or regarded as embryonic thyroid tissue – had also been removed. Kocher would later be awarded the Nobel Prize in physiology or medicine for his work on the physiology, pathology, and surgery of the thyroid gland. As for the parathyroid glands, they are now known to regulate the level of calcium in the body. Overactive parathyroids produce too much hormone, leading to high levels of calcium in the blood, whereas underactive glands (or their surgical removal) lead to low blood calcium levels and to tingling, twitching, cramps, spasms, and convulsions.

It was Felix Semon (1849–1921), then an assistant physician in London and later knighted as the leading British laryngologist of the period, who first suggested that myxedema (the disorder due to thyroid atrophy), cachexia strumipriva (the disorder that follows surgical removal of thyroid tissue), and cretinism (the name used for centuries in parts of Switzerland for people having congenital underactivity of the thyroid) were all caused by loss of function of the thyroid.[23] His conclusion initially excited ridicule.[24] Nevertheless, it caused the Clinical Society of London – founded just fifteen years earlier and later to merge with the Royal Society of Medicine – to appoint a special committee to examine the matter in 1883. In the following year, Horsley was invited to join the committee and began to study the thyroid experimentally.[25] The committee endorsed Semon's suggestion in its final report.[26,27]

Horsley started his studies of the thyroid gland in Schäfer's laboratory at University College, where he worked with Rickman Godlee, another member of the committee, but – with his appointment to the Brown – he continued the work alone in the Wandsworth Road. The functions of the thyroid were still obscure when he began his studies. Some claimed with apparent sincerity that the thyroid cushioned the nerves and vessels in the neck from mechanical injury, and attributed the effects of surgical removal to damage of these nerves. Among the more credible hypotheses, it was held that the thyroid regulated the circulation of blood in the brain, that it secreted a mucinoid substance that was then resorbed by the lymphatic system, or that it played a role in the formation of blood cells.[28,29] Horsley surgically removed the thyroid gland in monkeys, cats, and dogs without damaging the nerves in the neck, and was able to reproduce the symptoms of myxedema.[28,29,30,31] After thyroidectomy, a monkey, for example, became "more imbecile and apathetic ... taking no notice of anything, in strong contrast to its customary vivacious state."[28] He also noted tremor and convulsions (presumably due to concomitant removal of the adjacent parathyroid glands), profound anemia, and the accumulation of mucin in the connective tissues of the body. The findings were influenced by the animals' age (with symptoms being more acute in the young), and the ambient temperature (an increase led to longer survival).

As Schiff had earlier, Horsley suggested that patients with hypothyroidism should be treated with grafts of thyroid tissue.[32] Then, in early 1891, Horsley was shipped some of Brown-Séquard's organ (testicular) extracts and literature on its use.[33] At about this time, he and George Redmayne Murray (1865–1939), one of his former students, discussed treating hypothyroid patients with subcutaneous injections of thyroid extracts,[34] an idea probably based on Brown-Séquard's approach.[17] Indeed, Brown-Séquard had instructed d'Arsonval on how to treat thyroid disease with tissue extracts.[35] Nevertheless, when Murray later in 1891 reported the successful treatment of hypothyroidism with subcutaneous injections of thyroid extract, he chose to make no mention of Brown-Séquard.[36] Murray's report was soon followed by others indicating that thyroid extracts taken orally were also beneficial, and a practical treatment for hypothyroidism was thus developed.

Curiously, with the exception of two short communications to the Royal Society, Horsley did not publish the results of his work on the thyroid gland in any scientific journal.[37] He mentioned them in his annual reports from the Brown Institution, and they eventually appeared in the report of the Committee on Myxoedema published in 1888.[26] Horsley's reluctance to publish may well have been due to the rather variable changes that occurred with removal of the gland, which would have deterred acceptance for publication in a scientific journal. In retrospect, this variability almost certainly depended on whether the parathyroid glands had also been removed. The effects of age that Horsley described may also have related to this, because in the young the parathyroids are closer to the thyroid gland and thus more likely to have been sacrificed.[37]

One side issue is whether Brown-Séquard's testicular extracts ever actually had any true biological activity. A report published more than one hundred years after the original claim suggests that they did not: the dose of testosterone administered through canine testicular extracts prepared by his technique was much less than that required for testosterone replacement in hypogonadal men.[38]

Mad Dogs, Englishmen, and the French: Rabies

Horsley's work on the thyroid gland was interrupted in 1886 when he was appointed secretary of a committee set up by parliament to investigate rabies and its prophylactic treatment by the method introduced by Pasteur in Paris. As an experimentalist, he had much to offer the committee. As superintendent at the Brown, he had personal experience of rabies as a devastating disease of animals and one that posed great risks to the human population. (In the nineteenth century, *rabies* was the term used to refer to the disease in animals, and *hydrophobia* to that in humans. In the present account, the designation *rabies* is used for both the animal and human illnesses.)

Rabies, a viral infection of the brain, was commonly fatal in the nineteenth century and generally leads to death even now if clinical signs develop before preventive treatment can be initiated. At present, between sixty and seventy thousand people die each year from the disease, mainly in Asia and Africa. Almost all human cases involve bites from infected dogs, the virus being in the animals' saliva. Other viral sources include bats, raccoons, skunks, wolves, and foxes.

The incubation period can be as short as a few days or exceed a year. Infected persons may experience pain or pins-and-needles where they were bitten and then develop a flu-like illness followed by anxiety, agitation, confusion, visual or auditory hallucinations, fear, behavioral changes, sensitivity to light, shortness of breath, difficulty in swallowing, hypersalivation, hydrophobia, sweating, and "goose bumps" (hair standing on end; piloerection). Hydrophobia is characterized by fear of swallowing, inspiratory muscle spasm, and painful laryngospasm, initially when attempting to drink but eventually with the slightest stimulus or even at the mention of water. Aerophobia – a terror of drafts, which similarly can induce painful pharyngeal spasms – may also occur. In contrast to this encephalitic ("furious") form, other patients develop paralysis starting at the site of infection and spreading to the rest of the body (paralytic or "dumb" form). Regardless, the course is progressive, leading to coma and death.

Even today, a diagnosis of rabies can only be made clinically after the start of symptoms and the sensitivity of any single diagnostic test for rabies is limited. The disease can often be prevented if an at-risk person exposed to the virus – following, for example, an animal bite – is treated with rabies vaccine and rabies immunoglobulin before symptoms develop.

For much of the nineteenth century, the cause of rabies was unknown. It was attributed by many to spontaneous generation of the causal agent. Louis Pasteur (1822–1895), the French microbiologist and chemist, disproved this concept, however, showing that fermentation and putrefaction relate to the growth of micro-organisms that do not arise spontaneously from inanimate matter but are ubiquitous. He believed that rabies was due to an acquired infection. He also showed that the virulence of microbes could be attenuated by passage in special culture conditions and is credited with having developed the first vaccines for rabies and anthrax. As noted earlier, however, William Greenfield, one of Horsley's predecessors at the Brown, actually prepared an effective vaccine against anthrax by repeated subculture in vitro before Pasteur, an accomplishment for

which he has never received proper credit. In any event, it was Pasteur in Paris who came up with an effective treatment to protect humans or animals from becoming infected with the rabies virus and to prevent the occurrence of the disease in those already infected.

It is not easy to appreciate the extent to which rabies was feared in the late nineteenth century, much as infection with human immunodeficiency virus (HIV) was dreaded in the last quarter of the twentieth century. Patients experienced uncontrollable physical and mental anguish, while their caregivers faced personal danger and upheavals as they witnessed the disintegration of those they loved. Claims of successful cures were confounded by the fact that there was no sure means of diagnosis – many dogs with suspected rabies, for example, almost certainly did not have the disease – and in some patients symptoms after a dog-bite may have been psychogenic, brought on by anxiety that they might have contracted the disease that so alarmed the public. Rabies was sometimes confused with tetanus despite their clinical differences.[39] Most treatments were symptomatic but typically included some form of physical restraint, and sedation with opiates or chloroform. Other approaches to treatment included the use of various stimulants, tobacco, oil of turpentine, the salts of various metals, intravenous injections of warm water, electricity and galvanism, hot vapors and hot air baths, cupping and bleeding, the application of leeches, and even the poison of a viper. In advanced cases, doctors were rumored to resort to euthanasia by smothering their patients.[40]

In April 1886, a committee was established in Britain by the government, with Horsley as its secretary, to "enquire into M. Pasteur's treatment of hydrophobia [rabies]." Sir James Paget, the distinguished surgeon and pathologist, was its president, and the other committee members were Dr. George Fleming (principal veterinary surgeon to the army), Sir Joseph Lister (pioneer of antiseptic surgery), Sir Lauder Brunton (the physician who introduced amyl nitrite to relieve angina pectoris), Dr. Richard Quain (physician to Benjamin Disraeli, physician-extraordinary to Queen Victoria, best remembered for his *Dictionary of Medicine*), Sir Henry Roscoe (the chemist and member of parliament), and John Burdon Sanderson (the physiologist). Any suggestion that the committee should include an

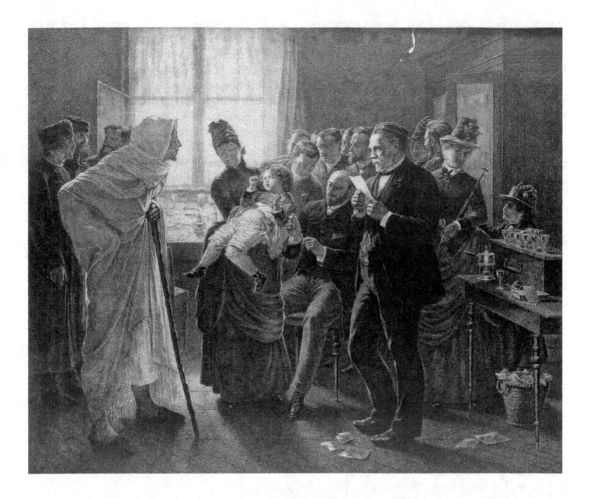

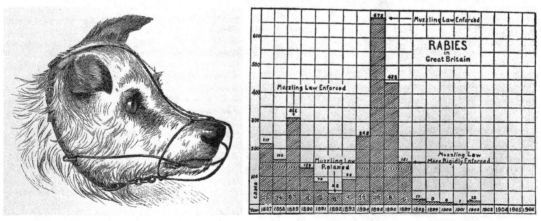

Figure 3.2 *Top,* Rabies vaccination in Pasteur's clinic in Paris. Pasteur is on the right foreground, holding a document. (Lithograph by F. Pirodon after L-L Gsell.) *Bottom left,* Dog with a muzzle of the sort used to prevent the spread of rabies. *Bottom right,* Chart showing the effect of muzzling on the spread of rabies in Britain. When the muzzling law is relaxed, the incidence of rabies increases; when it is strictly enforced, the incidence declines. (Images from the Wellcome Collection, London; chart from Paget S: *Sir Victor Horsley: A Study of His Life and Work.* Constable: London, 1919.)

antivivisectionist was declined. Several members of the committee, including Horsley, Roscoe, Brunton, and Burdon Sanderson, spent Easter in Paris meeting with Pasteur, observing his treatment, and following-up a number of the patients whom he had inoculated. They were initially skeptical about his claims, and at their first meeting Pasteur appeared irritable and distracted, which did not help. Their investigations were decisive, however, and they returned home convinced that his claims were justified. Horsley himself spent longer in Paris and then hurried back to London to study the issues further at the Brown.

In particular, Horsley undertook a series of experiments to examine the effects of Pasteur's inoculations in animals,[41,42] funded by fifty pounds from the committee and additional support from Roscoe. Two rabbits infected with the virus by Pasteur were taken from Paris to the Brown Institution for this purpose. They both developed rabies – after their death, crushed portions of their spinal cord were injected through small holes in the skull into the space under the fibrous dural covering of the brain in anesthetized rabbits and dogs. Horsley confirmed that extracts of the spinal cord of a rabid animal produces the disease when injected into a previously healthy animal. Indeed, the laboratory diagnosis of the disease in animals with few or no signs came to depend on experimental inoculation in this manner. The incubation period varied depending on the mode of infection, the age and condition of the animal, and certain other circumstances. However, by first preparing the spinal cord in the manner described by Pasteur "in a pure and dry atmosphere at a temperature of 20°C," the rabies virus was weakened, and injection into a healthy animal then failed to produce the

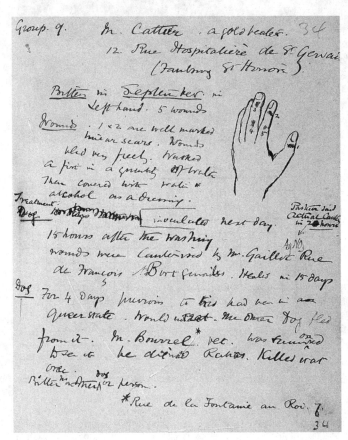

Figure 3.3 Page from the notebook that Horsley compiled when, as secretary of the commission of enquiry into Pasteur's treatment of hydrophobia, he visited Paris and followed up some of Pasteur's treated cases. His notes describe the bite-wound of a patient, the treatment received, and the details of the involved dog. (Image from the Wellcome Collection, London.)

disease. Furthermore, with serial inoculations on successive days using the virus from a spinal cord dried for progressively shorter periods, animals became protected from rabies, regardless of the source of infection.

Pasteur had come to believe that an unprotected person bitten by a rabid animal might be helped – and the disease prevented – by a series of similarly progressive inoculations. He had therefore treated in this way a large number of persons using either a standard treatment schedule or a more intensive one in which larger quantities of the inoculum were administered after being dried for shorter periods. The committee – with Pasteur's full cooperation – attempted to determine the success of the approach, and Horsley personally investigated a number of the cases that Pasteur had treated.

It concluded that his treatment did indeed prevent the occurrence of rabies in a large proportion of those who were bitten by rabid animals and who, without therapy, would have died from the disease.[43]

Horsley, like Pasteur, found no evidence that the disease ever arose spontaneously. It therefore became necessary for the committee to consider – as Pasteur urged – whether rabies could be prevented in an island such as Britain. This might be achieved, for example, by requiring the inoculation of all dogs but would involve the destruction of certain ownerless animals; by placing in quarantine or preventing the import of dogs from areas with endemic rabies; or by the compulsory muzzling of dogs in areas with endemic rabies. Pasteur awaited the report of the committee with impatience for he faced opposition not only in France but also in many other European countries.

In Britain during the year 1887, rabies affected more than two hundred dogs as well as livestock and, exceptionally, a large number of deer in Richmond Park. This royal park with its ancient trees and streams on the outskirts of London is a national nature reserve that has been managed as a deer park since the seventeenth century. In 1886, about twelve hundred fallow or red deer lived in the park, going about in herds of about one or two hundred. In September, a doe, which was suckling a fawn, was observed to be staggering about and had to be killed. A few days later other deer in the same herd began to behave erratically, constantly rubbing their heads against trees or posts until bald, biting themselves, tearing out their hair, and charging aggressively at other deer. A toxic cause was suspected but none could be identified. There were no poisonous foods or plants in the pastures. The disease spread slowly throughout the herd, about four animals dying each week after becoming paralyzed. An affected buck and a fawn were taken to the Royal Veterinary College for evaluation. The fawn died a few hours later; the buck survived for two days but became so violent that it could not be controlled. Portions of the lower brain (the medulla) or spinal cord of the animals were taken to Horsley at the Brown and inoculated into rabbits, which died of rabies, thereby enabling a firm diagnosis of the disease in the affected deer. The herd in Richmond was placed in an enclosure, and any animal with any sign of disease was shot, as were the members of a second herd that developed the disease. In the end, some two hundred and sixty-four animals died before the disease was eradicated.[44]

Despite the report of the committee and the role played by Horsley in establishing the cause of the illness affecting the deer at Richmond, the lay public and even members of the medical and veterinary professions refused to accept Pasteur's views and treatment. The issue had been confounded by the fury of the antivivisectionists at animal experimentation and the unnecessary extermination of animals, by the interests of those promoting alternative treatments, and by those whose own experience of infectious diseases made it difficult to accept the emerging view, particularly given an incubation period that varied from a few days to months or even years. An acrimonious correspondence between a certain Thomas Dolan, physician to the Halifax Fever Hospital, and Horsley continued for several years in various British medical journals.[45] Dolan also published books on the nature and treatment of rabies, but his unnecessarily emotive rhetoric eclipsed the cogent points he raised:

Whole hecatombs of animals have been ruthlessly sacrificed in the quest after the virus, ... [the slaughter] has taken place without, as we assert, benefit to the human race, nay, even to its injury. A new terror is now added to the bite of the dog.[46]

Between January 1886 and April 1887, Pasteur treated one hundred and thirty persons sent to him from all parts of Britain.[47] His opponents seized upon any failure as evidence against his whole approach, although neither Pasteur nor Horsley had ever claimed that treatment would be successful in all cases.

Ironically, one treatment failure involved Joseph Green, a laboratory assistant at the Brown Institution, who was bitten deeply in several places in the hand by a rabid cat. The wounds were immediately cleaned and cauterized and a few hours later were excised while the patient was anesthetized. He was then treated by Pasteur in Paris, but got drunk every day, on one occasion nearly drowning when he fell into the Seine. He suffered with exposure also on the return cross-Channel trip to England, and over the following days developed abdominal and then back pains, and subsequently a variety of constitutional symptoms and an ascending paralysis of the limbs without sensory loss, but with difficulty in swallowing. He gradually became stuporous and then comatose, dying about seven weeks after the original bite with either paralytic rabies, an inflammatory disorder of the nerves (Guillain–Barré syndrome, then referred to as Landry's paralysis), or both. Inoculation of his crushed spinal cord into rabbits confirmed the diagnosis of rabies.[48,49] Perversely, when treatment failures occurred, as in this instance, they were attributed by many antivivisectionists to the inoculations that the patients had received at Pasteur's hands, in other words to "rabbit hydrophobia."[50]

Other treatments continued in vogue. One popular approach was with the hot-air bath, the so-called Bouisson remedy that was supposed to allow toxic substances in the body to be "sweated out." Horsley evaluated the method in rabid rabbits because it had received so much support by "antivivisectionist agitators."[51] As might have been anticipated, he found, with some satisfaction, that it was useless – a result that the antivivisectionists chose to ignore.

Pasteur's work and its confirmation by Horsley helped to spur efforts to eliminate the disease in Britain, where in England alone an average of forty-three people a year died of rabies during the ten years ending in 1885.

An obvious approach in locations with endemic rabies was to muzzle all dogs for long enough for the disease to declare itself in infected animals, which could then be destroyed. In London, where twenty-seven people died from rabies in 1885, a muzzling order was issued and no-one bitten after that time died from the disease during the following year. In August 1886, however, a Dog Owners Protection Association was created in the metropolis to protect dogs from the cruelty of muzzling by those who believed that the registration and licensing of dogs would ensure the desired vigilance of dog-owners to the health and safety of their pets. In response, in September several physicians, surgeons, and veterinarians came together with a group of peers and gentlemen to form the Society for the Prevention of Hydrophobia and Reform of the Dog Laws, aiming to educate the public and lobby for parliamentary action.[47] The general committee of the society was chaired by Horsley.

The success in London of the muzzling order led to its suspension, following which there was a gradual increase in deaths until, in 1889, ten people died.[39] Proponents of muzzling believed that the disease could be eliminated in Britain – an island – by muzzling all dogs throughout the land for a few months, although this would also require the quarantining of dogs entering the country from overseas. Those concerned with the comfort of their dogs, however, opposed muzzling with an unreasoning passion.[52] Some even deluded themselves into believing that muzzling a dog could make it rabid. Queen Victoria's veterinary surgeon is said to have believed that rabies was hereditary and that the irritation of a muzzle activated the dormant disease.[53] Horsley's view was expressed quite succinctly – "putting a muzzle on a dog can no more produce rabies than tying a bib round a baby's neck can give it hydrophobia."[54]

In July 1889, James Whitehead, the Lord Mayor of London – who earlier in the year had visited Pasteur and his laboratories in Paris[55] – held a meeting to hear statements concerning the recent increase in rabies in Britain and about the efficacy of Pasteur's treatment. Because of his support, he received an enormous number of anonymous abusive letters. Horsley and other members of the original investigative committee attended the meeting. A letter from Pasteur was read out – apparently, over seven thousand patients had now been treated in his laboratory in Paris, including two hundred and fourteen from England. Of sixty-four English persons bitten by mad dogs during 1888 and 1889 and treated in Paris, not one had succumbed despite serious or extensive bites.[56,57] At the mayor's suggestion, a fund was initiated to support the Pasteur Institute in Paris (rather than attempting to start one in London, which might have hindered efforts to stamp out the disease) and the sum of two thousand pounds was eventually sent to Paris. The fund was also to underwrite the costs of treatment there for those otherwise unable to afford it. Horsley was one of a number of distinguished men (who included Thomas Huxley, James Paget, Henry Roscoe, Joseph Lister, and Ray Lankester) who served on the Mansion House Committee, chaired by Whitehead.

At its last meeting, the mayor expressed his sadness that the committee's work was drawing to a close. C. S. Roy (formerly at the Brown and now professor of pathology at Cambridge) then brought up once more the idea of establishing an institute of preventive medicine in England.[58] His powers of persuasion were such that a committee was created for this purpose. It consisted of twenty-one members and included Horsley. Whitehead served briefly as chair, but ill-health caused him to be replaced by Joseph Lister.[59] Roy and Dr. Sydney Turner, the secretary of the Mastiff Club (a dog-lovers' association) were asked to draw up plans and the British Institute of Preventive Medicine was incorporated in July 1891 and eventually established in its own premises on the Chelsea Embankment in London. Its aims were to foster fundamental scientific disease-related research and to develop and produce protective or restorative treatments. It was later renamed the Lister Institute of Preventive Medicine, but financial difficulties in the 1970s led to the closure of its research laboratories and production facilities. It is now a charity that supports young medical researchers by awarding competitive financial grants.

In 1889, the Society for the Prevention of Hydrophobia sent a deputation – including Horsley – to meet with the president of the Board of Agriculture, Walter Long (1854–1924), an amiable squire and rising Conservative politician. Horsley pointed out that if compulsory muzzling was adopted throughout the country for twelve months and all imported dogs were quarantined, rabies would be eradicated from the country. The minister initially was unsure how to proceed, believing instead that it would be adequate to require muzzling only in certain districts where the disease was long-standing rather than throughout the country. In any event, over the following decade and after much debate, false starts, reversals, re-emergence of the disease when temporary controls were lifted, and yet further discussions and committee hearings, the muzzling order was eventually extended to the whole country. Stray dogs were destroyed, quarantine regulations were put in place, and cases of rabies ceased to occur.[60] The regulations were then applied successfully to Ireland, where rabies was rife. It had been a long and difficult battle, with claims that the anti-rabies regulations were based on incomplete or misleading information, that they were discriminatory against the working classes, and that they were an infringement on civil liberties. Much of the credit for success belongs to Walter Long.

Britain was declared free of rabies in 1902. Five years later, in November 1907, Horsley appeared before the Royal Commission on Vivisection and was able to state:

> England today is, I believe, one of the few European countries of importance that is spared a Pasteur Institute [for the treatment of rabies], and in England there is no rabies . . . . Now the freedom of England from rabies I take to be one of the great achievements of modern science, and we owe it entirely to M. Pasteur.[61]

In fact, Horsley himself – as well as many others – also deserves credit for the eradication of rabies from the British Isles. Unfortunately, further outbreaks occurred when military personnel who were returning from World War I smuggled dogs with latent infection back to Britain. The country was declared rabies-free again in 1922 after compulsory quarantine for dogs limited the entry of infected animals, although rare infection with a rabies-like virus still occurs in the native bat population. The vaccination of all susceptible animals has led to an easing of restrictions concerning their entry, but certain unvaccinated animals are still quarantined before they can enter the United Kingdom.

Horsley's involvement with the eradication of rabies in Britain had a profound impact on him personally. Rather than being dismayed by the angry controversy surrounding the issue and by the discord and bitter disagreement that developed with a large segment of the general public – the antivivisectionists; the anti-muzzlers and animal welfare groups; the working classes, farmers, and many of the landed gentry; and certain members of the medical and veterinary professions – he seemed almost to welcome the excitement of the dispute, and enjoyed the camaraderie and competitiveness that it engendered. He relished the fight to impose on others his own beliefs for their welfare, based on a scientific appraisal of the evidence. His behavior was sometimes outrageous, as when he attended a meeting of the Dog Owners Protection Association that he packed with a group of medical students. The students heckled the speakers, and he then proposed a motion of his own to support muzzling that passed because of his student accomplices.[62]

The eradication of rabies was one of many causes that he was to take to heart, and this experience must surely have led him on the path to becoming a political social reformer. He found that he could impose on others his personal beliefs on various issues by harnessing support from influential national organizations or government agencies. His approach was not that of conciliation and compromise but rather to do battle with those who challenged his beliefs. He was already beginning to turn from surgeon-scientist to a man of the people, but on his own terms and always convinced of the correctness of his own beliefs.

Horsley and Cerebral Localization

Horsley began his important neurophysiological work on the cortical localization of functions at University College with Professor Edward Schäfer, but much of the work was undertaken at the Brown in collaboration with Charles Beevor and Felix Semon. The work not only established him as an experimental neurologist but honed his clinical skills in neurological diagnosis and localization. It also gave him the experience with intracranial surgery in animals that allowed him to develop into a pioneering neurosurgeon. This work is considered in detail in Chapter 4.

Canine Chorea

Canine chorea is characterized by rapid, shock-like, often rhythmic, involuntary muscle contractions, and usually follows distemper. It lacks the spontaneous fidgety movements and incoordination of human chorea. Pathological changes occur primarily in the spinal cord, cerebellum, and medulla.[63] While professor-superintendent at the Brown Institution, Horsley was required to provide clinical care to sick animals and he devoted two of his 1886 Brown lectures to canine chorea. He emphasized that the focus of the disease was on the motor nerve cells of the spinal cord but that its precise pathophysiology was not understood.[64] He attempted to define some of the factors influencing the disease and its clinical manifestation. Canine chorea is now thought to represent an immune-mediated inflammatory response to a preceding viral infection (postinfectious encephalomyelitis) and, despite its name, is unrelated to chorea in humans, a disorder that Horsley attempted to treat surgically in 1908 and thereafter.

Horsley's Resignation

In 1890, Horsley resigned from the Brown Institution. The Wandsworth Road was out of his way, and the post of superintendent was too demanding of his time despite the annual salary of three hundred pounds. He preferred to devote himself to his new laboratory at University College, but he did accept an appointment at the Royal Institution, founded in 1799 to advance public education in science. The appointment, as Fullerian professor of physiology and comparative anatomy,[65] came with a stipend of one hundred pounds annually and was particularly gratifying, for the same chair had been occupied a quarter-century earlier by his mentor, John Marshall. His successor at the Brown was Charles Sherrington, a future Nobel laureate, with whom Horsley later was to exchange angry words about scientific priority.

Notes

1. Wilson G: The Brown Animal Sanatory Institution. *J Hyg (Camb)* 1979; **82**: 155–176; 337–352; 501–521 (three parts).

2. Anon: *University of London: the Historical Record (1836–1912): Being a Supplement to the Calendar.* pp. 177–179. University of London Press: London, 1912.

3. Sykes AH: Thomas Brown and his Animal Sanatory Institution. *J Med Biogr* 1994; **2**: 151–155.

4. Burdon-Sanderson J (ed): *Handbook for the Physiological Laboratory.* J & A Churchill: London, 1873.

5. MacNalty AS: Sir John Burdon Sanderson. *Proc R Soc Med* 1954; **47**: 754–758.

6. Romano TM: *Making Medicine Scientific: John Burdon Sanderson and the Culture of Victorian Science.* pp. 139–154. Johns Hopkins University Press: Baltimore, 2002.

7. Tiggertt WD: Anthrax. William Smith Greenfield, M.D., F.R.C.P., Professor Superintendent, the Brown Animal Sanatory Institution (1878–81). Concerning the priority due to him for the production of the first vaccine against anthrax. *J Hyg (Camb)* 1980; **85**: 415–420.

8. Roy CS, Adami JG: Contributions to the physiology and pathology of the mammalian heart. *Philos Trans R Soc Lond B* 1892; **183**: 199–298.

9. de Bordeu T: *Recherches sur les Maladies Chroniques, leurs Rapports avec les Maladies Aigues, leurs Periodes, leur Nature: et sur la Manière dont on les Traite aux Eaux Minerales de Bareges, et des Autres Sources de l'Aquitaine.* Ruault: Paris, 1775.

10. Berthold AA: Transplantation der Hoden. *Arch Anat Physiol Wissensch Med* 1849; **42**–46. Translated by Quiring DP: The transplantation of testes. *Bull Hist Med* 1944; **16**: 399–401.

11. Benedum J: The early history of endocrine cell transplantation. *J Mol Med* 1999; **77**: 30–35.

12. Aminoff MJ: *Brown-Séquard: An Improbable Genius Who Transformed Medicine.* Oxford University Press: New York, 2011.

13. Rolleston HD: *The Endocrine Organs in Health and Disease with an Historical Review.* pp. 1–22. Oxford University Press: London, 1936.

14. Brown-Séquard CE: On a new therapeutic method consisting in the use of organic liquids extracted from glands and other organs. *Br Med J* 1893; **1**: 1145–1147 and 1212–1214.

15. Brown-Séquard CE: Des effets produits chez l'homme par des injections sous-cutanées d'un liquide retiré des testicules frais de cobaye et de chien. *C R Soc Biol (Paris)* 1889; **41**: 415–419.

16. Brown-Séquard CE: Note on the effects produced on man by subcutaneous injections of a liquid obtained from the testicles of animals. *Lancet* 1889; **2**: 105–107.

17. Borell M: Organotherapy, British physiology, and discovery of the internal secretions. *J Hist Biol* 1976; **9**: 235–268.

18. Brown-Séquard CE, d'Arsonval A: Recherches sur les extraits liquides retirés des glandes et d'autres parties de l'organisme et sur leur emploi, en injections sous-cutanées, comme méthode thérapeutique. *Arch Physiol Norm Pathol* (5th Series) 1891; **3**: 491–506.

19. Brown-Séquard CE, d'Arsonval A: De l'injection des extraits liquides provenant des glandes et des tissues de l'organism comme méthode thérapeutique. *C R Soc Biol (Paris)* 1891; **43**: 248–250.

20. d'Arsonval A: Letter to Brown-Séquard, March 24, 1891. In: Delhoume L :*De Claude Bernard à d'Arsonval.* pp. 377–380. Baillière: Paris, 1939.

21. Schäfer EA: Address in Physiology: On internal secretions. *Lancet* 1895; **2**: 321–324.

22. Schiff M: Résumé d'une nouvelle série d'expériences sur les effets de l'ablation des corps thyroïdes. *Rev Méd Suisse Romande* 1884; **4**: 425–445.

23. Semon F: A typical case of myxoedema. *Br Med J* 1883; **2**: 1072.

24. Medvei VC: *A History of Endocrinology.* pp. 248–249. MTP Press: Lancaster, UK, 1982.

25. Sawin CT: Victor Horsley (1857–1916). *Endocrinologist* 1991; **1**: 207–208.

26. Ord WM: Report of a committee nominated December 14, 1883, to investigate the subject of myxoedema. *Trans Clin Soc Lond* 1888; **21**(suppl): 1–215.

27. Ord WM: Conclusions of the Myxoedema Committee. Clinical Society of London. Friday May 25th, 1888. *Br Med J* 1888; **1**: 1162–1163.

28. Horsley V: On the function of the thyroid gland. *Proc R Soc Lond* 1884; **38**: 5–7.

29. Horsley V: Further researches into the function of the thyroid gland and into the pathological state produced by removal of the same. *Proc R Soc Lond* 1886; **40**: 6–9.

30. Horsley V: Remarks on the function of the thyroid gland: a critical and historical review. *Br Med J* 1892; **1**: 215–219 and 265–268.

31. Horsley V: An address on the physiology and pathology of the thyroid gland. *Br Med J* 1896; **2**: 1623–1625.

32. Horsley V: Note on a possible means of arresting the progress of myxedema, cachexia strumipriva, and allied diseases. *Br Med J* 1890; **1**: 287–288.

33. Brown-Séquard CE: Four letters to d'Arsonval, February 17 to 22, 1891. In Delhoume L :*De Claude Bernard à d'Arsonval.* p. 365. Baillière: Paris, 1939. That d'Arsonval did as requested by Brown-Séquard and sent samples of the fluids to Horsley and others is documented in his letter to

Brown-Séquard, February 25, 1891. In Delhoume L: *De Claude Bernard à d'Arsonval.* pp. 366–367. Baillière: Paris, 1939.

34. Paget S: *Sir Victor Horsley: A Study of His Life and Work.* pp. 65–66. Constable: London, 1919.

35. Brown-Séquard CE: Letter to d'Arsonval, March 27, 1891. In Delhoume L : *De Claude Bernard à d'Arsonval.* pp. 383–384. Baillière: Paris, 1939.

36. Murray GR: Note on the treatment of myxoedema by hypodermic injections of an extract of the thyroid gland of a sheep. *Br Med J* 1891; **2**: 796–797.

37. Sharpey Schafer E: Victor Horsley Memorial Lecture on the relations of surgery and physiology, delivered on October 25, 1923. *Br Med J* 1923; **2**: 739–744.

38. Cussons AJ, Bhagat CI, Fletcher SJ, Walsh JP: Brown-Séquard revisited: A lesson from history on the placebo effect of androgen treatment. *Med J Aust* 2002; **177**: 678–679.

39. Romanes GJ: Hydrophobia and the muzzling order. pp. 226–253. In Morgan CL (ed): *Essays by George John Romanes.* Longmans, Green: London, 1897.

40. Pemberton N, Worboys M: *Mad Dogs and Englishmen: Rabies in Britain, 1830–2000.* pp. 16–19. Palgrave Macmillan: New York, 2007.

41. Horsley V: Appendix. A. – Abstract report of Mr. Horsley's experiments. *Vet J Ann Comp Pathol* 1887; **24**: 88–92.

42. Horsley V: On rabies: its treatment by M. Pasteur, and on the means of detecting it in suspected cases. *Br Med J* 1889; **1**: 342–344.

43. Paget J, Lauder Brunton T, Fleming G, Lister J, Quain R, Roscoe HE, Burdon Sanderson J, Horsley V: Report of Committee of Enquiry into M. Pasteur's treatment of hydrophobia. *Vet J Ann Comp Pathol* 1887; **24**: 82–88.

44. Cope A, Horsley V: *Reports on the Outbreak of Rabies among Deer in Richmond Park during the Years 1886–7.* Her Majesty's Stationery Office: London, 1888.

45. Dolan TM: Horsley V (Correspondence). *Br Med J* 1886; **2**: 475–476, 573, 602–603, 654–655, 892; *Lancet* 1890 2: 205, 258, 371.

46. Dolan TM: *Pasteur and Rabies.* pp.77–78. Bell: London, 1890.

47. Nicols A: Dogs, and dog legislation. *Time* 1887; **6**: 407–419.

48. Bristowe JS, Horsley V: A case of paralytic rabies in man, with remarks. *Trans Clin Soc Lond* 1888; **22**: 38–47.

49. Bristowe JS, Horsley V: A case of paralytic rabies. *Lancet* 1888; **132**: 966 and *Br Med J* 1888; **2**: 1110–1111.

50. Anon: Notes and Notices. *Zoophilist* 1886; **6**: 138–139.

51. Horsley V: On hydrophobia and its "treatment": especially by the hot-air bath, commonly called the Bouisson remedy. *Br Med J* 1888; **1**: 1207–1211.

52. Anon: The muzzling order. *Law J* 1889; **24**: 700.

53. Pemberton N, Worboys M: *Mad Dogs and Englishmen: Rabies in Britain, 1830–2000.* p. 139. Palgrave Macmillan: New York, 2007.

54. Kerslake F: *Hydrophobia; Its Cause and Its Prevention by Muzzling.* p. 45. Society for the Prevention of Hydrophobia: London, 1890.

55. Pasteur L: Letter to Sir Henry Roscoe dated May 15, 1889. pp. 321–322. In Roscoe HE : *The Life and Experiences of Sir Henry Enfield Roscoe, D. C.L., LL.D., F.R.S. Written by Himself.* Macmillan: London, 1906.

56. Pasteur L: Letter to The Right Hon. The Lord Mayor, Mansion House, E.C. *Nature* 1889; **40**: 225–226.

57. Anon: The Pasteur Institute. *Lancet* 1889; **134**: 38.

58. Drury AN: The Lister Institute of Preventive Medicine. *Proc R Soc Lond B* 1948; **135**: 405–418.

59. In addition to Whitehead, Lister, and Horsley, the members of the committee to consider establishing an institute of preventive medicine in England, were Sir Andrew Clark, Sir Spencer Wells, Sir Henry Roscoe, Sir James Crichton Browne, Sir Jacob Wilson, Dr. Bridgewater, Dr. Fleming, Mr. Ernest Hart (editor of the *British Medical Journal*), Dr. Holman, Professor Huxley, Mr. Hutchinson, Mr. Lee, Mr. Everett Millais, Dr. MacAllister, Professor Penberthy, Professor Roy, Mr. Walter Gilbey, and Dr. Ruffer. Further details are available in the editorial on The Mansion House Pasteur Committee. *Br Med J* 1889; **2**: 1363.

60. Ritchie J: Rabies symposium: IV. The veterinary profession and rabies control in Great Britain. *J Small Anim Pract* 1964; **5**: 433–441.

61. Horsley V: *Royal Commission on Vivisection. Appendix to Fourth Report of the Commissioners. Minutes of Evidence, October to December, 1907.* p. 119. His Majesty's Stationery Office: London, 1908.

62. Pemberton N, Worboys M: *Mad Dogs and Englishmen: Rabies in Britain, 1830–2000.* p.144. Palgrave Macmillan: New York, 2007.

63. Gowers WR, Sankey HRO: The pathological anatomy of canine "chorea." *Med Chir Trans* 1877; **60**: 229–248.

64. Anon: Abstracts of the Brown Lectures delivered at the University of London by Victor Horsley, M.B., B.S., F.R.C.S. Lecture IV and V. Canine chorea. *Lancet* 1886; **127**: 54–56.

65. John Fuller (1757–1834) was a member of parliament and a major patron of the Royal Institution, founding professorships in chemistry (1833) and then in physiology and comparative anatomy (1834).

Chapter

4

Dividing the Indivisible:
The Localization of Cortical Functions

In the latter half of the nineteenth century, there was growing interest in the operation of the nervous system in health and disease. University professors studied different aspects of neurological form and function. On the clinical side, several new hospitals devoted to the nervous system were established in the British capital (see Chapter 5), and an insane asylum in the north of England became a leading center for research into mental and neurological disorders. In Paris, the large Salpêtrière Hospital was converted from a hospice for destitute, chronically ill, or supposedly immoral women to a hospital with a primary focus on neurological disease. Patients were examined, symptoms and signs were analyzed, distinct diseases were identified, and treatable disorders were managed appropriately. Patients were also photographed, and some were studied by electrical techniques and even by muscle biopsy. Neurology was emerging as a distinct discipline of medicine. Important centers for neurological and psychiatric diseases were established at many other Parisian institutions including the famous Pitié, Bicêtre, and Sainte Anne hospitals. The neurosciences also flourished in Vienna, and clinical research at the Charité Hospital in Berlin and at other polyclinics and medical centers in the German-speaking world added to the breadth of clinical neurology. In North America, the Civil War stimulated the development of the specialty at the Turner's Lane Hospital in Philadelphia, where the clinical observations of Silas Weir Mitchell and his colleagues on the burning pain that sometimes follows nerve injury (causalgia; reflex sympathetic dystrophy) and on phantom sensations following war wounds were particularly important.

For much of the nineteenth century, the cerebral hemispheres were considered to be beyond study because of their supposed insensitivity to experimental stimulation. The cerebral cortex – the wrinkled outer layer of the hemispheres – had

generally been dismissed as consisting largely of glandular tissue or blood vessels, or serving a protective function, despite the seventeenth-century writings of the influential English physician Thomas Willis, who assigned it an important role in storing memories and initiating movement.[1] A few authors in the eighteenth century – the French military surgeon François Pourfour du Petit and the Swedish philosopher-scientist Emanuel Swedenborg, among others – also conceived of the cerebral cortex as involved in movement or cognition, but they had little lasting impact on contemporary biological thought.

It was the phrenologists in the early nineteenth century who assigned distinct functions to different regions of the brain, based on the shape and bumps of the head. They thought that the size of these bumps reflected different personality traits, mental faculties, and moral attributes. A bump at the base of the head behind the ears, for example, supposedly marked the site in the underlying brain – actually, the cerebellum (see Chapter 6) – of "amativeness" or sexual appetite. Despite the apparent absurdity of their specific concept, their legacy was immense in suggesting that different regions of the brain have different functions and in stimulating the correlation of anatomical and clinical abnormalities. Nevertheless, even at mid-century, the twinned cerebral hemispheres – the repository of thoughts, memories, actions, and reactions – were still regarded as homogeneous in their function, so that damage or disease of a localized cortical region caused only a diminution of the function of the whole. It was the clinical study of patients that first revealed otherwise.

Language and its Disturbance
Modern concepts of cortical localization began when the French surgeon-anatomist and

anthropologist Paul Broca (1824–1880) reported in 1861 to the Société d'Anthropologie in Paris his postmortem findings in a fifty-one-year-old man with epilepsy, weakness of the right arm and leg, and progressive loss of the ability to speak over many years. The speech disturbance was his major clinical deficit, for the only word that he could utter was "Tan," which he often uttered twice, accompanied by expressive gestures. It was therefore by this name that the patient was known throughout the hospital, although his real name was Leborgne. His comprehension was normal and he responded appropriately to commands. Tan died several days after he was admitted to Broca's surgical service at the Bicêtre Hospital in Paris with cellulitis and gangrene of the leg. Autopsy revealed that parts of the second and especially the third frontal convolution of the left cerebral hemisphere were destroyed.[2,3]

Similar postmortem findings were noted by Broca in a second patient with an inability to speak, this time resulting from a stroke.[4] Broca then collected other cases of abnormal speech production, now termed motor aphasia. In every instance, the lesion involved the same circumscribed region of the left cerebral hemisphere,[5] suggesting that this was a distinct speech center in the human brain.

Marc Dax, an obscure country doctor living near Montpellier, France, had earlier noted a relationship between certain speech disturbances and abnormalities of the left cerebral hemisphere, but not to so localized an area within it. In 1865, additional papers – two by Marc Dax and his son Gustave, and the other by Broca – confirmed that the left and right cerebral hemispheres are functionally distinct, based on the speech disturbances that followed localized disease.[6,7]

Broca's aphasia is characterized by lack of speech expression, with difficulty in naming objects and repetition. There is an impaired ability to write or read aloud, but the understanding of language is preserved. By contrast, the comprehension of language was later found by the Prussian physician Carl Wernicke (1848–1905) to depend on the integrity of a different cortical region located within the left temporal lobe, which lies under and to the side of the rest of the cerebral hemisphere. Its destruction was associated with a failure of language comprehension accompanied by the production of profuse but meaningless speech. With time, other brain regions

also came to be recognized as having a substantial role related to language.

The recognition that the two sides of the brain differ in some of their functions led to differences among clinicians and scientists in interpreting these distinctions. In London, the kindly but austere Hughlings Jackson (see Chapter 5) used his clinical expertise to derive fundamental scientific principles. He concluded on the basis of his bedside observations that the left hemisphere served particularly the voluntary use of words, whereas the right was concerned more with their automatic use (that is, with the involuntary, spontaneous but recurring utterance of words such as "yes" and "no").[8,9,10] He also emphasized that localizing the damage that destroys speech is not the same as localizing speech.[9]

Others hesitated to attribute disturbances of language to discrete areas of the brain. The eccentric physiologist Charles Édouard Brown-Séquard, for example, reported that in some aphasic patients, Broca's area (the third left frontal convolution) was unaffected, that lesions in Broca's area were not accompanied in all instances by major deficits of language, and that causal lesions in aphasic patients sometimes were localized to other cerebral regions. Moreover, he pointed out, aphasia could occur in certain right-handed patients with disease of the right (rather than the left) hemisphere ("crossed aphasia").[11] Some of these discrepancies now can be explained. In some patients with aphasia similar to that of Broca, for example, the pathology indeed spares the third frontal convolution but it involves neighboring areas, thereby isolating Broca's area from other cortical regions important for speech (a mixed transcortical aphasia or transcortical motor aphasia).

In any event, the new concept that certain functions are localized within the cortex of the cerebral hemispheres was seductive enough that it was soon applied in other contexts.

Activation of Movement

Broca's work on speech led neurologists and physiologists to localize other functions in different cerebral regions. Much of human behavior involves motor activity - movement - and this is controlled by the brain, which has to determine the muscles to be activated to make a particular movement, and the order and extent of their activation, guided by sensory information (e.g., the position of the limb to be moved, the location of the target, the speed of a moving target, and so on). Not surprisingly, then, attention was soon focused on involvement of the brain in generating motor activity.

Jackson noted that convulsive seizures involving one side of the body relates to disease of the opposite cerebral hemisphere. He thus concluded that the part of the brain that activates movement is on the opposite side to that being moved.[12,13] He went further, describing the sequence of muscle activation or movement that occurs during focal motor seizures and using this to localize the discharging lesion more precisely in the brain. He inferred that different cortical regions are involved depending on the nature and type of movements that occur, and that these regions are arranged in an orderly manner. His observations of these and other clinical phenomena, and his subsequent lengthy ruminations seeking some underlying guiding principle concerning the operation of the nervous system, provided strong support for the localization of functions in different cortical regions.

In 1870, the physiologist Gustav Theodor Fritsch (1838–1927) and neuropsychiatrist Eduard Hitzig (1838–1907) reported the results of their experiments on dogs, performed on a dressing table in Hitzig's Berlin home because adequate university facilities were not available to them. Muscle contractions in a limb followed galvanic (continuous direct-current) stimulation of specific regions of the opposite (contralateral) frontal cortex.[14] Weak stimuli produced more localized responses, and surgical excision of the responsive cerebral areas led to weakness of the opposite limbs. Thus, it seemed clear that the cerebral cortex was excitable and that functions were localized within it so that only certain parts of the hemispheres were concerned with movement.

Why these two young Berliners undertook their studies is unclear. It is said, however, that Fritsch, who had once worked as a military surgeon, had noticed that the opposite limbs twitched when he inadvertently stimulated the brain mechanically while dressing an open head wound. As for Hitzig, he had apparently observed eye movements when treating patients by cranial stimulation with galvanic current.[1,15] Regardless,

their findings were startling and their conclusions were not generally accepted, at least initially. There were concerns, for example, that the stimulating current had spread to deeper parts of the brain known to be associated with motor activity or that the motor activity was secondary to sensory stimulation of the cortex.

The studies performed in the home of Herr and Frau Hitzig attracted the interest of David Ferrier (1843–1928), a reserved and dapper Scotsman who, utilizing the facilities in the newly established laboratory at the West Riding Lunatic Asylum (later the Stanley Royd hospital, closed in 1995), attempted to corroborate the theoretical deductions of Jackson concerning cortical localization. The asylum, at Wakefield in the north of England, had opened in 1818 and expanded rapidly to accommodate eventually more than one thousand patients. In 1866, James Crichton-Browne became its director and turned it into a very active center for research into mental and brain disorders. Its *Medical Reports* were published annually between 1871 and 1876, and included articles by a number of clinician-scientists who became highly respected in their field. (In 1878 Crichton-Browne joined with others to found the journal *Brain* as successor to the *Medical Reports*, and it remains one of the leading neurological journals in the world.)

Ferrier's initial studies on cortical localization were performed at the asylum and published in its *Reports*. Crichton-Browne not only provided the facilities but also "a liberal supply of pigeons, fowls, guinea-pigs, rabbits, cats, and dogs for the purposes of my [Ferrier's] research."[16] He also held medical conversaziones (best regarded today as conferences) in the magnificent main hall, with lectures, demonstrations, and the opportunity for dialogue between professional colleagues while refreshments were served and music was played by the asylum band.[17]

Ferrier lectured and gave a demonstration on the localization of function in the brain at the conversazione held in the asylum in November 1873.[17] He had electrically stimulated the brains of a variety of different animals, using faradic (interrupted direct-current) rather than galvanic (continuous direct-current) stimulation, and also excised localized portions of their brains, with results that supported Jackson's concept of motor centers and suggested that sensory centers could also be localized in the cerebral cortex.[16,18]

The excisions were necessary to support any conclusions derived from the stimulation experiments, helping to exclude the possibility that motor activity following cortical electrical stimulation was reflex or the "result of some conscious modification incapable of being expressed in physiological terms." He was able to produce convulsions and reproduce in the laboratory certain epileptic phenomena, further confirming Jackson's clinical speculations. He also produced precise movements of individual muscles and groups of muscles by the electrical stimulation of localized cortical regions in different small animals.

In a second paper published in the following issue of the *Medical Reports*, Ferrier showed the clinical relevance of his research by reference to the case books and pathological records of the asylum.[19] The former were often vague in their detail, whereas the latter were remarkably accurate. Regardless, Ferrier attempted clinicopathological correlations in five cases and found that the site of pathology and nature of any symptoms matched expectations from his experiments in animals. He also took the opportunity to rebut objections to his experimental studies. The differential effects of anesthesia on the cerebral cortex and deeper structures, the reproducibility of the responses to cortical stimulation, the focal nature of cortical regions from which specific responses were elicited, and the fact that stimulation of adjacent cortical regions gave different results, all suggested that his results did not relate to spread of current to subcortical structures.[19]

His work was communicated to the Royal Society of London, which awarded him funds to extend it to monkeys.[20] He later went on to report his studies on both monkeys and dogs in a paper submitted to the society for publication, but the referees adjudicating its suitability were concerned that he had not given proper credit to Fritsch and Hitzig. When his revised paper still failed to satisfy them, Ferrier limited it to his new experiments on monkeys[21,22] to avoid making further changes.[20] The work was important because monkey brains closely resemble the human brain. However, certain parts of the brain were either not explored by Ferrier or yielded negative results, and the results of experiments in which parts of the brain were destroyed were more ambiguous.[23]

Ferrier summarized his experimental findings in his 1876 monograph, *The Functions of the Brain*, which was dedicated to Jackson:

> To Dr Hughlings Jackson who from a clinical and pathological standpoint anticipated many of the more important results of recent experimental investigation into the functions of the cerebral hemispheres, this work is dedicated as a mark of the author's esteem and admiration.[18]

Perhaps wisely, he made it clear that all his experiments were performed on anesthetized animals, anticipating the outrage that would follow from the antivivisectionists. His experimental findings were startling, caused much excitement, but did not meet with immediate acceptance.

Ferrier, himself a competent physician, went on to hold appointments at King's College Hospital and its medical school and at the National Hospital for the Paralysed and Epileptic (Queen Square) in London, where he is said to have been one of the last physicians to do ward rounds wearing the traditional silk top hat and black tailcoat.[24] He made his name, however, by his expertise as an experimental physiologist.

The Confrontation between Goltz and Ferrier

In 1881, a famous confrontation between Ferrier and Friedrich Goltz (1834–1902) occurred at the glittering International Medical Congress held in London under the patronage of Queen Victoria.[25] Goltz, an illustrious physiologist from Strasbourg who opposed the concept of cortical localization, considered the stimulation experiments inconclusive because it was uncertain what was being stimulated, particularly as the stimuli may well have spread to different sites in the brain to cause the observed effects. Moreover, the known ability of other brain regions to take over the functions of excised areas, that is, the plasticity of the brain, seemed to conflict with the concept of functional specialization of the cerebral cortex. He believed instead that any loss of function following cortical excision related to the amount of cortex removed rather than the site of cortical damage. At the congress, he exhibited a dog from which a large portion of the cortex had been removed without producing much loss of sensorimotor function, seemingly in conflict with the concept that these functions were dependent on the cortex. Ferrier and his Irish colleague Gerald Yeo (1845–1909), professor of physiology at King's College, London, then reported that excision of a restricted part of the motor cortex in a monkey had caused paralysis of the opposite limbs precisely as they had predicted. The animals were exhibited later that day at King's College. The dog, though seemingly aimless and unresponsive to threatening gestures, was able to run and jump about, its tail wagging. When the hemiplegic monkey was shown, its leg weak, its arm powerless and bent at the elbow, Charcot, the celebrated French neurologist, was heard to exclaim, "C'est un malade."

Given the differences in motor abnormalities, it became important to determine whether the extent of cortical damage corresponded to that intended. The two animals – the dog and the monkey – were therefore sacrificed and their brains examined by three independent scientists, namely, Klein, Schäfer, and J. N. Langley of Cambridge University, whose work was to lead to a greater understanding of the function of the autonomic nervous system. Their reports were published in preliminary form that same year and in detail in 1883,[26,27,28] preceded by an account taken from the *Transactions of the Congress* of the condition of the two animals after placement of the lesions.[29] They found that the dog's lesion was smaller than Goltz had believed, so that remaining cortical areas could have accounted for its retained motor ability, whereas the monkey's lesion was as intended. Thus, Ferrier's views received formal endorsement.

As an aside, it is of interest that a few months later, Ferrier was charged in the Bow Street magistrate's court with having violated the Cruelty to Animals Act of 1876 because – without the required governmental license – he had operated on an animal, probably caused it pain, and then failed to euthanize it. Happily, all charges were dismissed when it became known that Ferrier had merely witnessed the experiments, which were actually performed at King's by Yeo, who was indeed licensed, followed all legal requirements in performing the experiment, used appropriate anesthesia, and possessed the required certificate to keep the animal alive thereafter.[30] Ironically, the notoriety of the case led to an immediate increase in Ferrier's clinical practice – as his obituarist pointed out, the public presumably reasoned that

"an authority persecuted for experimenting on the brain must possess knowledge about it worth consulting."[31]

Horsley's Involvement in Studies of Cortical Function

Schäfer now became increasingly interested in the localization of functions in the cerebral cortex, probably because of the Goltz–Ferrier controversy and his own role in examining the brain of Ferrier's monkey. When he succeeded Burdon Sanderson in the Jodrell chair of physiology at University College in 1883, he decided to extend the work on cortical localization. Given his own rather limited surgical experience with Listerian techniques, he asked Horsley, already a talented surgeon with a demonstrated interest in physiology, to collaborate with him.[23] Horsley and Schäfer worked together for almost three years, studying various animals including nonhuman primates. With time and changing circumstances, Horsley continued the experiments independently of Schäfer, working at the Brown Institution – with Charles Beevor (1854–1908) to study the cortical motor areas of the monkey and orangutan, and with Felix Semon (1849–1921) to identify the cerebral centers controlling the larynx.

Beevor was a gentle, thoughtful man, a graceful and musical soul who had known Horsley for years, for he had been the house physician to Bastian and Jenner when Horsley, a medical student, was their clinical clerk. At the Brown, their work together was often demanding but Horsley valued it deeply because of "the special charm of his [Beevor's] manner."[32] Semon was born in Prussia, studied medicine in Germany, and during the Franco-Prussian war served with a Prussian cavalry regiment and took part in the siege of Paris. He moved to London in the mid-1870s and became a famous laryngologist. William Gladstone and several other former or future prime ministers (Salisbury, Rosebery, Campbell-Bannerman, and the young Winston Churchill) were among his patients, as were many of the crowned heads of Europe, including Queen Victoria and King Edward VII. He was a courtly, cultured man and a fine pianist, and was much in demand at court as "a witty raconteur, an excellent bridge player, and a good shot – three qualifications that counted very highly with the king."[33] The three clinician-scientists – Horsley, Beevor, and Semon – became colleagues on the staff at the National Hospital in Queen Square.

Working with Horsley could be taxing. As Schäfer commented:

> He was too energetic. He would think nothing of performing several operations at a sitting, and acquired so much skill at them that they occupied a relatively small amount of time. But the operation was one thing, the study of the

symptoms quite another. Now it takes a long time to make a thorough investigation of symptoms in the human subject – although in this case the subject himself can give much assistance. But when it comes to making the same kind of investigation in animals, and especially in monkeys, which are often wild, and the attention of which it is always difficult to fix, an unconscionable amount of time has to be devoted each day to each case. It so happened that just about this time Horsley was leading an extremely busy life. . . . The result of all this was that most of the

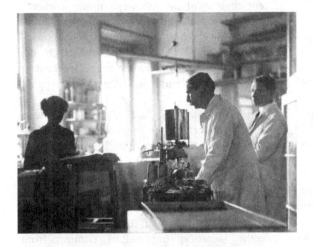

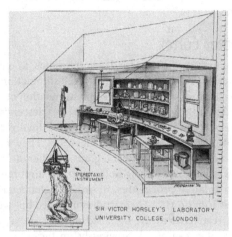

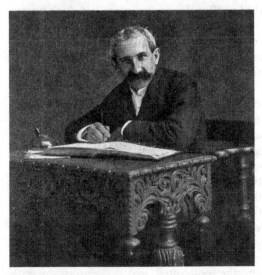

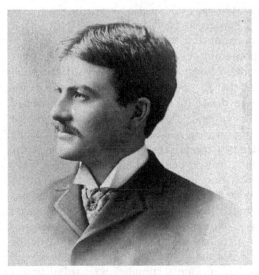

Figure 4.1 *Top left*, Horsley and colleagues in his laboratory at University College and, *top right*, drawing of the laboratory in about 1904, as reconstructed by H. W. Magoun and Ernest Sachs. *Bottom left*, Felix Semon, aged about fifty-five. He collaborated with Horsley in studies on the cortical representation of the laryngeal muscles and became one of the most famous laryngologists in Britain. Among his patients were several prime ministers, Queen Victoria, and King Edward VII. *Bottom right*, George Washington Crile worked with Horsley in the laboratory as a young man and later co-founded the Cleveland Clinic in the United States. (Image at top left from the Queen Square Archives; others from the Wellcome Collection, London.)

observations on the operated animals had to be made by his colleague . . .[23]

Indeed, Horsley and Schäfer appear to have had something of a falling out, probably because of Horsley's impatient approach to experiments, his inability to contribute fully because of competing clinical demands on his time, and the similar studies he undertook independently at the Brown Institution. It cannot have pleased Schäfer that much of their joint work, which he had initiated, appeared in print only after Horsley had published with Beevor.

Motor Cortex

The first studies of Horsley and Schäfer, to characterize the motor system, involved stimulation of the cerebral cortex, followed by stimulation of the underlying white matter with its descending motor fibers, the spinal cord, and finally the motor fibers in the spinal nerves.[34] They then studied different cortical regions in different species of monkeys, using both electrical stimulation and ablative procedures, in order to characterize their functions.[35] Their studies included but were not restricted to the so-called motor cortex, and they also examined previously unstudied areas, such as those on the medial aspects of the hemispheres.

They largely confirmed the findings of Ferrier concerning the motor cortex, publishing maps representing the responses to stimulation of different portions of this region. They stressed, however, that the distinct subdivisions of the motor region shown on these maps actually overlapped to a variable degree. They obtained motor responses with stimulation on either side of the rolandic (central) fissure, which separates the frontal from the parietal lobe of the brain. They demonstrated that the motor cortex was not restricted to the convexity of the hemisphere but extended to its medial surface, and emphasized that a lesion of the motor cortex was not necessarily accompanied by a loss of sensation in the paralyzed limb. The extent to which any slowed reaction to external stimulation related to diminished sensibility (as opposed to weakness) could not be determined. They could not elicit motor responses from the so-called prefrontal cortex, which covers the anterior part of the frontal lobe, confirming the experience of Ferrier and

Yeo.[36] This part of the brain is now thought to be involved with emotional, cognitive, social, behavioral, and other executive and goal-directed processes.

With Beevor, Horsley catalogued the movements of the different parts of the upper limb elicited by stimulation of localized regions of the motor cortex in the monkey, and thereby provided more topographic detail of this cortical region.[37] They then determined the primary movement, spread, and character of the movements following low-intensity stimulation of different regions of the monkey's motor cortex,[38] and the arrangement of the motor fibers descending from the cerebral cortex to the spinal cord.[39] Similar experiments were undertaken in the orangutan: motor points were found in front of and behind the rolandic fissure, with overlapping of cortical areas.[40]

Over the following decade, conflicting views emerged concerning the function of the perirolandic cortex – that it was purely motor, purely sensory, or sensorimotor. Horsley originally believed the area to be purely motor, but came round to the view that the motor cortex is actually a sensorimotor structure, "of which the motor element is the principal funnel-like outlet for afferent [sensory] impressions coming from many parts."[41] He also came to accept that "so-called volitional movements are not alone generated from the brain through the 'motor' area or pre-central gyrus, but must also be subserved by other parts."[41] These views received support from later studies by others.

The subsequent work of Sherrington (with Grünbaum; Chapter 8) led to the concept of a prerolandic (precentral) motor cortex separate from a postrolandic (postcentral) sensory area.[42,43,44] With the weak electrical stimuli that they used, motor responses were not elicited from behind the rolandic fissure. Most textbooks still show such a rigid functional demarcation, although this is somewhat misleading as the two areas are so integrated. Rather, the perirolandic region has both sensory and motor functions.[45,46] Motor responses, for example, can be elicited from the postcentral gyrus ("sensory cortex") even after removal of the perirolandic and supplementary motor areas. Similarly, sensory responses have been recorded from both the precentral and postcentral cortex. This and other evidence that has accumulated over the last one hundred years

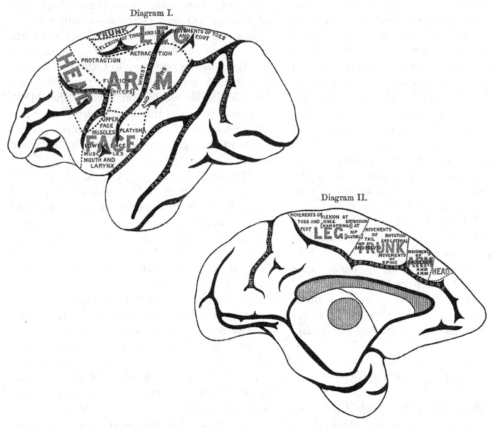

Figure 4.2 Results of electrical stimulation of the lateral (*Diagram I*) and medial surface (*Diagram II*) of the brain of a monkey. The muscles or movements activated are shown. (From Horsley V, Schäfer EA: A record of experiments upon the functions of the cerebral cortex. *Philos Trans R Soc Lond* B 1888; 179: 1–45.)

suggests a broad and overlapping cortical representation of sensorimotor function. Moreover, several discrete but interconnected cortical motor areas exist and contribute to different aspects of movement, with subcortical regions involved in feedback loops. It has been shown that there are multiple cortical outputs to the individual lower motor neurons that supply different muscles, that individual cortical cells commonly project to more than one muscle, typically to a particular set of muscles, and that there is extensive overlapping of the cortical output to different lower motor neurons (muscles). These features are important in allowing functionally relevant movements based on the cooperative interaction of several muscles to occur.[47,48] The motor cortex itself is best viewed as simply the output region for various complex neural systems.

Laryngeal Motor Cortex

Semon and Horsley collaborated for some four years in studying the control by the brain of the laryngeal muscles, which are activated during phonation (vocalization) and respiration. They had met previously when Semon first suggested that myxedema, cachexia strumipriva, and cretinism represented different phases of a single pathological process (hypothyroidism), a suggestion ridiculed by some but which Horsley was able to confirm experimentally (see Chapter 3). Semon had become interested in the position of the vocal cords in various circumstances – they are separated (abducted) to widen the airway during inhalation and brought together (adducted) to permit vocalization. He and Horsley now studied the representation of the larynx in the cerebral cortex and the pathway of the fibers running from there to the brainstem.[49]

Phonatory adductor movements of the vocal cords occurred bilaterally with stimulation of a localized cortical area in each cerebral hemisphere.[50] By contrast, abduction of the vocal cords (a respiratory movement) could not be elicited by cortical stimulation in monkeys or dogs, the main neural regulation being from the brainstem. Extrinsic (vertical) movement of the larynx as when swallowing occurred only with stimulation just in front of or just behind the rolandic fissure (upward or downward movement, respectively). This separation of the intrinsic and extrinsic laryngeal representation in the cortex has since been confirmed by others.

The cortical representation of the laryngeal muscles is important, bearing on the control of the voice, as in speech and song. The work by Semon and Horsley did not receive the attention it merited when first reported. Increasing attention is only now being directed at the anatomy and connectivity of the laryngeal motor cortex and at its variation between human and nonhuman primates.[51]

Gotch and the Croonian Lectures

Horsley collaborated with Francis Gotch, his brother-in-law, for much of the 1880s. Gotch had been a fellow student at University College, London, where he became a protégé of John Burdon Sanderson. When Burdon Sanderson became the first holder of the Waynflete chair of physiology at Oxford, Gotch moved with him and assisted in organizing the new department. He then briefly held the chair of physiology in Liverpool before returning to Oxford as Burdon Sanderson's successor. The work of the two brothers-in-law was summarized in their 1891 Croonian lecture at the Royal Society.[52] This lecture, delivered annually since 1738, is regarded as the most prestigious lectureship in the biological sciences in Britain.

Working mainly at Oxford, they used a capillary electrometer[53] to record the impulse generated in the sciatic nerve of the anesthetized rabbit, cat, and monkey by a single stimulus, using an induction coil to stimulate the nerve. The responses were small but consistent, and were "due to the electromotive change which accompanies the propagation of an excitatory state along the mammalian nerve when this state is evoked by the application of a single stimulus."[54] This seems to have been the first occasion in which a single nerve impulse (a nerve action potential) was actually recorded.[55] It was a remarkable achievement given the equipment available at the time, but Horsley's efforts were focused more on the central nervous system.

Horsley and Gotch showed that electrical currents could be recorded from different parts of the mammalian brain. They used the capillary electrometer to detect electrical activity in one part of

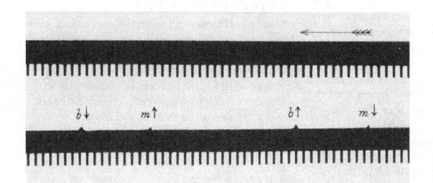

Figure 4.3 Nerve action potentials recorded by Gotch and Horsley. Tracings were recorded from the sciatic nerve, and should be read from right to left (top arrow). The cut end and the surface of the nerve was connected with the electrometer. The time marker at the bottom of each trace indicates one tenth of a second. The two prominences, *m* and *b*, in the lower trace reflect a make and break induction shock, and the arrows indicate the direction of the exciting induction current through the nerve. The effect is always in the same direction and is such that the electrode on the surface of the nerve becomes negative to that on the cut section. (From Gotch F, Horsley V: Observations upon the electromotive changes in the mammalian spinal cord following electrical excitation of the cortex cerebri. Preliminary notice. *Proc R Soc Lond* 1888: 45: 18–26.)

the nervous system following stimulation of a distant part.[54] They thus demonstrated that conduction occurs in the spinal cord and traced neural pathways in the central nervous system, such as the connectivity of the posterior and lateral columns of the spinal cord, which are the main avenues by which sensory information is conveyed to the brain. They stimulated the peripheral nerves and recorded from the spinal cord, and vice versa, and also stimulated the cerebral cortex to observe the responses obtained. No further advances in work of this sort could really occur until the invention of amplifiers.

Electrical Activity of the Cerebral Cortex

Despite their real achievements, certain claims by Gotch and Horsley were surprising, especially those relating to the electrical activity of the cerebral cortex. Richard Caton (1842–1926), the first professor of physiology in the University College of Liverpool, discovered in 1875 the "spontaneous" electrical activity of the brain (the electroencephalogram or EEG), and showed that it could be used to localize sensory function.[56] When both recording electrodes were placed on the cortex, he was able to record a rhythmic waxing and waning electrical potential, namely the "brain waves," which changed with sensory stimulation:

> Feeble currents of varying direction pass through the multiplier when the electrodes are placed on two points of the external surface, or one electrode on the grey matter, and one on the surface of the skull. . . . When any part of the grey matter is in a state of functional activity, its electric current usually exhibits negative variation. . . . Impressions through the senses were found to influence the currents of certain areas; e.g., the currents of that part of the rabbit's brain which Dr. Ferrier has shown to be related to movements of the eyelids, were found to be markedly influenced by stimulation of the opposite retina by light.[56]

The work, which had been supported by a grant from the British Medical Association, was presented at the annual meeting of the Association in 1875 but received only passing attention. It is unfortunate that his findings were not reported to the Royal Society, despite the encouragement of Burdon Sanderson, then the society's vice president, for they would undoubtedly have aroused more interest.[57] As it was, they were soon forgotten.

Adolf Beck (1863–1942) of Cracow, Poland, subsequently reported similar findings – the presence over the cerebral hemispheres of spontaneous electrical activity that became attenuated with sensory stimulation – in his doctoral thesis (written in Polish). He published a brief account in the German-language *Centralblatt für Physiologie*, not knowing about Caton's work.[58,59] Others soon claimed priority for the same discovery. The Viennese physiologist Fleischl von Marxow (1846–1891) – a brilliant, handsome, but tormented man who became addicted to heroin and morphine and died young – wrote to the *Centralblatt* pointing out that he had deposited a sealed letter with the Imperial Academy of Sciences in Vienna in 1883. Such sealed letters typically reported an important but incompletely delineated and unpublished observation; they were used to establish priority for the discovery when later this was disputed. Fleischl von Marxow's letter described his experimental findings that electrical activity could be recorded from different regions of the cerebral cortex in various animals in response to specific sensory stimuli (such as light, pain, sound, and touch).[60] This electrical activity could even be recorded over the dural membrane covering the hemispheres or from over the skull. He did not describe the spontaneous rhythmic activity found by Caton.

Beck responded courteously that the priority for a discovery should be given to the one who has revealed a secret of nature without creating another secret under the seal of the Imperial Academy of Sciences in Vienna. He nevertheless felt that any squabble over priority was unnecessary in the present instance, for the application of an old technique to a new question could hardly be rated as a discovery.[57,59,61] A letter from Gotch and Horsley was published in *Centralblatt* shortly thereafter, however, claiming priority over both Beck and von Marxow.[62] Their letter was unfortunate, for the writers apparently failed to see the difference between recording the spontaneous electrical activity of the brain and recording the responses to electrical stimulation of the brain.[59] It has been pointed out that in the many experiments described in their Croonian lecture, published later that same year, only one actually involved recording from the brain following retinal stimulation, with "capricious results." None of the experiments involved the electroencephalogram, and as only one of the recording electrodes was on the cerebral cortex, it seems that they were recording demarcation (or injury) potentials.[59]

The somewhat discreditable controversy was brought to a close when early in 1891 the journal published a letter from Caton in England, pointing out that it was he who first reported the presence of electrical currents on the surface of the cerebral hemispheres in 1875.[63] Curiously, Gotch and Horsley seemed unaware of Caton's contribution when first they wrote, but they made sure to include his name in their lengthy Croonian lecture. And ironically, in this same year, Gotch was appointed to the chair of physiology in Liverpool, succeeding the very Caton whose work was apparently unfamiliar to him.

Studies of the Human Brain

The human brain was also explored in the latter half of the nineteenth century. Roberts Bartholow (1831–1904), one of the founding physicians of the American Neurological Association, of which he became president in 1881, attempted to do so in Cincinnati. In 1874 he electrically stimulated localized regions of the cerebral hemisphere of one of his patients – a terminally ill, "rather feeble-minded," thirty-year-old housemaid who had voluntarily consented to the procedure – using needle electrodes insulated to near their tips and inserted through a cancerous skull defect directly into her brain.[64] This enabled him to induce muscle contractions or sensory phenomena in the contralateral limbs of the ailing woman. His report raised public concern about the ethics of human experimentation, however, especially when the patient had a seizure after one of his sessions, became comatose, and died, probably from venous sinus thrombosis unrelated to the experimental intervention.[64,65] Bartholow was subsequently criticized on ethical grounds for his experiments and publicly expressed his "regret that facts which I hoped would further, in some slight degree, the progress of knowledge, were obtained at the expense of some injury to the patient."[66]

Subsequent work on the brain in humans was largely confined to electrical stimulation for localization purposes at the time of surgery in conscious subjects, as in cases described by Horsley in London, William Keen (1837–1932) in Philadelphia, and Feodor Krause (1857–1937)

in Germany. Later, electrical stimulation came to be utilized extensively by Wilder Penfield (1891–1976) and his colleagues in Montreal during the 1930s.[67,68] Penfield had studied mammalian physiology under Sherrington at Oxford and went on to make important studies of functional localization in the human brain during the surgical treatment of epilepsy. The experimental work in animals and early studies in humans had led to these later, detailed stimulation studies. They had shown that the cerebral cortex is excitable, that the results of stimulation experiments in nonhumans can legitimately be extended to humans, and that there is indeed a certain localization of cortical functions, with more anterior cortical regions generating motor responses and posterior regions, sensory responses. The early experimental observations of Ferrier, Schäfer, Horsley, Sherrington, and others also provided support for Jackson's concepts of cerebral organization. The definition of the anatomical basis of various cerebral activities – and thus the ability to localize intracranial lesions by the symptoms and signs that they cause – led directly to successful intracranial surgery long before radiographic and other imaging procedures became available to guide the surgeon.

These early studies led also to considerations of the mind–brain issue. Ferrier and many contemporary neuroscientists came to relate the neural events associated with electrically evoked motor and sensory responses to the natural occurrence of voluntary motor activity or sensory perceptions. They held that the cortical motor center, for example, initiated voluntary activity because the activity generated by its electrical stimulation was sometimes coordinated and seemingly purposive. Indeed, they speculated further: "It must follow from the experimental data that mental operations in the last analysis must be merely the subjective side of sensory and motor substrata."[69] The melancholy Jackson took a different approach, claiming that it is impossible to localize mental function.[70,71] He believed that the nervous system is an explicitly sensorimotor machine, that the mind is a completely separate entity, and that neither causes the other to act in any way.[70] "We do not say that psychical states are functions of the brain ... but simply that they occur during the functioning of the brain."[70] Yet other neuroscientists, for example, the intuitive Brown-Séquard, were disturbed by the localization of complex functions to discrete cortical regions simply because apparently similar responses were elicited from these regions by focal electrical stimulation, holding that even "simple" functions depended on the complex interactions of several neurological systems. As for Horsley, when asked to examine pathologically the brain – preserved in alcohol for many years – of the brilliant mathematician Charles Babbage (1791–1871), a music-hating misanthrope who invented the prototype of the modern computer, he commented that it was still "impossible to make deductions of scientific value on the relation between special mental characteristics and cerebral development."[72]

It has become clear over the years that the brain is not to be viewed as the collection of independent centers for different functions as was once believed, but rather as a complex organ that functions as an integrated unit, with excitatory and inhibitory influences from many parts affecting the activity of a localized region. In the first quarter of the twenty-first century, complicated task-specific cortical networks are being mapped in healthy humans using advanced neuroimaging techniques. Indeed, using multimodal magnetic resonance images and a neuroanatomical approach that takes structure, function, and connectivity into account, a new map produced in 2016 delineated one hundred and eighty different regions.[73]

It was David Ferrier, in particular, who urged his surgical comrades to venture past the dura mater – the tough membrane covering the brain – and utilize the information gained from experimentation in animals to localize and remove focal abnormalities in the human brain. Victor Horsley, so familiar with the necessary procedures because of his own experimental studies in animals, heeded that call and helped to establish the modern field of neurosurgery. He was appointed consultant neurological surgeon at the National Hospital for the Paralysed and Epileptic (see Chapter 5) in early 1886, the first appointment of its kind in the world, and this was where he now focused his attention, as discussed in later chapters.

Notes

1. Gross CG: The discovery of motor cortex and its background. *J Hist Neurosci* 2007; **16**: 320–331.

2. Broca P: Perte de la parole, ramollissement chronique et destruction partielle du lobe antérieur gauche du cerveau. *Bull Soc d'Anthropol (Paris)* 1861; **2**: 235–238.

3. Broca P: Remarques sur le siège de la faculté du langage articulé, suivies d'une observation d'aphémie (perte de la parole). *Bull Soc Anat (Paris)* 1861; **6** (2nd series): 330–357.

4. Broca P: Nouvelle observation d'aphémie produite par une lésion de la moitié postérieure des deuxième et troisième circonvolutions frontales. *Bull Soc Anat (Paris)* 1861; **6** (2nd series): 398–407.

5. Broca P: Localisation des fonctions cérébrales. Siége du langage articulé. *Bull Soc d'Anthropol (Paris)* 1863; **4**: 200–204.

6. Finger S, Roe D: Gustave Dax and the early history of cerebral dominance. *Arch Neurol* 1996; **53**: 806–813.

7. Buckingham HW: The Marc Dax (1770–1837)/ Paul Broca (1824–1880) controversy over priority in science: Left hemisphere specificity for seat of articulate language and for lesions that cause aphemia. *Clin Linguist Phon* 2006; **20**: 613–619.

8. Head H: Hughlings Jackson on aphasia and kindred affections of speech. *Brain* 1915; **38**: 1–27.

9. Jackson JH: On the nature of the duality of the brain. *Brain* 1915; **38**: 80–86. [Reprinted from Medical Press & Circular, January 14, 1874]

10. Jackson JH: On affections of speech from disease of the brain. *Brain* 1888; **2**: 203–222.

11. Aminoff MJ: *Brown-Séquard: An Improbable Genius Who Transformed Medicine*. Oxford University Press: New York, 2011.

12. Jackson JH: On the anatomical and physiological localisation of movements in the brain. [In several parts.] *Lancet* 1873; **1**: 84–85, 162–164, and 232–234.

13. Taylor J (ed): *Selected Writings of John Hughlings Jackson. Volume 1. On Epilepsy and Epileptiform Convulsions*. Hodder & Stoughton: London, 1931.

14. Fritsch G, Hitzig E: Über die elektrische Erregbarkeit des Grosshirns. *Arch Anat Physiol (Lpz)* 1870; **37**: 300–332.

15. Walker AE: The development of the concept of cerebral localization in the nineteenth century. *Bull Hist Med* 1957; **31**: 99–121.

16. Ferrier D: Experimental researches in cerebral physiology and pathology. *West Riding Lunatic Asylum Medical Reports* 1873; **3**: 30–96.

17. Spillane JD: A memorable decade in the history of neurology 1874–84. *Br Med J* 1974; **4**: 701–706.

18. Ferrier D: *The Functions of the Brain*. Smith, Elder: London, 1876.

19. Ferrier D: Pathological illustrations of brain function. *West Riding Lunatic Asylum Medical Reports* 1874; **4**: 30–62.

20. Young RM: *Mind, Brain and Adaptation in the Nineteenth Century*. pp. 234–240. Clarendon: Oxford, 1970.

21. Ferrier D: Experiments on the brains of monkeys – No. 1. *Proc R Soc Lond* 1875; **23**: 409–430.

22. Ferrier D: The Croonian Lecture: Experiments on the brain of monkeys (second series) *Philos Trans R. Soc Lond* 1875; **165**: 433–488.

23. Sharpey Schafer E: The Victor Horsley Memorial Lecture on the relations of surgery and physiology. *Br Med J* 1923; **2**: 739–744.

24. Clark E: Ferrier, David. pp. 593–595. In Gillispie CC (ed): *Dictionary of Scientific Biography*. Scribner's: New York, 1971.

25. Tyler KL, Malessa R: The Goltz–Ferrier debates and the triumph of cerebral localizationalist theory. *Neurology* 2000; **55**: 1015–1024.

26. Klein E: Report on the parts destroyed on the left side of the brain of the dog operated on by Prof. Goltz. *J Physiol* 1883; **4**: 310–315.

27. Schäfer EA: Report on the lesions, primary and secondary, in the brain and spinal cord of the macacque monkey exhibited by Professors Ferrier and Yeo. *J Physiol* 1883; **4**: 316–326.

28. Langley JN: Report on the parts destroyed on the right side of the brain of the dog operated on by Prof. Goltz. *J Physiol* 1883; **4**: 286–309.

29. Klein E, Langley JN, Schäfer EA: On the cortical areas removed from the brain of a dog, and from the brain of a monkey. *J Physiol* 1884; **4**: 231–247.

30. Anon: The charge against Professor Ferrier under the Vivisection Act: Dismissal of the summons. *Br Med J* 1881; **2**: 836–842.

31. CSS [Sherrington CS]: Sir David Ferrier. *Proc R Soc Lond B* 1928; **103**: viii–xvi.

32. Horsley V: Obituary. Charles Edward Beevor, M. D., F.R.C.P (Lond.). *Br Med J* 1908; **2**: 1785–1786.

33. Lee S: *King Edward VII: A Biography*. Volume II. p. 63. Macmillan: London, 1927.

34. Horsley V, Schäfer EA: Experiments on the character of the muscular contractions which are evoked by excitation of the various parts of the motor tract. *J Physiol* 1886; **7**: 96–110.

35. Horsley V, Schäfer EA: A record of experiments upon the functions of the cerebral cortex. *Philos Trans R Soc Lond B* 1888; **179**: 1–45.

36. Ferrier D, Yeo G: A record of experiments on the effects of lesion of different regions of the cerebral hemispheres. *Philos Trans R. Soc Lond* 1884; **175**: 479–564.

37. Beevor CE, Horsley V: A minute analysis (experimental) of the various movements produced by stimulating in the monkey different regions of the cortical centre for the upper limb, as defined by Professor Ferrier. *Proc R Soc Lond* 1886; **40**: 475–476 [Abstract]; *Philos Trans R Soc Lond B* 1887; **178**: 153–167.

38. Beevor CE, Horsley V: A further minute analysis, by electric stimulation, of the so-called motor region of the cortex cerebri in the monkey (*Macacus sinicus*). *Proc R Soc Lond* 1887; **43**: 86–88 [Abstract]; *Philos Trans R Soc Lond B* 1888; **179**: 205–256.

39. Beevor CE, Horsley V: An experimental investigation into the arrangement of the excitable fibres of the internal capsule of the Bonnet monkey (*Macacus sinicus*). *Philos Trans R Soc Lond B* 1890; **181**: 49–88.

40. Beevor CE, Horsley V: A record of the results obtained by electrical excitation of the so-called motor cortex and internal capsule in an orang-outang (*Simia satyrus*). *Philos Trans R Soc Lond B* 1890; **181**: 129–158.

41. Horsley V: The Linacre Lecture on the function of the so-called motor area of the brain. *Br Med J* 1909; **2**: 121–132.

42. Grünbaum ASF, Sherrington CS: Observations on the physiology of the cerebral cortex of some of the higher apes. *Proc R Soc Lond* 1901; **69**: 206–209.

43. Grünbaum ASF, Sherrington CS: Observations on the physiology of the cerebral cortex of the anthropoid apes. *Proc R Soc Lond* 1903; **72**: 152–155.

44. Leyton ASF, Sherrington CS: Observations of the excitable cortex of the chimpanzee, orang-utan and gorilla. *Q J Exp Physiol* 1917; **11**: 135–222.

45. Rathelot JA, Strick PL: Muscle representation in the macaque motor cortex: An anatomical perspective. *Proc Natl Acad Sci U S A* 2006; **103**: 8257–8262.

46. Hatsopoulos NG, Suminski AJ: Sensing with the motor cortex. *Neuron* 2011; **72**: 477–487.

47. Humphrey DR: Representation of movements and muscles within the primate precentral motor cortex: Historical and current perspectives. *Fed Proc* 1986; **45**: 2687–2699.

48. Lemon R: The output map of the primate motor cortex. *Trends Neurosci* 1988; **11**: 501–506.

49. Semon F, Horsley V: An experimental investigation of the central motor innervation of the larynx. *Philos Trans R Soc Lond B* 1890; **181**: 187–211.

50. Semon and Horsley found that in monkeys, phonatory adductor movements of the vocal cords occurred bilaterally when they stimulated a localized cortical area just posterior to the lower end of the precentral sulcus at the base of the third frontal gyrus.

51. Kumar V, Croxson PL, Simonyan K: Structural organization of the laryngeal motor cortical network and its implication for evolution of speech production. *J Neurosci* 2016; **36**: 4170–4181.

52. Gotch F, Horsley V: Croonian Lecture: On the mammalian nervous system, its functions, and their localisation determined by an electrical method. *Philos Trans R Soc Lond B* 1891; **182**: 267–526.

53. The capillary electrometer was a simple but robust device for measuring small differences in electrical potential between two points based upon change of surface tension between mercury and a dilute solution of sulphuric acid in the capillary tip of a tube containing mercury.

54. Gotch F, Horsley V: Observations upon the electromotive changes in the mammalian spinal cord following electrical excitation of the cortex cerebri. Preliminary notice. *Proc R Soc Lond* 1888; **45**: 18–26.

55. McComas AJ: *Galvani's Spark: The Story of the Nerve Impulse*. pp. 63–64. Oxford University Press: New York, 2011.

56. Caton R: The electric currents of the brain. *Br Med J* 1875; **2**: 278.

57. Cohen, Lord, of Birkenhead: Richard Caton (1842–1926): Pioneer electrophysiologist. *Proc R Soc Med* 1959; **52**: 645–651.

58. Beck A: Die Bestimmung der Localisation der Gehirn- und Rückenmarksfunctionen vermittelst der elektrischen Erscheinungen. *Centralbl Physiol* 189: **4**: 473–476.

59. Brazier MAB: *A History of the Electrical Activity of the Brain: The First Half-Century*. pp. 4–63. Pitman Medical: London, 1961.

60. Fleischl von Marxow E: Mittheilung, betreffend die Physiologie der Hirnrinde. *Centralb Physiol* 1890; **4**: 537–540.

61. Beck A: Die Ströme der Nervencentren. *Centralbl Physiol* 1891; **4**: 572–573.

62. Gotch F, Horsley V: Ueber den Gebrauch der Elektricität für die Lokalisirung der Erregungserscheinungen im Centralnervensystem. *Centralbl Physiol* 1891; **4**: 649–651.

63. Caton R: Die Ströme des Centralnervensystems. *Centralbl Physiol* 1891: **4**: 785–786.

64. Bartholow R: Experimental investigations into the functions of the human brain. *Am J Med Sci* 1874; **66**: 305–313.

65. Harris LJ, Almerigi JB: Probing the human brain with stimulating electrodes: The story of Roberts Bartholow's (1874) experiment on Mary Rafferty. *Brain Cogn* 2009; **70**: 92–115.

66. Bartholow R: Experiments on the functions of the human brain [letter to the editor]. *Br Med J* 1874; **1**: 727.

67. Penfield W, Boldrey E: Somatic motor and sensory representation in the cerebral cortex of man as studied by electrical stimulation. *Brain* 1937; **60**: 389–443.

68. Jasper H, Penfield W: *Epilepsy and the Functional Anatomy of the Human Brain*. Little Brown: Boston, 1954.

69. Ferrier D: *The Functions of the Brain*. p. 256. Smith, Elder: London, 1876.

70. Jackson JH: Remarks on evolution and dissolution of the nervous system. *J Ment Sci* 1887; **32**: 25–48.

71. York GK, Steinberg DA: The philosophy of Hughlings Jackson. *J R Soc Med* 2002; **95**: 314–318.

72. Horsley V: Description of the brain of Mr. Charles Babbage, F.R.S. *Philos Trans R Soc Lond B* 1909; **200**: 117–131.

73. Glasser MF, Coalson TS, Robinson EC, et al: A multi-modal parcellation of human cerebral cortex. *Nature* 2016; **536**: 171–178.

The Making of a Specialty

James B. was a Scottish lad of twenty-two with focal epilepsy when he entered into the medical history books. He had been run over by a cab when seven years old, sustaining a depressed, compound skull fracture to the left of the vertex that led to a loss of brain substance and local infection. He developed seizures at the age of fifteen, and these became increasingly frequent and sometimes occurred in flurries such that he experienced as many as three thousand fits over a two-week period. They most commonly started in the right leg:

> The right lower limb was tonically extended, and the seat of clonic spasm. The right upper limb was then slowly extended at right angles, to the body, the wrist and fingers being flexed; the fingers next became extended, and clonic spasms of flexion and extension affected the whole limb, the elbow being gradually flexed. By this time, spasms in the lower limb having ceased, but those in the upper limb continuing vigorously, spasm gradually affected the right angle of the mouth, spreading over the right side of the face, and followed by turning of the head and eyes to the right.
>
> To sum up, the parts affected were so in the order of lower limb, upper limb, face, and neck; the character of the movements was, first, extension, then confusion, finally, flexion, showing clearly that *the focus of discharge was situated around the posterior end of the superior frontal sulcus* [italics added].[1]

The epileptic focus was thus localized based on principles derived from experiments in animals, and its site coincided with that of a scar on the scalp and an associated bony defect in the skull.

On May 25, 1886, Horsley operated. He removed the bone around the site of the old injury and then the matted fibrous membranes overlying the brain. This revealed a vascular, reddened scar in the brain that was about three centimeters long and two centimeters wide, that is, about the size of a half-penny coin or twenty-five cent piece. The brain itself looked more yellow than normal. He carefully cut away the scar and adjacent brain tissue. The wound healed in a week, but James was left with weakness or paralysis of the right hand and forearm and with some loss of feeling. Fortunately, he regained all these functions over the following two months, and had no further seizures.

The operation was watched by Hughlings Jackson and David Ferrier, as well as by many other colleagues. The tension was relieved toward the end of the procedure when Jackson turned to Ferrier and mournfully intoned "Awful, awful." The Scottish physiologist was astonished: "Awful? The operation was performed perfectly." "Yes," came the response, "but he opened a Scotsman's head and failed to put a joke in it."[2]

This was neither the first operation on the human brain nor the first attempt to localize clinically a cerebral abnormality based on the knowledge gained experimentally of the brain's motor and sensory areas. It occurred almost two years after Rickman Godlee's successful removal of a brain tumor, discussed later. Even earlier, in 1876, William Macewen (1848–1924) in Glasgow had localized correctly an abscess in the left frontal lobe in an eleven-year-old boy, based on the new principles of cerebral localization. The boy's parents would not consent to surgery, but the site of the lesion was verified with anatomical precision at autopsy, "giving poignancy to the regret that the operation had not been permitted during life."[3]

In 1879 at a meeting of the Glasgow Pathological and Clinical Society, Macewen had demonstrated two patients with intracranial pathology on whom he had operated successfully. One patient had a blood clot pressing on the brain (a subdural hematoma) and the other a benign tumor (probably a meningioma) in the left frontal region. In these cases, however, the site of surgery

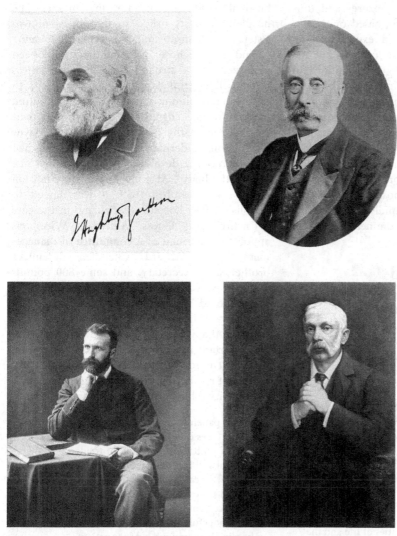

Figure 5.1 *Top left*, John Hughlings Jackson, father of British neurology, who developed a hierarchical concept of brain function and dysfunction. *Top right*, David Ferrier, the experimental neurologist whose work on the localization of cortical functions complemented that of Jackson. It permitted the clinical localization of cerebral lesions and thus allowed their surgical treatment. *Bottom left*, William Macewen, who preceded Horsley in operating successfully on intracranial and extradural spinal lesions. *Bottom right*, Rickman Godlee, who first successfully removed a brain tumor after its clinical localization. The patient died four weeks later from infection, perhaps because of inadequate preoperative preparation. Godlee went on to become a distinguished thoracic and general surgeon. (Images from the Wellcome Collection, London.)

had been determined at least in part by the presence of skin or bone changes.[4],[5] Macewen was a thorough and capable surgeon, a pioneer in the field, and an early advocate for the use of antisepsis and aseptic protocols, but he was a somewhat solitary figure who failed to leave a great school of neurosurgery as his legacy. Francesco Durante, a Sicilian who directed a surgical clinic in Rome, also preceded Horsley, having successfully removed in 1884 a benign intracranial tumor (meningioma) from the left anterior fossa in a thirty-five-year-old woman with loss of the sense of smell and a displaced left eye, but again the surgery was not based on studies of cortical function.

It was the operation performed by Horsley in 1886, therefore, that captured the attention of the medical world. He had localized the brain lesion responsible for the patient's seizures and thus focused his surgical approach, based on principles derived from localization experiments in animals. Moreover, the operation was but the beginning of Horsley's many contributions to the field of neurosurgery, underpinned by his devotion to the experimental studies on which neurosurgery came to be based. The company in which the surgery was performed and, perhaps more importantly, the setting in which it was undertaken must also have given the operation a particular appeal, for the surgery was undertaken at a small hospital in Queen Square, London, that was rapidly becoming the center for clinical studies of the nervous system in imperial Britain.

The National Hospital

Set in the Bloomsbury region of London, Queen Square is famous now for the various hospitals that came to be located there in the middle of the nineteenth century. It was the site, also, of the St. John's Nursing Services established by Florence Nightingale, the social reformer and nursing pioneer, famous as "the Lady with the Lamp" to the wounded during the Crimean War. Robert Louis Stevenson described the square as

> a little enclosure of tall trees and comely old brick houses, easy enough to see into over a railing at one end but not very easy to enter for all that, unless the visitor has profound knowledge or the instincts of an arctic explorer. It seems to have been set apart for the humanities of life and the alleviation of all hard destinies. As you go around it, you read upon every second door-plate, some offer of help to the afflicted. There are hospitals for sick children where you may see a little white-faced convalescent on the balcony talking to his brothers and sisters and the baby, who are below there, on a visit to him and obstruct your passage not unpleasantly . . . [2,5]

The square remains a tranquil refuge from the noise and bustle of the city, its center consisting of ordered gardens containing an imposing statue of Queen Charlotte, wife of King George III. It was in this square that a new hospital for patients with disorders of the nervous system opened in 1860, at a time when facilities in London for the care of the neurologically disabled consisted primarily of long-stay poor-law

hospitals and asylums for the insane. The hospital owed its origin to the efforts of two sisters – Louisa and, especially, Johanna Chandler – whose grandmother had been paralyzed by a stroke. The Chandler sisters began selling trinkets and small ornaments to raise money, aiming to establish an institution to care for the chronically disabled, and their efforts aroused the interest of the Lord Mayor of London, Alderman David Wire, who had himself recently developed weakness down one side of the body.[6] At a meeting in the Mansion House in November 1859, it was agreed to establish a new hospital specializing in the care of neurological illness. Alderman Wire was appointed chairman of a committee of management, with Edward Chandler, Johanna's brother, as its secretary, and some 800 pounds were soon received in public subscriptions to the proposed hospital.[2]

Wire – unlike the Chandler sisters – realized, however, that if the new hospital were to become an important institution and make its mark on society, it needed to become a center for active treatment rather than simply another board-and-care facility. Thus it was resolved that

> indoor patients will be, exclusively, those persons whose cases do not appear to be incurable. For these a probationary period of residence in the hospital will be granted; but if at the expiration thereof, or earlier if such persons shall be considered incurable, they will be removed in order to make room for others whose cases may be more hopeful. The persons so removed will still be eligible to become outdoor patients.[2]

The first order of business was to acquire suitable premises for the new institution. Early in 1860, the house at No. 24 Queen Square was rented for 110 pounds annually. Its front and back parlors were converted into a consulting (examining) room and waiting room for outpatients, and the butler's pantry became the dispensary. There was also accommodation for eight inpatients. The hospital opened in the spring, and patients were admitted at once. Over the next few years, the lease of the building was purchased, the adjacent building was acquired, and the property extended at the back, so that the hospital was able to accommodate some sixty-four patients by 1870.[5]

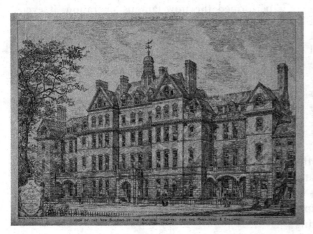
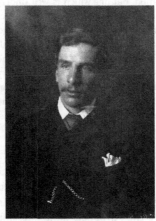

Surgeons.

1. The Surgeons shall attend at the Hospital at least once weekly at an appointed time, and shall give the requisite attention to any patients referred to them by the Physicians or Assistant-Physicians. They shall perform operations when necessary.

2. They shall communicate with the Board of Management or House Committee, through the Secretary and General Director, concerning absence from the Hospital, affecting the regular performance of their duties, and notifying a substitute.

I undertake to perform the duties of surgeon in conformity with the Rules set forth above.

12th. Febry, 1886. *Victor Horsley*

Figure 5.2 *Top left*, The National Hospital for the Paralysed and Epileptic at Queen Square, London. (Process print 1884 after J. W. Simpson, 1883); *Top right*, Victor Horsley. *Bottom*, Surgeons' rules at the hospital. Horsley signed his acceptance of these rules on February 12, 1886, stating: "I undertake to perform the duties of surgeon in conformity with the rules set forth above." (Top images from the Wellcome Collection, London; bottom image from the Queen Square Archives.)

Other Neurological Hospitals in Mid-Century London

Curiously, several other hospitals for neurological disorders were established in the metropolis at about the same time. The London Galvanic Hospital was founded in 1861 by Harry Lobb, a licentiate of the Society of Apothecaries, apparently because he could not obtain facilities at any established hospital in the metropolis to "treat suitable cases with the aid of galvanism."[7]

His hospital, in Cavendish Square, was therefore dedicated to "the treatment, with the aid of Electricity, of all forms of Nervous and Muscular Diseases, for which this force is particularly adapted."[8] It provoked the ire of the editor of the *Lancet*:

One gentleman, as though the whole range of diseases had been exhausted, founds an hospital which he conducts for carrying on a special form of treatment; not a new method, certainly not a universal method, but one which is well understood by the profession; which has been the subject of innumerable essays, papers, and books; and which is practised within its proper limits at all our hospitals. This institution is denominated the Galvanic Hospital and is conducted by Mr. Harry Lobb. Next may come a Quinine Hospital, an Hospital for Treatment by Cod-liver Oil, by the Hypophosphites, or by the Excrement of Boa-Constrictors.[9]

The hospital eventually foundered despite the attraction it held for the wealthy and titled, and regardless of its claims for therapeutic success in treating patients with certain neurological disorders, particularly the "dropped hands" resulting from lead poisoning (due to weakness of the wrist extensor muscles).[10]

Another hospital, the London Infirmary for Epilepsy and Paralysis, was opened in 1866, largely at the instigation of Julius Althaus (1833–1900), an émigré physician from Germany who was interested in the brain and believed in the use of electricity to manage various disorders of the nervous system and muscles.[11] His prolific writings included a popular *Treatise on Medical Electricity*, which went into several editions and was translated into three languages, as well as his well-known *On Failure of Brain Power*. The new hospital thrived, moved to larger premises next to Regent's Park after a few years, and changed its name to the Hospital for Diseases of the Nervous System to distinguish it from the National Hospital. It was at this hospital that, for the first time, a brain tumor was localized correctly and removed successfully by operation. The surgeon was Rickman Godlee, a senior colleague of Horsley's at University College Hospital and the nephew of Joseph Lister, and the operation was performed on November 25, 1884 in the presence of Hughlings Jackson, David Ferrier, and Horsley. Ironically enough, given the surgeon's relationship to the pioneer of antisepsis, the patient died four weeks later from infection, perhaps because of inadequate preoperative preparation. The localization of the tumor was only possible because of the clinical studies of Jackson and the experiments in animals performed by Ferrier, who had served as physician to outpatients at the hospital in Regent's Park before resigning in 1880 when appointed to the National Hospital.[12] Godlee went on to become a distinguished thoracic and general surgeon. As for the hospital where he had

performed the now-famous operation, it eventually moved to Maida Vale, amalgamated with the National in 1948, and was closed in 1983.

In 1878, a fourth hospital to serve the same branch of medicine was founded in London, this time by Herbert Tibbits, a fellow of the Royal College of Physicians of Edinburgh, who also was interested in the application of electrotherapy to neurological disorders. The West End Hospital for Diseases of the Nervous System, Paralysis, and Epilepsy survived for many years, moving to different premises about the capital as it expanded and then was damaged during World War II, finally closing in 1972.

Back to the National Hospital at Queen Square

Despite this competition from several new hospitals devoted to the nervous system and the disapproval of the contemporary medical establishment, which viewed the founding of specialist hospitals as a means of unseemly self-advertisement, the hospital at Queen Square flourished and there was much competition for appointments to its staff. Such appointments were based on the marriage of clinical and scientific expertise, and thus added to the aura of austere intellectualism that came to envelop the institution.

It was to the staff of this hospital that Horsley was elected unanimously in 1886,[13] and he remained active there for the remainder of his professional life. Letters in support of his election included one from Schäfer, who extolled his surgical and technical skill and his extensive knowledge of the structure and functioning of the nervous system.[14] Jean-Martin Charcot wrote from Paris. The magisterial professor of disorders of the nervous system at the Salpêtrière Hospital, on whose clinical service Horsley had spent some time a few months earlier, commented on his extensive theoretical knowledge and clinical experience.[15] His operative skill and scientific achievements were already widely known, however, and such testimonial letters simply added a layer of legitimacy to the appointment. Horsley thus joined a remarkable group that included John Hughlings Jackson (1835–1911) and William Gowers 1845–1915), the two greatest clinicians in contemporary British neurology.

Jackson's contributions to neurology are immense – he provided insights into the hierarchical organization of the nervous system, the nature of epilepsy, the somatotopic representation that underlies the spread or "march" of focal seizures (so-called Jacksonian seizures), and the manifestations of what came to be called temporal lobe or complex partial seizures. He wrote on disorders of language, on consciousness, and on the cerebellum, and he developed general concepts about the working of the brain from his descriptive analyses of neurological disorders. Gowers – also on staff at University College Hospital – was quite different; a superb clinician and showman when he so chose, he extended Jackson's thoughts into the clinical realm. Articulate, authoritative, and at ease in putting his thoughts to paper, he was renowned as a teacher whose *Manual of Diseases of the Nervous System* became the standard reference book for generations of neurological trainees.

Horsley was not the first surgeon to be appointed to the National Hospital, but he was the first neurological surgeon on its staff. There was already an orthopedic surgeon (William Adams), as well as a consulting general surgeon (Sir William Ferguson) who lent his name rather than his technical expertise to the young institution.

Thus it was at the National Hospital that Horsley operated on James B. on that day in May 1886. He used an antiseptic technique, with the patient prepared carefully for surgery. The head was shaved, washed, marked up with the probable site of the lesion, and then covered with lint soaked in a solution of carbolic acid for some twelve hours prior to the operation. The patient was anesthetized with chloroform for the operation, after an initial injection of morphine that, based on Horsley's experience with monkeys, caused a "well-marked contraction of the arterioles of the central nervous system" and hence reduced bleeding.[1] (The use of morphine was subsequently abandoned in this context because it depressed respiration.) Horsley made a semilunar incision into the scalp rather than utilizing the cruciform cut generally preferred at the time, keeping intact the blood supply to the skin flap. His surgical technique was described in clear terms – removal of the bone, opening of the subjacent dura mater (the tough outer membrane encasing the brain and spinal cord),

treatment of the brain itself, and wound closure. Postoperatively, he followed strict Listerian principles in managing the wound, freely using a carbolic spray and dressings of carbolic gauze.[1]

Horsley gave an account of his operation on James B. at the annual meeting of the British Medical Association in 1886, and described two other patients on whom he had operated successfully for a focal cerebral lesion (one, a tuberculoma, the other a posttraumatic cystic abnormality). Prior to surgery, all three patients had experienced recurrent seizures, the character of which suggested – by analogy to experimental studies in animals – that they originated in a specific part of the brain, and this permitted their successful surgical treatment. In other words, the site of the abnormality was localized on purely clinical grounds, which permitted Horsley to operate. Postoperative neurological deficits (weakness or paralysis and sensory abnormalities) were present in all three, but resolved almost completely within a few days or weeks.

His report caused enormous excitement and Horsley was congratulated on all sides, including by both Hughlings Jackson and Charcot. Not long afterwards, he performed another, more dramatic operation – hailed as the first of its kind – at the National.

Spinal Surgery

In 1884, shortly after a road traffic accident in which his wife was killed and he saved himself only by jerking abruptly backwards, Captain Gilbey, a forty-three-year-old businessman, began to develop pain in his upper back, just below the left shoulder-blade. The pain gradually worsened, was aggravated by activity, was accompanied by vague symptoms in his legs, and fluctuated in severity over the next two or three years; at times, it was so severe that he could barely walk. He was seen by a number of physicians, given many different diagnoses including "hypochondriacal insanity," and – because he seemed mad and there was doubt that he had any organic disease – told to go on a sea voyage or travel abroad, take Turkish baths, and take the waters at Aix-la-Chapelle. In February 1887, however, he developed increasing weakness, first in the left leg and, after a few weeks, in the right. His condition worsened until there was complete loss of power and sensation in the legs, occasional extensor spasms, and urinary retention; he also had severe girdle pain around the chest at the level of the sixth and seventh thoracic segments.

In early June he consulted William Gowers who, just a few years earlier, had published a monograph on diseases of the spinal cord. Gowers diagnosed a tumor compressing the spinal cord a little above the mid-thoracic region and wondered about surgical intervention, an unprecedented approach to an otherwise fatal disorder. Sir William Jenner – Gowers' former chief – was consulted and "sanctioned" the surgery. Horsley saw the patient on June 9 at the National, and operated on him two to three hours later assisted by Charles Ballance (who was himself later appointed surgeon to the hospital).

Unroofing the fourth to sixth thoracic vertebrae disclosed no abnormality, and extension of the laminectomy by one segment at each end still failed to reveal the cause of mischief. At the urging of Ballance, Horsley then extended the laminectomy upwards for yet another segment and this revealed beneath the dura a benign tumor (fibromyxoma) on the left, attached to the fourth thoracic nerve root and compressing the spinal cord. The tumor was removed completely. The patient gradually improved, regaining control of his bladder, sensation in the legs, and eventually full strength so that he was able to go dancing and walk three miles daily. Within a year, he was working full-time, and he lived for another twenty years before dying of an unrelated cause.

Horsley gave an account of the reasoning that had led to the surgery, as well as of the operation itself, at a meeting of the Royal Medical and Chirurgical Society in June 1888, and this caused quite a stir. The operation excited the medical community, and the case became a celebrated one. The tumor was at a somewhat higher level than had been anticipated, but its approximate clinical localization had allowed it to be removed. Horsley's skill, his prior experience with similar operations on animals for experimental purposes, and his use of antiseptic precautions had shown that the procedure was both feasible and less dangerous than previously believed, and therefore opened up a new realm of surgery. Appended to his case report was an analysis of fifty-seven previously published cases – all died, whereas surgery

might well have saved most of them.[16] William Osler, the regius professor of medicine at Oxford, remarked that it was "an epoch-making case, and one is at a loss which to admire more – the brilliant diagnosis of Gowers or the matchless technique of Horsley."[17]

Interestingly, this was the first time that an intradural spinal tumor (that is, a tumor within the dural membrane) had been removed, although spinal surgery for extradural compressive tumors had earlier been reported by others. In May 1883, William Macewen in Glasgow had removed a "fibrous neoplasm" that lay between the bone and dura, attached to the dura and compressing the mid-thoracic spinal cord in a nine-year-old with paralyzed and senseless legs and incontinence of urine and feces for the preceding two years. Within a few days sensation and then power of the legs began to recover and he regained control of his sphincters. Six months later he could get about without support and after five years he could walk three miles to visit his doctor.[3] Macewen described three other cases in which he had been successful in restoring function by removal of compressive extradural lesions, and two others who had failed to improve and eventually died.[3,18,19] In these six cases undergoing laminectomy, he summarized, four "completely recovered and two have died, one from extension of tubercular disease months after the operation, and after the wound had healed, leaving one in which the operation possibly hastened the death of a patient who was otherwise in such a helpless and hopeless condition." And he continued, "Such operations are now beginning to be practiced by others. Mr. Horsley a few months ago published a successful case in which a somewhat similar operation had been performed for the removal of a small tumour of the theca diagnosed by Dr. Gowers."[3]

As with the intracranial surgery referred to earlier, Macewen had preceded Horsley but he is not always accorded the recognition that he clearly merits. Horsley recognized his contribution and was one of those who signed their support of his candidacy when he was elected to fellowship of the Royal Society of London.[20]

Subsequent Developments

Horsley did not have admitting privileges to the hospital beds at Queen Square. Patients were

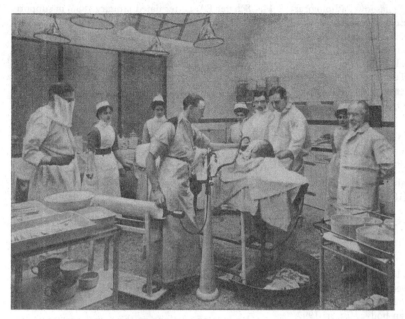

Figure 5.3 The operating room at the National Hospital (Queen Square), London, in 1906. Horsley, masked, stands at the extreme left. If he appears more bulky than usual, it is because he is wearing a large antiseptic dressing on his abdomen in preparation for the planned appendicectomy he was to undergo on the following day. Emil Theodor Kocher, a visiting Swiss surgeon and later Nobel laureate for his work on the thyroid gland, is on the extreme right. (From Horsley V: On the technique of operations on the central nervous system. *Br Med J* 1906; 2: 411–423.)

therefore admitted under the care of one of the physicians on staff, who assumed responsibility for their care and referred them to Horsley when surgery was deemed necessary. Requests by Horsley to admit patients under his own name were turned down by a medical staff anxious to safeguard its own privilege and to avoid setting any precedent that might later be regretted. Gowers was the exception – he allowed Horsley free access to the limited number of beds nominally under his own (Gowers') name and otherwise advised him to borrow another physician's beds "in silence" when necessary.[21] As for the facilities available to Horsley, at first he had only a kitchen in which to operate.[22] Later, two small surgical wards and an operating room were carved out of an existing ward, providing together some seven or eight beds, but the obvious inadequacy of this arrangement led to the opening of a new operating theater in 1904.

Horsley was invited to speak at the first Congress of American Physicians and Surgeons in Washington, D.C., in September 1888, where he discussed the physiological aspects and clinical implications of cerebral localization.[23] By 1890, he was able to report to the International Medical Congress in Berlin the results of forty-four cases in which he had operated on the brain.[24] Considering that he was treating patients with a grim outlook if surgery had not been undertaken and the fact that surgery of this sort carried very high risks, the death of only ten of his patients has to be considered something of a triumph. Horsley had shown that surgery on the nervous system was feasible and – with the proper techniques of anesthesia and antisepsis or asepsis – could be undertaken with acceptable morbidity and mortality rates. The new specialty of neurosurgery was born.

Notes

1. Horsley V: Brain surgery. *Br Med J* 1886; **2**: 670–675.

2. Holmes G: *The National Hospital, Queen Square.* Livingstone: Edinburgh, 1954.

3. Macewen W: An address on the surgery of the brain and spinal cord. *Br Med J* 1888; **2**: 302–309; also published in *Lancet* 1888; **132**: 254–261.

4. Anon: Reports of Societies. Glasgow Pathological and Clinical Society. Tuesday, November 11th, 1879. *Br Med J* 1879; **2**: 1022; also published with more detail in Reports of hospital and private practice. Glasgow Royal Infirmary: From Dr. Macewen's wards. Tumour of the dura mater – convulsions – removal of tumour by trephining – recovery. *Glasgow Med J* 1879; **12**: 210–213.

5. The Chartered Society of Queen Square: *Queen Square and the National Hospital 1860–1960.* Edward Arnold: London, 1960.

6. Critchley M: The beginnings of the National Hospital, Queen Square (1859–1860). *Br Med J* 1960; **1**: 1829–1837.

7. Lobb H: Special hospitals – The London Galvanic Hospital. [Letter to the editor.] *Lancet* 1863; **81**; 219.

8. Advertisement for the London Galvanic Hospital. Electrician v (1863), between pp. 120 and 121. Cited by Morus IR: The measure of man: technologizing the Victorian body. *Hist Sci* 1999; **37**: 249–282.

9. Anon: Editorial: The march of specialism. *Lancet* 1863; **81**: 183.

10. Lobb H: Uses and value of galvanism and electricity in general practice. Harveian Society of London, February 19, 1863. *Med Times Gaz* 1863; **1**: 493.

11. Bladin PF: Julius Althaus (1833–1900). Neurologist and cultural polymath; founder of Maida Vale Hospital. *J Clin Neurosci* 2008; **15**: 495–501.

12. Feiling A: *A History of the Maida Vale Hospital for Nervous Diseases.* Butterworth: London, 1958.

13. Anon: Minuted note (unsigned) dated February 9, 1886 regarding Horsley's election to the staff of the National Hospital. QSA/2147, Queen Square Archives (London, UK).

14. Schäfer EA: Letter dated January 1886, in support of the appointment of Victor Horsley to the surgical staff at the National Hospital. QSA/2152, Queen Square Archives (London, UK).

15. Charcot JM: Letter dated January 1886, in support of the appointment of Victor Horsley to the surgical staff at the National Hospital. QSA/2141, Queen Square Archives (London, UK).

16. Gowers WR, Horsley V: A case of tumour of the spinal cord: Removal: Recovery. [Abstract] *Br Med J* 1888; **1**: 1273–1274; Tumour of spinal cord, with removal and recovery. [Abstract] *Lancet* 1888; **131**: 1194; A case of tumour of the spinal cord. Removal; recovery. *Med Chir Trans Lond* 1888; **71**: 377–428.

17. Osler W: Some personal appreciations. *Br Med J* 1916; **2**: 165.

18. Macewen W: Trephining of the spine for paraplegia. *Glasgow Med J* 1884; **22**: 55–58.

19. Macewen W: Two cases in which excision of the laminae of portions of the spinal vertebrae had been performed in order to relieve pressure on the spinal cord causing paraplegia. *Glasgow Med J* 1885; **25**: 210–212.

20. Bowman AK: *The Life and Teaching of Sir William Macewen: A Chapter in the History of Surgery.* pp. 24–25. Hodge: London, 1942.

21. Gowers WR: Letter to Victor Horsley dated November 16, 1891. Section E4/7, Horsley Papers, Special Collections, UCL Library Services (London, UK).

22. Ballance C: Remarks and reminiscences. *Br Med J* 1927; **1**: 64–67.

23. Horsley V: Discussion on cerebral localization. *Trans Cong Am Phys Surg* 1889; **1**: 340–350.

24. Horsley V: Remarks on the surgery of the central nervous system. *Br Med J* 1890; **2**: 1286–1292.

The Grammar of Neurosurgery: Technical Underpinnings

Horsley's first brain operation for the treatment of posttraumatic epilepsy in May 1886 was followed rapidly by others: by the end of the year he had operated on the brain in ten cases, and by the end of the decade in forty-four.[1] His technical facility in handling the brain had been developed through his experimental studies in animals and by his experience as a pathologist. His skill, self-confidence, anatomical knowledge, and ambidexterity allowed him to operate with enormous speed, thereby lessening the very real risks of anesthesia, and his adherence to the new principles of antisepsis, which many of his surgical contemporaries initially rejected, reduced the complication rate from infection. Working primarily at the National Hospital assured him of a plentiful supply of patients requiring neurosurgical intervention. Localization of the pathological abnormality was by clinical methods alone.

A major issue faced by Horsley was the variability between specific sites in the brain and the external markings on the skull and scalp, that is, the surface anatomy of the head. He summarized his experience in 1887 based on his experimental studies in nonhuman primates as well as his as-yet limited clinical experience with ten patients.[2] His aim was to aid less experienced surgeons when "called upon to explore the cranial cavity" by providing them with a "topographical guide to definite portions of the brain."[2] The relationships between scalp markings and underlying brain he regarded as provisional, however, until more information accumulated to support or extend them. This variability eventually was to lead Horsley to collaborate with Robert Clarke in developing an instrument for localizing the deeper structures of the brain, the Horsley–Clarke stereotactic apparatus (discussed later). Modifications of this apparatus are used widely today in clinical neurosurgery.

Horsley's underlying belief concerning the role of surgery was expressed in a letter he wrote to Gowers – his former teacher and now his colleague at University College Hospital and at Queen Square – in December 1894: "I am averse to performing operations in so-called medical conditions if there is any medical procedure yet untried."[3]

Before reviewing his individual experience and contributions, his cumulative clinical experience between 1886 and the end of the century merits consideration. His surgical results on charity patients treated at the National Hospital have been analyzed by the recent neurosurgical staff at that hospital.[4] Horsley's private patients were treated elsewhere – at private houses or nursing homes – and these records were therefore not available for analysis.

Among sixty-eight patients who underwent intracranial surgery for diverse reasons (tumor, seizures, trauma, infection, head or facial pain, or various structural abnormalities) during this time period, half were cured or improved, six worsened or were unchanged, and twenty-six died. Among forty-two undergoing spinal surgery, most often for spinal infection (usually tuberculous), twenty-three were cured or improved, nine died, and two worsened; the remainder were unchanged.[4] Horsley also undertook operative sectioning of various cranial or peripheral nerves, and some more general surgical procedures.

He often anesthetized the patients himself, especially when operating alone away from an established hospital and without junior assistants. He generally used chloroform combined, in his early cases, with morphine, but he subsequently advised against morphine because it depressed respiration.[5] He stressed that the level of anesthesia should vary depending on the stage of surgery: a greater concentration of chloroform was required when cutting sensitive structures such as the skin or the dural membrane enveloping the brain, whereas a lower concentration was

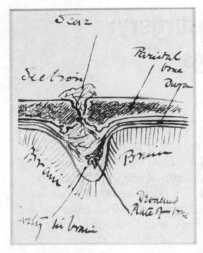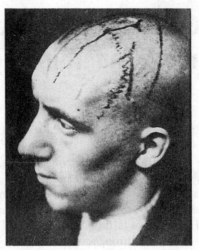

Figure 6.1 Horsley operated on GWJ, a twenty-four-year-old stable-help with posttraumatic seizures, in July 1886. The seizures began with abdominal discomfort and a sense of impending defecation, followed by tightness of the throat, deviation of the head and eyes to the right, jerking of the right arm, and loss of consciousness with the limbs generally flexed. Postictally the right arm was weak. The patient also had frequent headaches and a right-sided sensory loss. There were numerous scars about his head and a minute depression of a skull fracture to the left of the vertex. Based on localization experiments in animals, the clinical characteristics of the seizures led to a diagnosis of an irritative lesion in the posterior third of the superior frontal convolution, just under the depressed fracture. *Right,* Preoperative markings on the scalp. The serrated vertical line represents the coronal suture; other scalp markings show the position of the rolandic fissure and certain frontal sulci. *Left,* Diagram from the operative note showing the scar, depressed bone fragment, and a cavity in the brain, which were removed. The wound healed rapidly; weakness of the right arm developed one week postoperatively and gradually settled. The seizures ceased. The case is described in Horsley V: Brain surgery. *Br Med J* 1886; **2**: 670–675. (Images from the Wellcome Collection, London.)

generally sufficient at other times. He had taken a particular interest in the effects of anesthesia from his early days as a junior doctor, and he took an active role in the Special Chloroform Committee set up by the British Medical Association in 1901 to determine the minimal dose providing adequate anesthesia without endangering life.[6]

Horsley recognized that some of his surgical procedures were curative, whereas others were simply palliative, such as operations to reduce the pressure within the head and thereby prevent blindness in patients with brain tumors. For decompressive purposes alone, he favored a large craniotomy, opening the skull in the right basal temporal region if the underlying cause was not to be treated. With regard to the management of brain tumors, he concluded that surgery should be undertaken as early as possible and the tumor fully exposed and removed with surrounding tissue when feasible. If they could not be removed, he recommended that they be decompressed to provide symptomatic benefit.[5] When others

pointed out that operative treatment helped only a small minority of patients with brain tumors, Horsley retorted that this was because surgery had been delayed for too long and should have been used as a primary method of treatment rather than as a treatment of last resort.[7]

Neurosurgical Techniques

Based on his clinical experience and on his experiments in animals, Horsley provided a detailed account of his operative techniques, illustrated by three case reports, at the 1886 annual meeting of the British Medical Association, held in Brighton on the south coast of England.[8] He went on to update and extend these views based on his accumulated experience over the following twenty years in a lecture he gave in 1906 at the annual meeting of the association held on this occasion in Toronto, Canada.[5] His general operative approach, with antiseptic precautions,[9] is summarized in Appendix 1. In the present chapter, attention is confined to various specific contributions – of major importance – that he made.

Hemostasis

The oozing of blood from the well-vascularized diploe of the skull-bones posed a particular problem during intracranial operations, obscuring the operative field and contributing to blood loss. Contemporary techniques to control bleeding from small vessels by hot saline douches and packs[10] were not particularly successful in the case of bone, and the sources of bleeding, which were not compressible, could be neither tied off nor cauterized.

In the eighteenth and early nineteenth centuries, candle wax was used in rare instances to stop the oozing, particularly in Russia, but with suboptimal results given its poor malleability and the lack of sterility. In France, François Magendie, the physiologist who held the chair of medicine at the Collège de France, had sometimes used wax to close off the venous sinuses during his experiments on animals, and the Parisian surgeon Henri-Ferdinand Dolbeau (1840–1877) is said to have used it to limit bleeding when operating on the frontal bone.[11]

In his experiments on cerebral localization in animals, conducted primarily at the Brown Institution (see Chapter 3), Horsley also needed something to limit oozing of blood from bone. Remembering Magendie's technique, he smudged modeling wax on the cut and bleeding surface of the cranial bones in dogs, working it in until the bleeding stopped. When his attempts to prepare an antiseptic wax compound for use on humans were unsuccessful, he approached Mr. P. W. Squire of Oxford Street, who had been the pharmacist to the medical staff of the royal household since 1867 and would be knighted in 1918. Together, they came up with a product composed of beeswax (seven parts) and almond oil (one part), to which salicylic acid was added.[12] It had to be sterilized by boiling before use.

Horsley's bone wax, modified in one way or another and sometimes re-named, has been used successfully for the many years since then by surgeons. Certain authors have denied him credit for its introduction by pointing to its earlier use by others – as did Horsley himself – but it was he who improved on it, applied it to humans at almost the birth of neurosurgery, and popularized its use.

Despite his spectacular operative speed, Horsley took meticulous care to limit any bleeding regardless of its source. Blood vessels were tied

with fine horsehair or silkworm gut.[9] To control bleeding from the surface of the brain, he sprayed it with warm saline (at 110° to 115° F) and then applied gentle pressure with a sponge.[5] He also used muscle tissue to control bleeding from the brain (a forerunner of the modern Gelfoam, a commercially available, sterile, absorbable surgical sponge).[13] Harvey Cushing is sometimes credited for this latter approach, but Cushing himself indicated in 1911 that it was Horsley who had demonstrated "the haemostatic action of a fragment of muscle" on the exposed brain at a professional meeting in Britain.[14] Indeed, Horsley went on to publish a note on the technique and the research on which it was based, emphasizing that muscle was aseptic, adherent to the tissues to which it was applied (resisting systolic blood pressures of 60 to 80 mm Hg), and promoted clot formation.[15] Microscopic examination of the contact zone revealed profuse platelets and fibrin threads within a few minutes of muscle application.[15]

Finally, Horsley, in order to diminish the risk of bleeding, would also adjust the level of chloroform anesthesia:

> One of the most striking features of the physiological action of chloroform on the mammalian animal is that it soon (10 to 20 seconds) causes a marked fall in blood pressure. Consequently when a lesion is about to be extirpated, and there is reason to expect considerable oozing, or when the brain is obviously turgid with congestion, I always ask that the chloroform percentage should be raised for, say, a quarter to half a minute to 1 or 2 per cent. This at once induces a convenient, proportionate, and, of course, temporary anaemia.[5]

Regardless of its greater safety, he discouraged the use of ether for anesthesia during neurosurgical procedures both because of the hypertensive effects and increased risk of hemorrhage that he had noted during experiments in animals and because of the agitation that occurred during the recovery stage.[5]

Electrical Stimulation

Horsley was probably the first surgeon to stimulate the human brain electrically at operation, having done so in 1884 to distinguish between brain and other tissue and to determine the part of the brain that was displaced. The patient, a six-week-old infant, had a pendulous fluid-filled mass, some twelve inches in diameter, attached to the back of the head and covering much of the occipital bone. It was overlaid by skin that, over about one quarter of its surface, was hairy. A hole could be felt in the occipital bone from which solid tissue protruded into the mass. Firm pressure on the mass caused the infant to stop breathing, and pressure on the contained tissue led to a generalized convulsion. Electrical stimulation of the prolapsed brain tissue elicited eye movements, suggesting that a portion of the midbrain (the corpora quadrigemina) was involved.[16] Despite the attempted repair of the congenital abnormality, the infant died.

In his lecture on brain surgery at the British Medical Association in 1886, Horsley described three cases in which he had operated at the National Hospital. The first, that of James B., was described in Chapter 5. The second involved Thomas W., a twenty-year-old man with focal motor seizures that secondarily became generalized. The seizures began with focal twitching of the left thumb and forefinger; the muscle jerking then spread up the arm and to the face, to be followed by loss of consciousness and more generalized convulsive activity. There was no history of head trauma and thus no scarring to point to the site of the lesion, which was localized on purely clinical grounds. After he had removed a tuberculoma adherent to the dura, Horsley used an induction current to localize the center of the left thumb area of the motor cortex – the presumed epileptogenic area – which he then excised, as Hughlings Jackson had urged preoperatively.[8]

A year later, while referring in general terms to his experimental studies in nonhuman primates and relating them to clinical observations in humans, Horsley mentioned a case in which he applied faradic current to the cortical surface in order to define the representation of the face, a cortical area that he intended to excise.[2,17]

Intraoperative electrical stimulation techniques were soon adopted by others, most notably by Fedor Krause in Germany and William Keen in the United States, and later by Wilder Penfield and his group in Montreal, as discussed in Chapter 4. The motor and sensory maps of the human cerebral cortex constructed by Penfield are still in widespread use, and he also explored the functions of other parts of the cortex.

Other Technological Advances

With increasing experience in the operating room, Horsley came up with a number of technological advances to facilitate his surgical procedures. He adapted an electrical motor to work the trephine (a small circular saw used to remove a disk of bone from the skull), for example, and devised a rolandic-fissure meter (see Chapter 4) to determine the angle of the fissure, which he believed to vary with the shape of the head. He developed his own bone cutter, and a dural separator to part the membranous dura from overlying bone or to separate growths from brain tissue. He also introduced hand-held retractors of various sizes that could be shaped or modified based on need.[18] His most important accomplishment, however, was in helping to develop the stereotactic frame named after him.

The Horsley-Clarke Stereotactic Frame

The "little brain" or cerebellum, filling most of the posterior fossa of the skull, weighs about one tenth of the total weight of the brain but contains almost half of the brain's nerve cells. It has two hemispheres, separated by the worm-like vermis. The cerebellar surface is scored by numerous parallel, ravine-like fissures separating folds or folia that are arranged in several lobules, forming the anterior, posterior, and flocculonodular lobes. The interior of the cerebellum contains a central core of white matter composed of nerve fibers entering or leaving the cerebellum in the stalk-like superior, middle, and inferior peduncles connecting with the cerebral hemispheres, brainstem, and spinal cord, respectively. Within the white core are nests of neurons forming several relatively inaccessible nuclei. The function of the cerebellum is still being unraveled but it is clearly involved in modulating motor function and also affects cognition, behavior, and personality.

In the last few years of the nineteenth century, both Horsley and Sherrington independently reported that stimulation of the anterior lobe of the cerebellum, and especially the vermis, relieved (inhibited) the experimentally induced decerebrate rigidity (that is, rigidity with the limbs in extension and thrust backward) that occurs following removal of the cerebral hemispheres in animals.[19] Sherrington stimulated the cerebellar cortex while Horsley and his co-worker Max Löwenthal stimulated the subjacent white matter and the peduncles connecting the cerebellum to the brainstem.[20,21] These reports initially aroused little attention, but mark the beginning of a new line of approach in which the cerebellum was investigated by stimulation experiments,[22] and they provided the first clear evidence of functional localization within the cerebellar cortex.[23]

Horsley returned to the study of the cerebellum in a seminal paper with Robert Henry Clarke (1850–1926), published in 1908. They wished to study in monkeys, dogs, and cats the effects of lesioning the deep-seated cerebellar nuclei without damaging neighboring structures. With this aim in mind, they described a major methodological innovation, namely instrumentation to stimulate or place lesions very precisely in discrete regions within the depths of the brain for experimental purposes. The approach was actually conceived by Clarke, but at the urging and instigation of Horsley, with whom he worked at the Brown Institution and then at University College. The apparatus has since come to form the basis of modern stereotactic surgery.

Easy going and athletic, fond of the good life, and enjoying both tobacco and alcohol, Clarke became – somewhat surprisingly, as he was so unlike his colleague – a family friend and a favorite of the Horsley children. He had trained at St. George's Hospital in London, and then undertaken further surgical training in Glasgow before returning to London and research studies with Horsley. As they worked on the cerebellum, they came to realize the problems of attempting to stimulate or destroy deeply placed structures in the brain without damage to adjacent areas.

Accurate measurements cannot easily be made of the curved surface of an irregular sphere, such as the skull, especially when few consistent features exist to serve as fixed points and these points are anyway obscured by the skin and muscles that cover the head. Moreover, the variable thickness of the skull and its coverings compound the difficulties in localizing structures within the depth of the brain. A practical solution to this problem, they realized, could be reached by dividing the head into segments by three section planes perpendicular to each other (sagittal, horizontal, and frontal, defined later). Each segment then presents the three internal surfaces of a cube, and every point in it can be identified by measurements in a straight line from these internal boundaries. In other words, instead of attempting to project the detailed structure of the depths of the brain on to the surface of the head, the positions of the deep parts of the brain are determined by their relation to three defined planes.

Clarke accordingly set about devising an instrument that utilized three coordinates, supposedly doing so while he was in Egypt recuperating from a pneumonia that he attributed to the aspiration of an aspirin tablet.[24] Recognizing that there was a consistent relationship between certain landmarks of the skull, he planned to attach a rigid brass frame to the animal's head by bars clamped below the orbit of the eye and inserted into the external auditory meatus, and pins that are screwed in at the sides.[25,26] With the head thus fixed, an electrode could be passed through an opening in the skull to the target, the location of which was defined in three planes at right-angles to each other in space. No previous approach had used this Cartesian coordinate system.

A horizontal (axial) zero plane was represented by the line drawn from the center of the auditory meatus to the lowest margin of the bony orbit. It divided the brain into upper and lower segments. The depth of the target was defined by its location above or below the horizontal zero plane, which therefore served as zero for up and down measurements. The frontal (coronal) zero plane was the plane passing at right-angles from the vertex of the skull to the horizontal zero plane, passing through the center of the external auditory meatus on each side to divide the brain into front and back portions. The location of the target was defined along an anteroposterior direction from this plane. The sagittal zero plane passed through the head in the midline, bisecting it perpendicular to the other two planes to divide the brain into right and left halves. The brain was thus divided by the three zero section planes into eight segments (designated right and left frontal, occipital, temporal, and cerebellar); each segment had on its inner aspect three rectilinear surfaces corresponding to the three section planes – sagittal, frontal, and horizontal. The segments were then subdivided into slices or lamellae one millimeter thick in each plane, and each lamella was divided by lines parallel to the other two planes into millimeters.

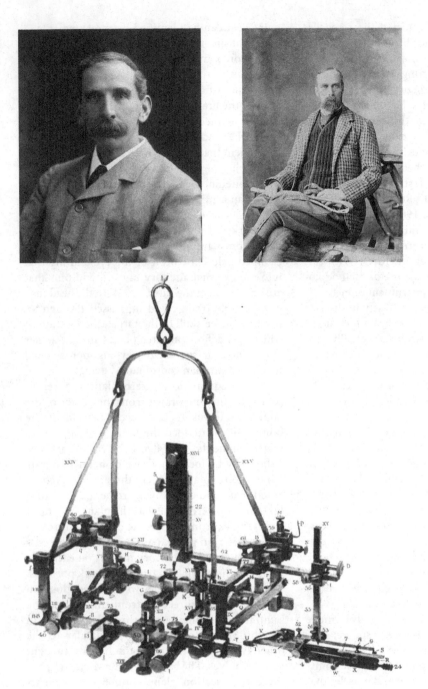

Figure 6.2 *Upper left*, Victor Horsley. (Image from the U.S. National Library of Medicine.) *Upper right*, the somewhat eccentric Robert Henry Clarke, who worked with Horsley and who designed the stereotactic apparatus for use in their animal experiments. (Image from the Wellcome Collection, London.) *Lower panel*, side view of Clarke's stereotactic apparatus for directing an insulated needle to intracerebral locations by graduated movement in three planes. (Further details and a full listing of the components are to be found in Horsley V, Clarke RH: The structure and functions of the cerebellum examined by a new method. *Brain* 1908; **31**: 45–124, from which the figure is taken.)

Clarke and Horsley created a stereotactic atlas of the monkey brain based on photographs of sections and these were used in conjunction with the instrument to stimulate or make lesions at any desired point of the brain in these animals. For this purpose, an electrode was supported on a longitudinal bar that could be moved laterally, the electrode holder being moveable in an anteroposterior and vertical direction – movement of the electrode was thus limited originally to these three planes at right angles to each other.[27] A localized target, defined by its location in three dimensions, could thus be approached with precision and without extensive injuries to other parts of the brain using this apparatus.

A prototype of the device, constructed by James Swift, a machinist at Palmer & Co. in London and costing three hundred pounds,[28] was demonstrated in 1906 by Horsley at the annual meeting of the British Medical Association,[29] and a detailed description of the apparatus was published in a lengthy (seventy-nine page) article in 1908.[26] In their report, Horsley and Clarke described how they evaluated several different methods of lesioning, that is, of destroying, a discrete region of the brain and the optimal parameters for their chosen method. They decided that the lesions were best made electrolytically, unaware that this approach had been used previously in St. Petersburg and in Bordeaux. They utilized a needle electrode that was insulated except at its tip. They also provided an atlas of the monkey brain, illustrating on a grid the relationship between landmarks and specific cerebral targets shown on brain sections.

The original apparatus was utilized for several studies that Horsley and Clarke undertook together. It was used subsequently by Ernest Sachs, the American surgeon who, under Horsley's guidance, studied the structure and function of a deeply placed neuronal structure (the thalamus) in the brain of cats and monkeys,[30] by the neurologist S. A. Kinnier Wilson for his studies of certain subcortical nuclei (the basal ganglia) of monkeys,[31] and finally by Frederick Barrington, a urogenital surgeon-scientist who studied the brain's control of urination in cats.[32] Thereafter it was little used despite various modifications to it by individual investigators until it inspired the systems now used in humans to treat certain movement disorders, notably Parkinson's disease, by stereotactic surgery.

As for the partnership between the two British investigators, their friendship dissolved for uncertain reasons and after 1909 they did not work together. This may have related to the differences that existed in their personalities, outlook, and interests.[33] It may be, also, that Clarke, a modest man, resented not receiving the credit that was his due for designing the system. Horsley received all the accolades even though he made a point of always referring to "Clarke's apparatus," and it was described thus in their original paper in the journal *Brain*.[26] Moreover, before that paper was published, Horsley requested that the order of the authors' names be reversed so that Clarke's came first, but the journal's editor responded that Clarke's name already appeared immediately below illustrations of the instrument, thereby giving him full credit for designing it.[34] Clarke is also said to have proposed the stereotactic approach as an aid to surgery in humans, particularly for treating brain tumors by electrical means or by radium implantation, and for relieving pain by coagulating pathways within the brain.[27,35] He was therefore annoyed that Horsley thought the idea impractical because the spatial relationships between cranial landmarks and cerebral structures were too variable.

Thus it was that Clarke alone applied for a patent for a device to be used in humans. He wrote to Swift in 1925 in connection with the manufacture of another apparatus: "I only patented the machine till I got the description published for I suffered from several attempts to pirate the invention ... I am afraid you will find it an expensive instrument to make."[36] Clarke himself became a general practitioner in Croydon, now a suburb of London, wintered in Italy to escape the cold of England, and died in Paris in 1926.[27]

The apparatus was copied and rebuilt at the Northwestern University Medical School in Chicago in the 1930s, and again at the University of Chicago, for experiments in animals. Various modifications allowed it to be used in different animals and subsequently also in humans through the use of intracerebral reference points visualized by imaging techniques that can define subcortical structures. A number of human brain atlases were published in the last half of the twentieth century. Frameless systems were devised. Stereotactic surgery was used to place lesions accurately – and later to place stimulating electrodes – for the relief of certain movement disorders and for pain relief. Stereotactic procedures came also to be used for psychoaffective disorders (psychosurgery) and for epilepsy and biopsy procedures, and show promise in developing techniques for the restoration of function in neurodegenerative disorders.[37] Various stereotactic radiosurgery programs are available commercially.

The stereotactic method was developed by Clarke and Horsley in the first decade of the twentieth century to allow experimental studies of brain function in animals. A century later, the approach is widely used in clinical neurosurgery. The use of a Cartesian coordinate system, as in the Horsley-Clarke frame, or the related polar coordinate system forms the basis of all modern stereotactic systems.

Notes

1. Horsley V: Remarks on the surgery of the central nervous system. *Br Med J* 1890; **2**: 1286–1292.

2. Horsley V: A note on the means of topographical diagnosis of focal disease affecting the so-called motor region of the cerebral cortex. *Am J Med Sci* 1887; **93**: 342–369.

3. Lyons JB: Correspondence between Sir William Gowers and Sir Victor Horsley. *Med Hist* 1965; **9**: 260–267.

4. Uff C, Frith D, Harrison C, Powell M, Kitchen N: Sir Victor Horsley's 19th century operations at the National Hospital for Neurology and Neurosurgery, Queen Square. *J Neurosurg* 2011; **114**: 534–542.

5. Horsley V: Address in surgery on the technique of operations on the central nervous system. *Lancet* 1906; **168**: 484–490; *Br Med J* 1906; **2**: 411–423.

6. The Special Chloroform Committee was chaired initially by Augustus Desiré Waller, the physiologist who discovered the electrocardiogram. In addition to Horsley, its other members were James Barr, later president of the British Medical Association; the anesthesiologists Dudley Buxton and W. J. McCardie; Charles Sherrington, the physiologist; a Dr. Walker; and the chemists A. Vernon Harcourt and Wyndham Dunstan. The committee continued for some years, its membership and activities changing with time.

7. Horsley V: Discussion on the treatment of cerebral tumours. Remarks on the surgical treatment of cerebral tumours. *Br Med J* 1893; **2**: 1365–1367 (additional discussion, 1369).

8. Horsley V: Brain-surgery. *Br Med J* 1886; **2**: 670–675.

9. Sachs E: *Fifty Years of Neurosurgery: A Personal Story*. pp. 38–39. Vantage: New York, 1958.

10. Northfield DWC: Sir Victor Horsley 1857–1916. pp. 43–48. In: Bucy P (ed): *Neurosurgical Giants: Feet of Clay and Iron*. Elsevier: New York, 1985; reprinted from *Surg Neurol* 1973; **1**: 131–134.

11. Steimle RH: A note on the use of wax for bone hemostasis. Henri-Ferdinand Dolbeau (1840–77). *J Hist Neurosci* 1993; **2**: 243–244.

12. Horsley V: Antiseptic wax. [Letter to the editor.] *Br Med J* 1892; **1**: 1165.

13. Bucy P: Editor's comments. pp. 49–50. In: Bucy P (ed): *Neurosurgical Giants: Feet of Clay and Iron*. Elsevier: New York, 1985.

14. Cushing H: The control of bleeding in operations for brain tumors: With the description of silver "clips" for the occlusion of vessels inaccessible to the ligature. *Ann Surg* 1911; **54**: 1–19.

15. Horsley V: Note on haemostasis by application of living tissue. *Br Med J* 1914; **2**: 8.

16. Horsley V: Case of occipital encephalocele in which a correct diagnosis was obtained by means of the induced current. *Brain* 1884; **7**: 228–243.

17. Vilensky JA, Gilman S: Horsley was the first to use electrical stimulation of the human cerebral cortex intraoperatively. *Surg Neurol* 2002; **58**: 425–426.

18. Assina R, Rubino S, Sarris CE, Gandhi CD, Prestigiacomo CJ: The history of brain retractors throughout the development of neurological surgery. *Neurosurg Focus* 2014; **36**: E8, 1–12.

19. Sherrington CS: On reciprocal innervation of antagonistic muscles. Third note. *Proc R Soc Lond* 1896; **60**: 414–417.

20. Sherrington CS: Decerebrate rigidity, and reflex coordination of movements. *J Physiol* 1898; **22**: 319–332.

21. Löwenthal M, Horsley V: On the relations between the cerebellar and other centres (namely cerebral and spinal) with especial reference to the action of antagonistic muscles. (Preliminary account.) *Proc R Soc Lond* 1897; **61**: 20–25.

22. Dow RS, Moruzzi G: p. 7. In: *The Physiology and Pathology of the Cerebellum*. University of Minnesota Press: Minneapolis, MN, 1958.

23. Dow RS, Moruzzi G: p. 51. In: *The Physiology and Pathology of the Cerebellum*. University of Minnesota Press: Minneapolis, MN, 1958.

24. Davis RA: Victorian physician-scholar and pioneer physiologist. *Surg Gynecol Obstet* 1964; **119**: 1333–1340.

25. Clarke RH, Horsley V: On a method of investigating the deep ganglia and tracts of the central nervous system (cerebellum). *Br Med J* 1906; **2**: 1799–1800.

26. Horsley V, Clarke RH: The structure and functions of the cerebellum examined by a new method. *Brain* 1908; **31**: 45–124.

27. Schurr PH, Merrington WR: The Horsley–Clarke stereotaxic apparatus. *Br J Surg* 1978; **65**: 33–36.

28. Fodstad H, Hariz M, Ljunggren B: History of Clarke's stereotactic instrument. *Stereotact Funct Neurosurg* 1991; **57**: 130–140.

29. Anon: Section of Physiology. Thursday, August 23rd, 1906. *Br Med J* 1906; **2**: 633.

30. Sachs E: On the structure and functional relations of the optic thalamus. *Brain* 1909; **32**: 95–106.

31. Wilson SAK: An experimental research into the anatomy and physiology of the corpus striatum. *Brain* 1914; **36**: 427–492.

32. Barrington FJF: The effect of lesions of the hind- and mid-brain on micturition in the cat. *Q J Exp Physiol* 1925; **15**: 81–102.

33. Tepperman J: Horsley and Clarke: A biographical medallion. *Perspect Biol Med* 1970; **13**: 295–308.

34. Head H: Letter to Victor Horsley dated May 22, 1908. Section E2, Horsley Papers, Special Collections, UCL Library Services (London, UK).

35. Clarke RH: Investigation of the central nervous system: Methods and instruments. pp. 16–17. In Clarke RH, Henderson EE : *Investigation of the Central Nervous System*. The Johns Hopkins Hospital Reports. (Special Volume). Johns Hopkins Press: Baltimore, MD, 1920.

36. Clarke RH: Letter to J. Swift dated December 13, 1925, reproduced by Schurr PH, Merrington WR: The Horsley–Clarke stereotaxic apparatus. *Br J Surg* 1978; **65**: 33–36.

37. Gildenberg PL: The history of stereotactic neurosurgery. *Neurosurg Clin N Am* 1990; **1**: 765–780.

7 The Neurosurgery of Specific Disorders

As Horsley's workload increased at the National Hospital, it became necessary to make new surgical appointments to support him. Charles Ballance (1856–1936) came on staff in 1891 but was somewhat overshadowed by Horsley – whom he had assisted in the famous operation on Captain Gilbey (discussed in Chapter 5) – and resigned in 1908. He became a celebrated aural and general surgeon in his own right. Donald Armour (1869–1933) and the technically brilliant Percy ("Pretty Percy") Sargent (1873–1933) both assisted Horsley in the early years of the twentieth century, became assistant surgeons at the hospital in 1906, and full surgeons three years later, after Ballance had resigned. All three made their mark in the field of surgical neurology, helping to establish the tradition of neurosurgical excellence at the hospital. But it was Horsley more than anyone who was responsible for advancing the emerging specialty of neurosurgery and who developed a school of followers that included Wilfred Trotter (p. 19), Armour, and Sargent in Britain, Ernest Sachs (p. 91) in the United States, Edward Archibald in Canada, Thierry de Martel in France, and Vilhelm Magnus in Norway. With Horsley's death, neurosurgery at the National Hospital went into something of a decline for the following quarter-century.

Horsley's surgical approach to various neurological disorders received enthusiastic support across the English Channel. Among the many visitors who came to see him in action was the Parisian surgeon Thierry de Martel (1875–1940), who spent a day in London every week for more than a year, watching him in the operating room.[1] De Martel and his rival, Clovis Vincent (1879–1947), were both protégés of the celebrated French neurologist Joseph Babinski and founded the French school of neurosurgery. They were a curious pair. The one, De Martel, a proud and aloof aristocrat, committed suicide when the Germans entered Paris during World War II.

The other, Vincent, was warm and approachable, a physician who became a neurosurgeon in his late forties and was the first chaired professor of clinical neurosurgery in Paris. During the German occupation he joined the Resistance, sheltering allied airmen shot down over France by putting them into his hospital beds, covered in bandages, until they could be sent back to England. Vincent learned his craft in part from De Martel (and thus indirectly from Horsley) and in part also from Harvey Cushing in America. Another European physician-turned-surgeon, Vilhelm Magnus (1871–1929), founded the Scandinavian school of neurosurgery in Oslo after having worked with Horsley in the operating theater and laboratory during part of 1903 and 1904.

Across the Atlantic, Edward Archibald (1872–1945) from Montreal trained with Horsley in 1906 and subsequently went on to publish a major monograph on neurosurgery. Although often regarded as Canada's first neurosurgeon, he later focused on the treatment of pulmonary tuberculosis – with which he himself was afflicted – as head of surgery at McGill University. William W. Keen (1837–1932), certainly the most influential exponent of neurosurgery in the United States during the last quarter of the nineteenth century, greatly admired Horsley, referred often to his surgical expertise and innovations, and followed his example, such as in utilizing intraoperative electrical stimulation to explore the brain.[2] By contrast, Cushing, who later had a major role in establishing neurosurgery as a specialty in America, viewed Horsley more unfavorably – but, then, there seemed to be an unnecessarily competitive edge in many of Cushing's utterances or writings regarding anyone who might be viewed as undermining his own position.

Horsley's pioneering experimental and clinical work in advancing the surgical treatment of various neurological disorders, known to past generations of neurosurgeons through his writings, is

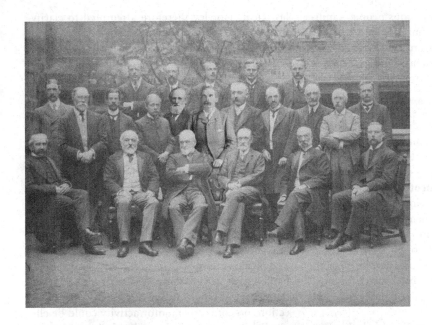

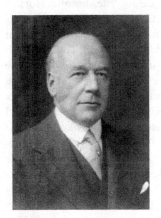
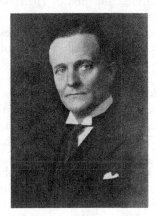

Figure 7.1 Staff at the National Hospital in about 1904. Horsley is in the second row, middle. To the left of him, William Gowers (bearded) stands behind Hughlings Jackson; to the right of Horsley, Charles Ballance is behind Charlton Bastian. In the front row, Felix Semon is at the extreme left, and David Ferrier is second from the right. Horsley's assistants are in the back row – Donald Armour at the extreme left, and Percy Sargent second from the right. (Image from the Queen Square Archives.) Bottom left, Donald Armour (photograph by J. Russell & Sons); *bottom right*, Percy Sargent. (Images from the Wellcome Collection, London.)

now largely forgotten or taken for granted. It is the focus of this chapter.

Epilepsy

Background

Epilepsy is an ancient disease that was wrapped for years in fear and mystery, its seizures attributed by the ancient Babylonians and later by the Romans to the god of the moon or to demonic possession, and by the ancient Greeks to a divine curse, sometimes associated with genius. It was not until Hippocrates (400 BC) that it came to be considered, at least briefly, a natural disease rather than a supernatural or divine phenomenon.[3] The disorder came to have religious implications in the Middle Ages and was related in the Christian world to an "unclean spirit" contracted by contact with an afflicted person. Indeed, in the early days of the church the possessed were separated from the faithful to prevent infection and desecration of holy objects. A number of famous people – military leaders, philosophers, church leaders, writers, painters, and musicians – are said to have had epilepsy, but in many instances the evidence is flimsy and alternative diagnoses cannot be excluded.

From the earliest times, epileptics faced discrimination and abuse: under the Babylonian code of ancient Mesopotamia (circa 1750 BC), for example, they could not marry, and until about seventy years ago, epilepsy remained a justification for annulment of a marriage in certain developed and developing countries. In the United States and Germany, people with epilepsy were sterilized well into the twentieth century. Some were thought to be of subnormal intelligence, mad, or dangerous. Happily, disability laws in many countries now restrict the mistreatment and stigmatization of epileptics, but misconceptions persist.[4]

John Hughlings Jackson provided the first modern insight into the disease, in the nineteenth century. He related seizures to excessive and disordered discharges of nerve tissue, and recognized that they can alter consciousness, motor activity, sensation, and behavior. Finally it became possible to deny any demonic influence and return to the Hippocratic concept of epilepsy as a brain disorder. Others with an influential role were Russell Reynolds, William Gowers, David Ferrier, and Victor Horsley.

Jackson had deduced in the 1870s that focal motor seizures arise in the cerebral cortex rather than in the lower brainstem, as previously had been the prevailing opinion. Thus it was that Horsley's first intracranial operation in 1886, for the treatment of focal motor seizures in a patient with posttraumatic epilepsy, was of especial interest to Jackson and David Ferrier, as was his second case in which he excised an epileptogenic area of the cerebral cortex after identifying it by electrical stimulation (see Chapter 6). Indeed, he can justly be considered a pioneer of the surgical treatment of epilepsy, a disorder on which he also focused experimentally.

Experimental Work and Its Clinical Application

Jackson came to believe that the auras that may precede generalized seizures have a cortical origin, but the basis of the seizures themselves was less clear. Horsley therefore attempted to clarify the neurological substrate for these, believing that both the loss of consciousness and convulsive motor activity arose in the cerebral cortex.[5]

Earlier investigators had attributed the motor accompaniments of generalized convulsions to brainstem (medullary or pontine) or even spinal lesions, or to a reduced blood supply to the brain. Since about 1885, while at the Brown Institution, Horsley had been investigating these phenomena by injecting intravenously into monkeys and other animals a small quantity of absinthe, which had a "most wonderful toxic effect on the central nervous system." Several seconds after injection, when the absinthe reached the brain, the monkey went through all the stages of a typical generalized seizure. The brain itself looked as if it were congested with blood rather than short of blood. Following spinal cord transection, no convulsive motor activity could be elicited by absinthe below the lesion. Horsley therefore concluded that the spinal cord conducts impulses from the brain during a seizure, but that it cannot itself initiate a convulsion. Together with Gotch, his brother-in-law, he showed that the pattern of impulses descending in the spinal cord following stimulation of the motor cortex "are of the characteristic form of tonus followed by clonus, and consequently we have now the proof that the 'motor' part of the epileptic disturbance is seated in the cortex of the hemispheres."[5,6] Slicing off the cerebral cortex itself altered the character of the motor activity elicited by electrical stimulation of the descending cortical fibers so that it no longer resembled a seizure.[7]

Electrical stimulation of the cerebral cortex on one side elicits generalized (bilateral) convulsions. When the limbs on both sides of the body are convulsing in this way, Horsley concluded that both hemispheres must be involved in the fit. He showed that division in dogs of the corpus callosum – the broad band of fibers that connects the two cerebral hemispheres – followed by unilateral cortical stimulation led to convulsive motor activity only opposite the stimulated side.[7] Similarly, after removal of the motor cortex from one hemisphere, absinthe led to convulsive motor activity only on the side corresponding to (that is, opposite) the uninjured cortex.[5] These findings suggested that the evoked seizure activity spread from the cerebral cortex on one side to that on the other via the callosal connections between them. Others repeated Horsley's experimental work but with conflicting results,[8] although experiments in monkeys confirmed that the corpus callosum played a role in seizure spread.[9]

Because seizures can spread in the brain via many different routes, it was only in the late 1930s that therapeutic callosal section was attempted in humans, and then based not on experimental evidence but on the clinical improvement occurring in epileptic patients with callosal tumors or vascular disease. Based on their experience in ten patients, Van Wagenen and Herren concluded:

> Section of the commissural pathways contained in the corpus callosum may be carried out without any untoward effect on the patient. Such a section may serve to limit the spread of an epileptic wave to the opposite hemisphere. When such limitation occurs, the patients do not seem to lose consciousness or have generalized convulsions.[10]

Their lead was not followed initially because other targets in the brain seemed also to be important, but callosotomy, combined with the sectioning of other fiber-tracts joining the two sides of the brain, was reintroduced some twenty years later for medically refractory epilepsy, with partial benefit. Several reports of the success of partial or complete callosotomy followed,[11,12,13] but not all patients became seizure-free and some had unilateral seizures.

Nevertheless, the accumulated experience over the last fifty years has shown that this approach helps some patients with frequent seizures that are poorly responsive to antiepileptic drugs, especially drop attacks (tonic and atonic seizures), although other types of seizures may also respond. It also has a palliative role in limiting the spread of convulsive discharges between the hemispheres in patients with widespread pathology affecting both hemispheres (secondary generalized epilepsy). In order to reduce the risk of postoperative behavioral disturbances resulting from the disconnection of one part of the brain from another, however, many surgeons limit the extent of the surgery.[14]

Modern evaluation of Horsley's experimental studies suggests that they were well planned and interpreted, and his conclusions are in keeping with modern concepts.[15] The number of animals studied was small, control observations were limited, and his published accounts were terse, but this was not uncommon in the late nineteenth century. Since then, Horsley's work has been extended and clarified. His insight had led him to recognize the importance of subcortical activity in the spread and maintenance of convulsive seizures once they had been generated cortically and was important in providing a theoretical basis for the development of modern epilepsy surgery.

Increased Intracranial Pressure

The pressure within the head is maintained normally at a fairly stable level. A change in the volume of one of the tissues and fluids contained within the rigid bones of the skull, however, is likely to cause an increase in intracranial pressure. This can have major clinical consequences and may require urgent treatment.

Experimental Aspects

For many years and, certainly, well before Horsley was born, the clinical manifestations of increased intracranial pressure were recognized by the *cognoscenti*. Such pressure increases were known to follow acute brain swelling as a result of injury, inflammation, or surgery; to accompany tumors or other lesions that occupied space within the cranial cavity; and to result from an increased volume or a disturbance in flow of the cerebrospinal fluid that surrounds the brain and spinal cord, separating them from the inner surface of the head and backbone. There was particular interest in the relationship between the intracranial pressure, heart rate, and blood pressure, which was studied experimentally in animals during the eighteenth and nineteenth centuries.[16]

In 1880, Ernst von Bergmann (1836–1907), a pioneer of asepsis and professor of surgery successively at the universities of Dorpat, Würzburg, and Berlin, reported that increased intracranial pressure led to slowing of the heart and irregular respiration, and then to an increase in blood pressure and to swelling and vascular congestion of the optic discs, that is, of the optic nerve at the back of each eye (papilledema). Patients developed headache, nausea, confusion, somnolence, visual disturbances, and eventually coma, all of which were attributed to reduced cerebral blood flow. Bergmann undertook systematic studies in dogs to clarify the underlying mechanisms.[17]

Horsley, in London, together with Walter Spencer, then an assistant surgeon at the Westminster Hospital, also studied the cardiovascular and respiratory effects of increased intracranial pressure in dogs and monkeys. They inserted a thin-walled, distensible rubber bag into the head through a hole that they then closed by a metal plate. A fine metal tube passed through the metal plate and connected the bag to a mercury-filled burette. When the burette was raised above the level of the bag, the bag became distended with mercury, compressing the cranial content; the reduction in cerebral volume was indicated by the amount of mercury that escaped from the burette. The height of the level of mercury above the surface of the brain reflected the degree of pressure involved, which could be increased slowly or rapidly depending on the experiment.[18] As the intracranial pressure increased, the heart slowed until it finally stopped, and respiration became irregular, slowed, and eventually ceased. The blood pressure response, however, was more variable and depended on the rapidity with which the intracranial pressure increased, the duration of the increase, and the animal studied. Their detailed report, published in 1891, was more than fifty pages long and acknowledged the work of earlier investigators including Bergmann, but it made rather dreary reading and no clear conclusions or advances emerged from it.

An American in Europe

Almost a decade later, Harvey Cushing, the young American surgeon from Johns Hopkins Hospital who was spending the 1900–1901 academic year in Europe, came under the influence of the surgeon Theodor Kocher in Bern, Switzerland. Kocher knew personally both Bergmann and Horsley and was familiar with their work. He suggested that Cushing study the effects of increased intracranial pressure on the blood pressure and cerebral circulation, using laboratory facilities provided by Hugo Kronecker (1839–1914), professor of physiology at the University of Bern. When Cushing left Bern after a few months, he continued the work in Turin, Italy, in the laboratory of Angelo Mosso, a former student of Kronecker.[19] They raised the intracranial pressure not only by inserting into the head

a rubber bag that could be filled with mercury, but also by injecting physiological saline into the subarachnoid space to cause a more diffuse rise in intracranial pressure.[19]

Cushing wrote up the results at Mosso's urging in June 1901, after he had returned to Bern but, believing that Mosso was going to present the findings at an international congress in Turin a few weeks later, he rushed into print himself in the pages of the *Johns Hopkins Hospital Bulletin*, with a footnote stating that the paper was reprinted from the *Archives Italiennes de Biologie* for 1901. In fact, the article never appeared in the Italian journal and Mosso appears to have had no further dealings with Cushing, who had included no co-authors so that the paper appeared under his name alone.

Cushing's paper was just three pages long, with two additional pages of illustrations, but its findings were clear, crisp, and unequivocal:

> As a result of these experiments a simple and definite law may be established, namely, that *an increase of intracranial tension occasions a rise of blood pressure which tends to find a level slightly above that of the pressure exerted against the medulla.* [Emphasis in original.] It is thus seen that there exists a regulatory mechanism on the part of the vaso-motor centre which, with great accuracy, enables the blood pressure to remain at a point just sufficient to prevent the persistence of an anaemic condition of the bulb, demonstrating that the rise is a conservative act and not one such as is consequent upon a mere reflex sensory irritation.[20]

Cushing subsequently published a more detailed, single-authored account after first, somewhat brashly, clashing with his mentor, Kocher, who had wished to write the paper himself. The article appeared in a German-language journal in 1902,[21] but it was followed by an appendix in which the editor, Bernhard Naunyn (1839–1925), a distinguished physician and chemical pathologist, pointed out that he himself had published similar findings twenty years earlier and was dismayed that Cushing had not acknowledged any earlier work. Naunyn returned to this same point in his memoirs, published in 1925.[16,19] It seems that he had published Cushing's paper not because it was particularly original but out of courtesy to his friend Kocher. In fact, similar findings had indeed been published by others, whose work Cushing chose simply to ignore, perhaps out of self-interest.

Probably in response to such criticism, Cushing, in his 1901 Mütter Lecture to the College of Physicians in Philadelphia, did credit several predecessors including a handful of his contemporaries, among whom were both Bergmann and Horsley.[22] He made little attempt to put his work into the context of the earlier work by others, although he did point out that the apparatus he used to produce local compression was similar to that of Horsley and that several of his findings confirmed those of Horsley.[22]

Regardless, it was Cushing's brief paper that emphasized concisely the clinical relevance of the observation, and the phenomenon he described has since been known generally as the Cushing reflex or Cushing's law. He and others regarded it as a final device to protect the brain by maintaining cerebral perfusion when its blood supply is failing.

Clinical Aspects

Horsley observed early on that parts of the brain could be displaced by pathological processes that increased the intracranial volume. In particular, part of the cerebellum could be pushed down through the foramen magnum and compress the lower brainstem and upper spinal cord. (The foramen magnum – Latin for large hole – is the hole at the base of the skull through which the brain connects with the spinal cord.) A fatal outcome would then result unless this herniation was relieved by a decompressive procedure. He studied experimentally the effect of cerebral compression by allowing a balloon inserted into the cranial cavity to expand slowly, as discussed in the preceding section. In addition, he had a good understanding of German and kept up with the European medical literature, so that he was probably well aware of the work of Bergmann and other surgeons who had made similar observations. These various considerations influenced particularly his management of patients with intracranial tumors.

Intracranial Tumors

Patients with suspected brain tumors or other space-consuming lesions were usually referred to Horsley only after their symptoms had progressed despite medical treatment, a practice that concerned him because of the resulting delay in their operative management. He therefore suggested that medical treatment should be limited to six weeks unless it led to striking symptomatic benefit.[23] The medical treatment to which he referred was not for tumors but for the localized inflammatory masses that may occur in the brain in syphilis (gummas) and tuberculosis (tuberculomas).[23]

Horsley did not advise surgical exploration and direct treatment of an underlying tumor unless patients had features suspicious for a localized space-consuming lesion, such as focal (Jacksonian) seizures or auras and focal or lateralized weakness or sensory deficits. He pointed out that bulging of the exposed brain into the wound when the dura was incised and a yellowish discoloration of the brain itself supported the belief that a tumor was present.[24] He regarded "innocent tumours which are encapsulated, and which shell out, such as fibroma," to be curable, but he was never sure that he had removed gliomas – brain tumors arising in the supporting cells that surround nerve cells – in their entirety, in part because patients were seen so late in the course of the disease. As for syphilitic or tuberculous lesions, they often did poorly because of surrounding inflammation, the presence of multiple lesions, and the difficulty in removing them.

The presence of headache, vomiting, and papilledema – evidence of increased intracranial pressure – helped to reinforce the clinical suspicion of an underlying tumor. In the absence of other features to guide operative intervention, Horsley advocated early decompressive surgery to relieve symptoms and preserve vision. In his own words, "The skull of course being a rigid box, it follows that making a fair-sized hole in it would afford a certain degree of release of pressure."[25] In most instances, simple opening of the skull was not sufficient, however, and he therefore also opened the membranous dura covering the brain.[25] This was best accomplished in the temporal region (with removal of the overlying bone) or "by trephining the occipital bone and prolonging the aperture into the foramen magnum." Tapping the lateral ventricles (the cavities containing cerebrospinal fluid that lie deep in each cerebral hemisphere) to reduce intraventricular pressure or draining the cerebrospinal fluid though lumbar puncture did not provide adequate or long-term relief.

Horsley pointed out that after palliative surgical decompression, papilledema generally subsided within three weeks unless the optic nerve showed early signs of damage (atrophy), in which case blindness typically developed.[23] Decompressive surgery helped also to reverse mental symptoms and relieve seizures, and sometimes ameliorated focal neurological deficits such as weakness. In those cases where the tumor was near the surface of the brain and close to the opening made in the skull, however, the tumor – covered by the layers of the scalp – would often grow through the opening (so-called hernia cerebri). In exceptional cases, it might even reach the shoulders. Regardless, the surgery permitted patients additional years of life by relieving intracranial pressure, but without necessarily relieving neurological deficits. Many such patients were sent to the Archway Hospital in North London for long-term care. (The hospital later became the Archway wing of the Whittington Hospital and then a teaching and research center before being sold for redevelopment in 2013.)

The long-term outlook for patients coming to operation for brain tumors was bleak during Horsley's time. Indeed, despite improvements in surgical technique and the development of other treatment modalities, it remains somewhat gloomy today, depending on the site and nature of the tumor. From a survey of the U.S. Surgeon General's Index catalogue for the years 1886 to 1896, it appears that in the decade following Horsley's initial report on brain surgery, more than five hundred different general surgeons reported operations performed on the brain. Over the following decade, however, the number of surgeons reporting such cases declined to less than eighty.[26] Many surgeons seemingly "gave it a go," but were daunted and disappointed by an initial lack of success. This was hardly surprising as they were without Horsley's experience, and may not have followed rigorous antiseptic procedures or utilized the other steps he described.

In any event, the prognosis of untreated brain tumors was and continues to be bleak in many instances. Treatment has evolved. Electrosurgery, suction, and other neurosurgical techniques have been developed; and depending on the surgeon, enucleation or radical excision of tumors, and wider approaches such as removal of the involved lobe of the brain or total or partial removal of the affected cerebral hemisphere (lobectomy or hemispherectomy) have been utilized as treatment strategies, together with radiation, chemotherapy, and newly developing molecular therapies. But the principles established by Horsley remain as relevant today as when first he advocated them. An early direct approach to the tumor is important if feasible; palliative treatment is also crucial, although decompressive surgery has largely been replaced by medical approaches with anti-edema agents to reduce brain swelling and intracranial pressure, and anti-epileptic medications to control seizures.

In his 1906 lecture in Toronto to the British Medical Association, Horsley re-emphasized his earlier beliefs and pointed out that unlike brain lesions, "tumours which, growing from the meninges, penetrate the brain, or which are encapsulated, such as fibromata, myxomata and endotheliomata, tuberculomata and gummata, can all be excised with a good permanent result."[27] Among twelve patients on whom he had operated for endothelioma or fibroma, only one had a recurrence and that was after three years. This contrasted with twenty of twenty-three cases of glioma or sarcoma in which recurrences occurred within two years of surgery.

The Localizing Value of Papilledema

It was Horsley's belief based on personal experience that the location or at least the side of an underlying intracranial tumor sometimes is suggested by the side on which vision first begins to fail. The important point, in his view, was not the severity of the papilledema as judged by differences in swelling of the optic discs but rather its duration as evidenced, for example, by the resulting damage to the optic nerve (optic atrophy). The localizing value of papilledema had, in fact, been a subject of controversy for some years.[28] Gowers was unsure about its value but had described a case of unilateral papilledema on the opposite side to an intracranial tumor; on the side of the tumor the optic nerve had atrophied due to direct compression by the tumor.[29] Horsley's early views on the topic were summarized in a lecture he gave at University College Hospital in 1910:

> One word finally must be stated concerning frontal tumours: they are often easy to diagnose because of the fact that their vertical pressure

causes a paralysis of the olfactory tract, and sometimes of an optic nerve. Hence, anosmia is very common, and may be unilateral. ... Pressure on the optic nerve causes an atrophy of the retrobulbar type, the field showing a central scotoma, whereas the opposite eye, of which the nerve sheath is not obstructed, exhibits papilledema or choked disc in the typical form.[30]

Such a finding is now widely accepted for certain tumors (frontal lobe or olfactory groove) and was later recorded more formally with pertinent case histories by Foster Kennedy, then a junior physician at the National Hospital in Queen Square, where his duties included assisting both Gowers and Horsley. Horsley had operated on the patient described by Gowers, but she died postoperatively. Kennedy later moved to the Neurological Institute of New York, where he saw five similar cases and, with Horsley's encouragement, published them.[28,31]

Horsley wrote to him from the Orkney Islands where he was vacationing in September 1910:

We are delighted to hear of so much good fortune attending your deserving work. ... I expect you will find an *embarras de richesse* in material for as I remember the Bellevue before any reforms occurred in it there was any amount unworked. Certainly, you ought to publish your thesis with any additional material you can get. Take warning and do not accumulate a lot of work but put it out at regular intervals.[32]

The Foster Kennedy syndrome now refers eponymously to the occurrence of compressive optic atrophy on the same side as a frontal lobe or olfactory groove tumor, with papilledema on the opposite side.

Horsley believed, however, that papilledema associated with increased intracranial pressure had a more general lateralizing value, appearing first or being more marked on the side of any intracranial tumor or other space-occupying lesion.[33] Most clinical neurologists today have difficulty in accepting this concept, however, and claims that papilledema generally appears first on the side with an underlying tumor are now forgotten.[34]

Posterior Fossa Tumors

The posterior fossa, the lower and back part of the cranial cavity, contains the brainstem and cerebellum. Only in the last years of the nineteenth century, largely due to the efforts of Jackson and Gowers in Britain and a number of prominent neurologists in continental Europe, was it possible to localize tumors in the posterior fossa with sufficient accuracy to permit their surgical treatment. A few cases came to operation but generally did badly.

Tumors in the posterior fossa commonly are located in the cerebellopontine angle, that is, between the cerebellum and a brainstem region known as the pons. Most of these tumors are benign. Charles Ballance in London may have been the first (in 1892) to remove successfully an acoustic neuroma – a tumor on the nerve passing from the inner ear to the brain – in this region, but the tumor on which he operated is now thought to have been a meningioma, a benign tumor of the fibrous membranes surrounding the brain. If so, credit for first successfully removing an acoustic neuroma properly belongs to Thomas Annandale, an Edinburgh surgeon. In 1895, he operated on a twenty-five-year-old pregnant woman who had become ataxic and deaf in the right ear. After he removed piecemeal a cystic tumor the size of a pigeon's egg, the patient recovered well, her symptoms cleared, and she was delivered of a healthy daughter.[35] Horsley was also successful in operating on acoustic neuromas, and one of the patients on whom he had operated in 1912 was presented at a meeting of the Royal Society of Medicine more than ten years later.[36] But the consistently successful management of these tumors really had to await the expertise of Harvey Cushing (subtotal removal) and his former student, Walter Dandy (total resection). Later, in the latter half of the twentieth century, came the translabyrinthine approach of William House, and later still the development of stereotactic (focused) radiosurgery.

Stereotactic Surgery

Horsley's contributions to the management of intracranial lesions continues even now, albeit more indirectly. Some thirty years after his death, stereotactic devices were developed for use in humans,[37] essentially being modifications and derivatives of the stereotactic apparatus that he had developed with Clarke. Their use and applications have expanded steadily since that time. They are used for obtaining a biopsy of suspected brain tumors and other lesions that are deeply placed or poorly defined and for treating those unlikely to benefit from resection, such as by implanting radioactive seeds, placing drug delivery devices, directing laser surgery, delivering various other therapies directly into the affected tissues, and allowing the development of localized radiation therapy (stereotactic radiosurgery).[38] Numerous adaptations to the original device have been made over the years and the various frames are named for their developers, but they often so resemble each other that they are sometimes hard to tell apart. They serve as a fitting memorial to the inventive genius of Horsley and Clarke.

The Pituitary Gland and Related Tumors

The pea-sized human pituitary gland weighs less than one-half of a gram. It is suspended beneath the brain from the hypothalamus and lies protected in a bony cave, the sella turcica, covered by a dural fold. The optic chiasm – where part of each optic nerve crosses from one side of the brain to the other – lies above it, the cavernous venous sinuses to either side of it, the sphenoidal air sinus beneath it, and the nasal passage in front of it. Its function remained unknown in the late nineteenth century.

The pituitary controls the secretions of the adrenal and thyroid glands, ovaries, and testes; the proper functioning of the breast, uterus, and kidneys; and the general state of bone, muscle, and fat. A mass in the sella may relate to one or another of several causes, such as a benign or malignant tumor, an abscess, or a cyst. A benign pituitary growth (adenoma) is the most common cause and may be functioning (that is, hormone secreting) or nonfunctioning. Excessive hormonal secretion can be devastating – excessive secretion of growth hormone, for example, leads to acromegaly. There is enlargement and coarsening of the face in adults, with overgrowth of the jaw and eyebrows, and enlargement of the hands and feet; gigantism occurs in children. Various metabolic disturbances, such as hypertension, diabetes, and heart disease, also occur. Arthritis is common.

Nonfunctioning pituitary tumors or intrasellar masses do not produce hormones and their detection is thus often delayed until they compress neighboring structures leading to headaches, characteristic visual field defects, or even blindness. Hormonal failure in such circumstances, resulting from damage to functioning pituitary tissue, may involve the loss of one, several, or all of the pituitary hormones. Hyposecretion of growth hormone, for example, leads to a decrease in muscle mass, an accumulation of fat, and reduced exercise capacity.

Horsley's Experimental Work

In 1886, Horsley removed the pituitary gland from two dogs and showed that they could survive for several months.[39] The function of the pituitary was then unknown, but he had previously noted that seizures often occurred with tumors of the pituitary, hence his interest in the consequences of their removal.[40] No neurological or other signs were noted in the animals, but stimulation of the cerebral cortex revealed a marked increase in the excitability of the motor region. Others subsequently repeated the experiments, some showing that animals could survive for long periods, others that they succumbed rapidly.

In conjunction with a Dr. Handelsmann, of whom little is now known, Horsley returned to the topic in 1911, studying fifty-four animals (cats, dogs, and monkeys) in which the gland was approached surgically.[41] Their results conflicted with the common belief that death followed within a few days of removal of the anterior portion of the pituitary, because three of their animals survived in good health despite removal of the entire anterior pituitary. Detailed experimentation since Horsley's time has confirmed that animals "deprived of their pituitaries do not die in a few days; their expectation of life is reduced by about half. No urgent disaster faces them."[42] Nevertheless, animals may die several days or weeks after removal of the pituitary, probably from adrenal or multigland failure, which Horsley erroneously attributed to "asthenia" from being in captivity.

It is unfortunate that Horsley's experimental work on the pituitary gland was not documented more fully. His early work while at the Brown Institution was reported in abstract form based on his annual lectures, but it left unanswered many queries. It is unclear whether his work with Handelsmann added to his experience at the Brown or simply incorporated it. He seemed not to have made detailed observations on animals in which some pituitary fragments remained, thereby losing the opportunity to study the effects of chronic hypopituitarism.[42] A more detailed report by Handelsmann was promised but apparently not delivered.

Pituitary Surgery in Humans

Horsley was the first to explore the pituitary gland surgically in humans, having done so in 1889 by lifting up the frontal lobe of the brain to find a pituitary tumor pressing on the optic chiasm.[27] To accomplish this, however, he tied off certain veins and he attributed to this the ischemic damage to part of the frontal lobe that was noted at autopsy some years later. He therefore preferred to approach the pituitary by elevating the temporal lobe when surgery was necessary to relieve mechanical pressure, prevent blindness from optic nerve compression, and remove an underlying tumor.[27,40] He operated in two stages: an initial craniotomy followed three to seven days later by dural incision and gradual elevation of the temporal lobe to expose the pituitary.

By 1906, Horsley had performed operations on the pituitary in ten cases, with two deaths.[27,40] Patients had visual impairment (typically a bitemporal hemianopia, an inability to see in the outer half of both visual fields), sometimes associated with other complaints such as reduced libido, a failure of menstruation, more marked visual loss, and symptoms of increased intracranial pressure, with headache, nausea, and declining memory and concentration. The only treatment possible was surgical.[43]

The technical details of Horsley's surgical approach were not specific to pituitary surgery and are summarized in Appendix 1. His speed was remarkable – he could apparently perform "a pituitary surgery" in just thirty-six minutes.[44] When a large pituitary adenoma was encountered, he scraped the tumor out of the sella in little pieces using a sharp spoon.[45] He gave few other operative details except to point out that, after removing the tumor, he was able to view several previously inaccessible parts of the brain and its associated nerves without resorting to excision of brain tissue. He similarly provided no pathological evidence regarding the nature of the pituitary lesions on which he had operated, possibly because of his premature death or his increasing non-medical activities, but the distinction between true adenomas and other neoplasms

was anyway ill-defined at that time. A later lengthy report from the National Hospital on intracranial tumors again fails to provide useful detail.[46]

Although Horsley performed his first pituitary surgery in 1889, he did not report his work until 1906. Meanwhile a general surgeon, Frank Thomas Paul (1851–1941) of Liverpool, England – after discussion with Horsley – removed a window of bone from the temporal region of the skull in a thirty-three-year-old acromegalic to relieve her symptoms of raised intracranial pressure, without attempting more radical surgery to remove the tumor because of her poor general condition.[47] This case report is the first published account, in 1893, of surgery for a pituitary tumor.

Horsley's work on the pituitary came to attract the young Giovanni Verga (1879–1923), an assistant at the Institute of Human Anatomy in Pavia, Italy. In 1911 he published a monograph, *La Patologia Chirurgica dell'Ipofisi* [Surgical Pathology of the Hypophysis], on surgical approaches to the removal of pituitary tumors. In his book, Verga included details of Horsley's unpublished cases.[48] Where and how the two met is unknown, but it seems to have been in London, and Horsley was hospitable and kind to the eager young man. The surgery was performed by Horsley at the National Hospital in four instances and in his private practice in eight.[45] The cases included ten pituitary tumors and two craniopharyngiomas, as judged by Verga's description and subsequent analysis.[45] Thus Horsley, in addition to being the first to remove the pituitary in animals and to operate on it in humans, was the first to operate on craniopharyngiomas. These are benign, slow-growing tumors derived from embryonic pituitary tissue that may cause increased intracranial pressure and compress the optic nerves or pituitary gland. In the first decade of the twentieth century, they were often mistaken for pituitary tumors or cysts.

Horsley's clinical approach is exemplified by his analysis of a boy who was referred to him from Chicago and became his second patient with a craniopharyngioma. The fourteen-year-old had experienced recurrent episodes of headache, nausea, and impaired consciousness, and then of transient weakness of one side of the body. He had delayed sexual development, with genitalia of infantile appearance and no axillary or pubic hair.

Examination by Horsley revealed a combination of findings that he attributed to a pituitary tumor (bilateral optic atrophy and visual loss on the right of the field of vision; delayed sexual development; enlargement on radiographs of the bony cave – the sella – at the base of the skull in which the pituitary rests), distension of the ventricular system in the brain (transient right-sided weakness attributed to pressure on the left cerebral hemisphere), and compression of the connections between the cerebellum and the brainstem (mild gait ataxia). Horsley had seen a similar radiographic appearance in his previous patient with craniopharyngioma ("cystic pituitary tumor"), the enlarged sella being accompanied by opaque shadows above the sella defining the tumor boundary and which he attributed to calcium spicules and concretions in the walls of the cyst, confirmed at operation. He performed a right temporoparietal craniectomy and, four days later, opened the dura and lifted the temporal lobe to find a large cystic tumor, which he drained. The boy's convalescence went well and he returned to Chicago. Horsley was frank when writing to the referring doctors about the prognosis:

> As regards now his future: of course, hemorrhagic cysts do not tend to fill again. Therefore, the pressure on the tracts ought to be relieved and the boy's sight saved. At the same time this is the first cyst (non-suppurative) that I have done and it is not possible to dogmatize on such a subject. If at any time there was evidence of re-established pressure it would be (now) quite possible to pass an aspirator needle with suitable precautions and very little risk into the cyst.[49]

As it happens, the subsequent course was stormy. A pulsating mass developed at the surgical site, apparently containing cerebrospinal fluid; the boy's parents would not allow further treatment or even aspiration, and he died eighteen months after his surgery from chronic hydrocephalus ("water-on-the-brain").

The case is complex but instructive in many ways. First, it shows Horsley's analytical skill in localizing the underlying abnormality, which resembles that of an experienced modern clinician. Second, it emphasizes his ready acceptance of new ancillary diagnostic approaches (in this instance, radiography) to confirm or support his clinical diagnosis and the clinical-radiological correlations that he attempted. Radiological changes in the sella had been described by the great German neurologist Hermann Oppenheim (1858–1919) just a few years earlier, in 1899. Third, it reflects his good sense in limiting the surgery to drainage of the cyst rather than attempting to remove it, for the cyst would probably have been adherent to adjacent vital structures. Finally, it demonstrates his frankness in considering the uncertain prognosis and in anticipating potential complications and their treatment.

Horsley's approach to the pituitary was complicated and did not receive general acceptance. His contribution has since been forgotten, especially as others appeared to have little success with his transtemporal exposure and as various simpler approaches through the nose and sphenoidal sinus were developed. Subsequent advances, namely the recognition of the endocrine function of the pituitary, the development of hormone assays and the ability to correct hormonal imbalances, the detection of pituitary microadenomas by new imaging techniques, and the development of pituitary microsurgical techniques led to an upsurge in pituitary surgery, but the introduction of antisecretory drugs has again limited the number of patients requiring operative treatment.

Pineal Tumors

Nestling near the center of the brain between the two cerebral hemispheres, the pineal gland was once regarded as the seat of the soul. Tumors of the pineal are rare and difficult to approach. Horsley seems to have been the first to attempt to remove one.

In discussing a report of three patients with these tumors presented at a meeting of the Royal Society of Medicine in 1910,[50] he pointed out that he had not only seen the cases himself but referred to yet another that he had seen earlier at University College Hospital. In addition to the symptoms and signs of increased intracranial pressure, vertical eye movements (especially upgaze) were impaired, and vertigo, an unsteady gait, and mental changes were sometimes present. He had previously approached the lesion subtentorially with results "that were far from favorable," but in the future planned a supratentorial approach, decompressing or removing these tumors by splitting the tentorium to expose the dura. No further clinical or surgical details were provided, and it is not even clear whether he had operated on one or more cases.

Movement Disorders

Various neurological disorders are characterized either by excessive involuntary repetitive movements or by a paucity of voluntary and automatic movements unrelated to weakness. The best known of these disorders is Parkinson's disease, a chronic neurodegenerative disease characterized by a combination of tremor, rigidity, slowness and poverty of movement, and postural imbalance, together with a variety of non-motor symptoms. Horsley came to believe that these disorders could be treated surgically, and in this respect he has had a considerable but indirect impact on the management of these diseases.

He was one of the first to treat torticollis (now called cervical dystonia) – an abnormal posturing of the head due to overactivity of certain neck muscles – by sectioning specific nerves to weaken or paralyze the affected muscles. He did so when there was no specific identifiable cause for the disorder, which, he realized, often arose centrally in the brain. In this regard he was following in the footsteps of others in America and Australia.[51] In a lecture to the Hunterian Society in February 1897, he stressed that for operative success it was important to determine whether, in addition to involvement of the main muscles in the neck, any other muscles were affected, and also that a large section of the divided nerves should be removed to prevent their reunion.[51]

In 1908, Horsley was asked to consider surgical treatment for a fourteen-year-old boy who had developed involuntary, slow, sinuous writhing movements (athetosis) of the left hand seven years earlier. These eventually developed into violent convulsive jerking movements of the entire upper limb, with the arm being strongly flexed and adducted across the trunk (so that it was clamped tightly to the side and bent at the elbow) or, more rarely, flung out away from the body in abduction. The abnormal movements were worse with activity or with stress. When the involuntary movements were absent, the limb was powerful and moved normally. There was no sensory or reflex deficit. Horsley had successfully treated similar involuntary movements in two earlier cases by excision of the motor cortex, so

he advised that the cortical arm area be defined by electrical excitation and removed. On March 20, 1908, the upper-limb area of motor cortex was excised. Postoperatively, the limb was motionless and flaccid; the abnormal movements were gone, but the arm was completely paralyzed and some sensory changes were present. One year later, voluntary movements had partially recovered so that the limb had regained useful but not perfect function, without involuntary movements.[52]

Over the following thirty years, Paul Bucy in Chicago and Ernest Sachs in St. Louis reported similar findings using Horsley's procedure, as did others,[53] but which fiber tracts were involved remained ambiguous.[54] Subsequent attempts by others to relieve movement disorders (Parkinson's disease, dystonia, athetosis, or tremor) by dividing the corticospinal tract in the upper cervical region[55] or by motor or premotor cortical excision[56,57] led to initial hemiplegia that often resolved partly with time; cortical excision sometimes led also to postoperative seizures. Other surgical procedures led similarly to profound motor disability, seizure disorders, or both, and thus failed to find favor. In order to reduce the complication rate of open surgery, stereotactic devices – modifications of the Horsley and Clarke apparatus – came to be used to make discrete lesions in deeper parts of the brain, with variable success. Then, in 1951, Irving Cooper (1922–1986), a neurosurgeon in New York, noted that accidental occlusion of the anterior choroidal artery in the brain helped parkinsonian tremor and rigidity; repetition of the operation yielded excellent results in several other instances, due to ischemic changes in part of the thalamus and globus pallidus (neuronal collections within the depths of the cerebral hemispheres), as well as in various efferent pathways.

Overnight Cooper became a sensation, and hordes of patients were referred to him for treatment. He subsequently abandoned ligation of the choroidal artery in favor of the direct surgical destruction of the target region. He went on to develop a cryogenic probe to make destructive lesions by freezing the tissues with liquid nitrogen.[58] Ablative surgery at the level of the basal ganglia (neuronal aggregates within the cerebral hemispheres) thus came to be used increasingly for the symptomatic relief of Parkinson's disease until the late 1960s, when the advent of levodopa and related medications was found to help the associated motor disturbance.

With the late failure of medical treatment and renewed interest in surgical therapy using modifications of Horsley and Clarke's stereotactic approach, operative treatment has once again become an important means of managing various movement disorders, notably classic Parkinson's disease, essential tremor, and certain forms of dystonia. Ablative surgery, with its higher complication rate, eventually ceded to brain stimulation techniques that render the stimulated target functionally inactive. The quality of life of carefully selected patients has been improved noticeably by so-called deep brain stimulation of targets selected on the basis of the patients' symptoms and localized using techniques first developed by Horsley and Clarke.

Intracranial Aneurysms

An aneurysm consists of a balloon-like bulging of the wall of an artery. Aneurysms may cause symptoms by pressure on neighboring anatomical structures or by their rupture, which leads to hemorrhage that often has a fatal outcome. Horsley is reputed to have been the first person to have ligated the common carotid artery in the neck for the treatment of an intracranial aneurysm, but the medical literature is conflicting about what he actually did and when, probably because individual authors failed to go back to the original sources.

In a discussion on intracranial lesions at a meeting of the New York State Medical Association in 1890, the great American neurosurgeon William Keen referred to a remarkable case of Horsley that involved an aneurysm at the base of the brain, pressing on the optic chiasm. Horsley, having exposed the pulsating mass, apparently ligated both carotid arteries, "a surgical feat only equaled in its daring by the brilliancy of the diagnosis, which was verified by the operation."[59] (It is not clear from Keen's account whether the arteries ligated were the internal, external, or common carotid arteries.) However, Horsley himself recounted that when the patient died some years later, the supposed aneurysm was found at autopsy to be a large "blood cyst" connected with the anterior part of the pituitary gland.[60] In the absence of any good explanation for its persistence for several years after operative treatment, some have concluded that the lesion

was indeed an aneurysm, but the issue remains unsettled.

On another occasion, possibly in 1902, while performing an exploratory craniotomy, Horsley encountered a large pulsating aneurysmal mass that measured almost two inches in diameter and arose from the right internal carotid artery. He ligated the right common carotid artery in the neck a few days later and the patient did well, being in good health for at least the following five years.[60]

Apart from these interventions, Horsley had little to contribute to the management of cerebral aneurysms, and indeed major advances had to wait until the widespread utilization of percutaneous cerebral angiography some thirty years after his death.

Spinal Surgery

An account was provided in Chapter 5 of the celebrated case of Captain Gilbey, on whom Horsley operated in 1887 for progressive paraplegia from a benign tumor attached to the fourth thoracic (T4) nerve root on the left and compressing the spinal cord. He removed the tumor completely and the patient made a good recovery. Macewen in Glasgow actually preceded Horsley in having performed similar surgery to remove spinal tumors in six patients, four of whom made good recoveries whereas two died.

By 1890, Horsley was able to report that he had "trephined the spine (opening the theca in six cases) nineteen times with one death, that is, from shock." He regarded such surgery as usually having few risks other than infection. Spinal injury with displacement carried the risk of spinal cord or nerve root compression and merited early consideration of surgery. "We ought to operate without delay in all cases where displacement or crepitus indicates compression, and where extension directly after the accident clearly fails to reduce the deformity."[61] Horsley also treated other spinal disorders surgically. In syringomyelia, he reported temporary benefit following tapping of the dilated cavity in the spinal cord, but he provided few details.[62]

Spinal Tuberculosis

Horsley urged treatment for tuberculous disease of the spine, if only to relieve pain, which was a prominent feature of the disease.[61] The standard approach to spinal tuberculosis at the time involved bedrest, tonics and food supplements such as iron, and, when deformity occurred, plaster jackets.[63] Horsley considered that the infection began in the bone, spread to involve the intervertebral disk, and led to the early formation of an abscess beneath the anterior common ligament. Angular deformity with vertebral destruction and sometimes paraplegia followed, especially when there was mechanical compression of the spinal cord by the bony deformity and, more particularly, by the inflamed tissues around – and involving – the dura (pachymeningitis).[64,65] For patients with tubercular spinal disease with paraplegia, his practice was to put the patient to bed and apply extension "by the elastic method" so that the whole body was in a straight line. If signs of cord compression developed, and especially if there was a mild fever, he explored the patient surgically, drained any abscess, and debrided bony lesions, but generally without opening the dura. He scraped the abscess out with a sharp spoon, rinsed the abscess cavity with a strong disinfectant solution, and ensured the cavity was drained and dressed so as to obliterate its sac.[64] Painful death often occurred in his experience if operative intervention was delayed.

Of seven patients with spinal tuberculosis on whom he operated in or before 1890, three showed complete or significant recovery of paraplegia or quadriplegia, two others showed slight improvement in paraplegia, and one was unchanged. The remaining patient, with complete paraplegia, had temporary relief of pain but died after six weeks from "exhaustion" and was found to have a residual abscess in front of the vertebral bodies. Given that they were obtained in the years before antibiotics and antituberculous agents were available, Horsley's results must be regarded as surprisingly good, although the long-term outlook was presumably poor.

Spinal Arachnoiditis

Localized or circumscribed arachnoiditis (that is, inflammation of the membranes surrounding the spinal cord and nerve roots) may masquerade as a compressive tumor, as shown in the first report of a case in 1903, by Spiller and his colleagues in Philadelphia.[66] A subsequent report from Germany by Fedor Krause of six cases was followed by a detailed description of a series of cases by Horsley in 1909 and this, in turn, led to the disorder being recognized as a distinct entity.[67] Some twenty-one patients had been referred to him with a diagnosis of spinal tumor. They had developed progressive weakness of the legs and a slight kyphotic curvature of the spine, but exploratory surgery failed to reveal any tumor; their disorder typically ended fatally. In many instances Horsley could find no specific underlying cause, but in some it was inflammatory (syphilitic) in origin.

Horsley had encountered his first case in 1899, a paraplegic patient of Gowers with a diagnosis of probable spinal tuberculosis. He operated to relieve spinal cord compression but found no tumor or evidence of bony disease. Instead, the thick dural sheath surrounding the spinal cord was distended and filled the lumen of the spinal canal and, when opened, revealed a flattened spinal cord and seeming excess of cerebrospinal fluid. Exploration with a probe up and down the neural canal for a distance of five or six inches revealed no other abnormality, and the wound was therefore closed. No definite diagnosis could be made at the time, but the patient's progressive disease was reversed by laminectomy, opening the dural sac and washing it out with mercurial lotion.[67] Indeed, the patient was eventually able to return to work at the stock exchange, from which he had previously retired on medical grounds.

It is now widely appreciated that spinal arachnoiditis may be associated with infective or inflammatory processes such as syphilis or tuberculosis, may relate to trauma or degenerative changes of the spine, or may occur for uncertain reasons.[68,69,70] In recent years, it has occurred also following exposure to certain radiological contrast materials, now used no longer.[68,69] It may be asymptomatic or associated with pain, disturbances of the bladder and bowels, and progressive weakness of the limbs; death may occur from systemic complications such as urinary and kidney infection. Treatment is of the underlying cause and of symptoms such as pain; the utility of surgery is unclear.

Trigeminal Neuralgia

The trigeminal nerve is the sensory nerve for the face. Lightning stabs of unilateral shock-like facial pain characterize trigeminal neuralgia and often occur in paroxysms separated, at least initially, by pain-free intervals. The disorder can be quite devastating; patients are afraid to wash, shave, blow their nose, or even eat for fear of precipitating pain. Even a slight draught of air may do so. The pain occurs particularly in the territory supplied by the middle or lower division of the nerve, and is felt most commonly shooting along the upper or lower jaw toward the ear or from the side of the nose toward the eye. It may be followed by a burning ache in the face. There is typically no sensory loss or weakness. The cause for the disorder was unknown until recently, as discussed later.

Medical treatment in the nineteenth century was unsatisfactory. In 1891 Horsley summarized the operative procedures performed over the years on the various branches of the nerve for relief of trigeminal neuralgia, namely nerve stretching, nerve division (neurotomy), excision of part of the nerve (neurectomy), and nerve avulsion.[71] He himself had removed various peripheral branches of the nerve (depending on the location of pain) in a number of patients with trigeminal neuralgia but a seemingly successful outcome was followed by recurrence of pain after two or three years in many instances.[72] In consequence, he concluded that, to be successful, surgery would have to be more radical.

Believing that complete removal of the gasserian ganglion (the sensory ganglion of the trigeminal nerve) risked hemorrhage from the adjacent cavernous venous sinus, in the wall of which it is partially embedded, he instead preferred to cut the sensory root extending behind the ganglion to connect it with the brainstem. The surgery was deliberately planned, based on feasibility studies he performed in monkeys and on a human cadaver. He exposed the temporal lobe and elevated it to reveal the trigeminal nerve, which he gently avulsed from its connection to the pons. The first patient who underwent the procedure – a frail old lady in a "desperate state" – died seven hours later, supposedly from "shock."[70,71] A similar procedure apparently was attempted independently and at about the same time by Macewen, with the same outcome.[71]

Subsequent refinements of the surgical approach to the gasserian ganglion by Frank Hartley (1857–1913) in America and Fedor Krause (1857–1937) in Germany, and then by others, had a major impact on the treatment of trigeminal neuralgia. Partial or complete removal of the ganglion or the section of its sensory root became the surgical treatment of choice, at least for some years. Horsley named the basic procedure after Hartley and Krause,[71] but his own fundamental contribution has never received the credit that is its due.[73] By the time of his death, he had probably gained more experience than anyone in removing the gasserian ganglion and its sensory root for trigeminal neuralgia, and he did so with extraordinary skill.[74] Among twenty-one patients on whom he had operated in this way by 1900, there were only two fatalities, one due to the surgery (in an eighty-year-old woman) and the other probably unrelated to it; in none of the survivors was there any recurrence of facial pain, in contrast to the old operation on peripheral branches of the nerve.[71] In many instances, these patients had tried every conceivable treatment for their facial pain, suffering agonies before Horsley operated on them with his seemingly magical touch.

Over the years, treatment evolved such that destructive agents (for example, alcohol) were injected percutaneously into the gasserian ganglion, but benefit was often accompanied by significant complications. In the latter half of the twentieth century, however, trigeminal neuralgia came to be attributed to compressive injury of the root entry zone of the trigeminal nerve by small blood vessels that are visible with the operating microscope, and this led to its novel surgical treatment by a microvascular decompressive procedure rather than by disruption of the nerve. The approach has been successful in providing long-lasting relief in most patients.

Peripheral Nerve Injuries

Horsley treated a variety of nerve injuries over the years and attempted to clarify experimentally the pathophysiological basis of some of the injuries that he encountered clinically. For example, he simulated accidents in which people are thrown out of moving vehicles and found that the resulting neurological deficit related to stretch injury of nerves. On one occasion, he hoisted a cadaver by its feet to the top of the postmortem room at University College, with the head tilted slightly, and then allowed it to fall to the floor – when it struck the ground, the head was forced in one direction and the shoulder in the other. This led to stretch of the fifth and sixth cervical nerve roots, accounting for the selective muscle weakness but minor sensory disturbance that is common with such injury.[75]

He summarized his clinical approach in a lecture that he gave at the National Hospital in 1899 and subsequently published.[75] He stressed the importance of distinguishing between transection, laceration, contusion, compression, and stretch injuries. Continuity of the nerve implied an excellent prognosis. Nerve stretch injuries typically recovered, generally within six months. The outlook after nerve contusion was less certain, and exploratory operation was sometimes required to distinguish such an injury from nerve transection: if the nerve remained in continuity, recovery was likely but could take several years. Transected nerves embedded in scar tissue generally failed to regenerate or did so poorly. The experience by others over subsequent years has confirmed these general principles.

As regards surgical technique for repairing severed nerves, the simplest method was by stitching the two ends together with horse-hair that only passed through the connective tissue (epineural) sheath around the nerve. When freeing a nerve from callus and scar tissue that made it difficult to distinguish the nerve with confidence, he advised that it be defined above the scar tissue and followed down while preserving its blood supply, thereby proceeding from the known to the unknown. Cut or crushed nerves require time to regenerate, and he urged that sufficient time be allowed for regeneration before any surgical intervention is contemplated. He had a number of surgical successes. For example, he reported a patient who was carving wood with a narrow chisel when it slipped and pierced the palm of her hand, cutting the nerve to various muscles, which were paralyzed and had wasted away when Horsley saw her. At exploratory operation the two ends of the nerve were reunited and she made a complete recovery over the following two years.

Horsley supported his approach by such anecdotal case histories, sometimes exotic, but often provided no reliable evidence to support his conclusions or clinical decisions. Follow-up was often insufficient to justify (or refute) his claims. Thus, he described a patient who was shot in the thigh by a Martini-Henry bullet in the Matabele campaign (in Rhodesia, now Zimbabwe), and presented with a paralyzed leg. Horsley questioned the diagnosis of a lacerated sciatic nerve because sensory loss in the foot was patchy and he therefore explored the nerve, which was found to be contused and embedded in scar tissue, but in continuity; he freed the nerve and the patient returned to Africa with every expectation of a good recovery in time, but was lost to follow-up.[75]

He also described the difficulties that arose in distinguishing between organic deficits and those due to malingering.[75] An especially curious case of malingering involved a man whose forearm had to be amputated below the elbow following an injury. He subsequently developed weekly swelling and inflammation of the stump that was prevented by sealing the arm in an impervious case. It thus came to light that, in order to maintain the compensation he was receiving, the patient was inducing the inflammatory reaction himself by the application of mustard to the stump.

Reflections on a Neurosurgeon

It is difficult to overemphasize the importance of Victor Horsley in the development of neurosurgery. He continues to serve as a role model for modern neurosurgeons, combining the diagnostic abilities of a competent neurologist with the outstanding technical and operative skills required for success in the operating room. He had an intuitive appreciation of the anatomy of the nervous system and of the manner in which it operates, buttressed by his experimental studies of different aspects of cerebral function in animals. With his scientific curiosity and surgical skills, he was able to explore novel surgical approaches to ancient diseases by experimenting on animals and human cadavers before operating on patients. Indeed, his laboratory work gave him an easy familiarity with the nervous system, and his early operative focus on the brain and spinal cord enabled him to operate safely but with remarkable speed and to devise new instruments and operative approaches to facilitate achievement of his surgical objectives. He showed that it was possible to operate safely on the central nervous system and that such surgery was often effective in alleviating otherwise incurable neurological disorders, as evidenced by the numerous procedures that he originated. His interest in pathophysiology helped him better to understand the impact of disease on neurological function. He was not simply a technician, but a surgical neurologist who thought deeply about matters of the brain.

Notes

1. Pecker J: Thierry de Martel 1875–1940. pp. 197–202. In: Bucy P (ed): *Neurosurgical Giants: Feet of Clay and Iron*. Elsevier: New York, 1985.

2. Stone JL: W.W. Keen: America's pioneer neurological surgeon. *Neurosurgery* 1985; **17**: 997–1010.

3. Magiorkinis E, Sidiropoulou K, Diamantis A: Hallmarks in the history of epilepsy: Epilepsy in antiquity. *Epilepsy Behav* 2010; **17**: 103–108.

4. De Boer HM: Epilepsy stigma: Moving from a global problem to global solutions. *Seizure* 2010; **19**: 630–636.

5. Horsley V: An address on the origin and seat of epileptic disturbance. *Br Med J* 1892; **1**: 693–696.

6. Gotch F, Horsley V: Croonian Lecture: On the mammalian nervous system, its functions, and their localisation determined by an electrical method. *Philos Trans R Soc Lond B* 1891; **182**: 267–526.

7. Horsley V: Abstract of the Brown Lectures delivered at the University of London. Epilepsy. *Lancet* 1886; **128**: 1211–1213.

8. Spiegel E: The central mechanism of generalized epileptic fits. *Am J Psychiatry* 1931; **87**; 595–609.

9. Erickson TC: Spread of the epileptic discharge. An experimental study of the after-discharge induced by electrical stimulation of the cerebral cortex. *Arch Neurol Psychiatry* 1940; **43**: 429–452.

10. Van Wagenen WP, Herren RY: Surgical division of commissural pathways in the corpus callosum. Relation to spread of an epileptic attack. *Arch Neurol Psychiatry* 1940; **44**: 740–759.

11. Bogen JE: The neurosurgeon's interest in the corpus callosum. pp. 489–498. In: Greenblatt SH, Dagi TF, Epstein MH (eds): *A History of Neurosurgery in its Scientific and Professional Contexts*. American Association of Neurological Surgeons; Park Ridge, IL, 1997.

12. Luessenhop AJ, dela Cruz TC, Fenichel GM: Surgical disconnection of the cerebral hemispheres for intractable seizures. Results in infancy and childhood. *JAMA* 1970; **213**: 1630–1636.

13. Wilson DH, Reeves A, Gazzaniga M, Culver C: Cerebral commissurotomy for control of intractable seizures. *Neurology* 1977; **27**: 708–715.

14. Asadi-Pooya AA, Sharan A, Nei M, Sperling MR: Corpus callosotomy. *Epilepsy Behav* 2008; **13**: 271–278.

15. Eadie MJ: Victor Horsley's contribution to Jacksonian epileptology. *Epilepsia* 2005; **46**: 1836–1840.

16. Bakay L: Ernst von Bergmann and the Cushing reflex. pp. 73–83. In: *Neurosurgeons of the Past*. Thomas: Springfield, IL, 1987.

17. Bergmann E von: Die Lehre von den Kopfverletzungen. Enke: Stuttgart, 1880.

18. Spencer WG, Horsley V: On the changes produced in the circulation and respiration by increase of the intra-cranial pressure or tension. *Philos Trans R Soc Lond B* 1891; **182**: 201–254.

19. Fodstad H, Kelly PJ, Buchfelder M: History of the Cushing reflex. *Neurosurgery* 2006; **59**: 1132–1137.

20. Cushing H: Concerning a definite regulatory mechanism of the vaso-motor centre which controls blood pressure during cerebral compression. *Bull Johns Hopkins Hosp* 1901; **12**: 290–292.

21. Cushing H: Physiologische und anatomische Beobachtungen über den Einfluss von Hirnkompression auf den intracraniellen Kreislauf und über einige hiermit verwandte Erscheinungen. *Mitteilungen aus den Grenzgebieten der Medizin und Chirurgie* 1902; **9**: 773–808.

22. Cushing H: Some experimental and clinical observations concerning states of increased intracranial tension. The Mütter Lecture for 1901. *Am J Med Sci* 1902; **124**: 375–400.

23. Horsley V: Discussion on the treatment of cerebral tumours. Remarks on the surgical treatment of cerebral tumours. *Br Med J* 1893; **2**: 1365–1367 [additional discussion, 1369].

24. Horsley V: Brain-surgery. *Br Med J* 1886; **2**: 670–674.

25. Horsley V: The operative treatment of optic neuritis. *Ophthalmoscope* 1908; **6**: 658–663.

26. Wilkins RH: Treatment of craniocerebral infection and other common neurosurgical operations at the time of Lister and Macewen. pp. 83–96. In: Greenblatt SH, Dagi TF, Epstein MH (eds): *A History of Neurosurgery in its Scientific and Professional Contexts*. American Association of Neurological Surgeons; Park Ridge, IL, 1997.

27. Horsley V: On the technique of operations on the central nervous system. *Br Med J* 1906; **2**: 411–423; Horsley V: Address in surgery on the technique of operations on the central nervous system. *Lancet* 1906; **168**: 484–490.

28. Demetriades A: Victor Horsley's contribution to the Foster Kennedy syndrome. *Br J Neurosurg* 2004; **18**: 371–374.

29. Gowers WR: A lecture on a case of unilateral optic neuritis from intracranial tumour. *Lancet* 1909; **174**: 65–68.

30. Horsley V: A lecture on the topographical diagnosis of tumours of the cerebral hemisphere. *Univ Coll Hosp Mag* 1910; **1**: 9–17.

31. Kennedy F: Retrobulbar neuritis as an exact diagnostic sign of certain tumors and abscesses in the frontal lobes. *Am J Med Sci* 1911; **162**: 355–368.

32. Butterfield IK: Appendix Papers. p. 83. [Letter of encouragement from Victor Horsley to Foster Kennedy dated September 10, 1910]. In: *The Making of a Neurologist: The Letters of Foster Kennedy M.D., F.R.S.Edin. 1884-1952 to his Wife.* Stellar Press: Hatfield, Hertfordshire, 1981.

33. Horsley V: A paper on "optic neuritis," "choked disc," or "papilloedema": Treatment, localizing value, and pathology. *Br Med J* 1910; **1**: 553–558.

34. Walsh FB, Hoyt WF: *Clinical Neuro-Ophthalmology.* 3rd edition. pp. 569–574. Williams & Wilkins: Baltimore, MD, 1969.

35. Ramsden RT: 'A brilliant surgical result, the first recorded': Annandale's case, May 3, 1895. *J Laryngol Otol* 1995; **109**: 369–373.

36. Cleminson FJ: Case of acusticus tumour (right); Operation by Sir Victor Horsley in 1912; removal of tumour; recovery. *Proc R Soc Med* 1923; **16** (Otol Sect): 31–32.

37. Spiegel EA, Wycis HT, Marks M, Lee AJ: Stereotaxic apparatus for operations on the human brain. *Science* 1947; **106**: 349–350.

38. Dagi TF: History of stereotactic surgery. pp. 401–437. In: Greenblatt SH, Dagi TF, Epstein MH (eds): *A History of Neurosurgery in its Scientific and Professional Contexts.* American Association of Neurological Surgeons; Park Ridge, IL, 1997.

39. Anon: Abstracts of the Brown Lectures delivered at the University of London by Victor Horsley, M. B., B.S., F.R.C.S. Lecture III. Functional nervous disorders due to loss of thyroid gland and pituitary body. *Lancet* 1886; **127**: 5.

40. Anon: British Medical Association Clinical and Scientific Proceedings. South-Western Branch, Diseases of the pituitary gland. [Report of an address by Sir Victor Horsley.] *Br Med J* 1906; **1**: 323.

41. Handelsmann, Horsley V: Preliminary note on experimental investigations on the pituitary body. *Br Med J* 1911; **2**: 1150–1151.

42. Jefferson G: Sir Victor Horsley, 1857–1916. Centenary Lecture. *Br Med J* 1957; **1**: 903–910.

43. Pollock JR, Akinwunmi J, Scaravilli F, Powell MPZ: Transcranial surgery for pituitary tumors performed by Sir Victor Horsley. *Neurosurgery* 2003; **52**: 914–925; comments 925–926.

44. Goodrich JT: Comments. *Neurosurgery* 2003; **52**: 926.

45. Pascual JM, Prieto R, Mazzarello P: Sir Victor Horsley: pioneer craniopharyngioma surgeon. *J Neurosurg* 2015; **123**: 39–51.

46. Tooth HH: Some observations on the growth and survival-period of intracranial tumours, based on the records of 500 cases, with special reference to the pathology of the gliomata. *Brain* 1912; **35**: 61–108.

47. Caton R, Paul FT: Notes of a case of acromegaly treated by operation. *Br Med J* 1893; **2**: 1421–1423.

48. Verga G: Cap. V. Sintomatologia. pp. 139–193. In: *La Patologia Chirurgica dell'Ipofisi.* Tipografia Cooperativa: Pavia, 1911.

49. Horsley V: Letter to Archibald Church, MD, dated May 7, 1907. Quoted in Church A: Pituitary tumor in its surgical relations. *JAMA* 1909; **53**: 97–105.

50. Horsley V: Discussion, p. 77. Howell CMH: Tumors of the pineal body. *Proc R Soc Med* 1910: **3**: 77–78.

51. Horsley V: Torticollis. *Clin J* 1897; **10**: 145–149.

52. Horsley V: The Linacre lecture on the function of the so-called motor area of the brain. *Br Med J* 1909; **2**: 121–132.

53. Gabriel EM, Nashold BS. Evolution of neuroablative surgery for involuntary movement disorders: An historical review. *Neurosurgery* 1998; **42**: 575–591.

54. Bucy PC: Relation to abnormal movements. pp. 397–399. In: Bucy PC (ed): *The Precentral Motor Cortex.* 2nd ed. University of Illinois Press: Urbana, IL, 1949.

55. Putnam TJ: Relief from unilateral paralysis agitans by section of the pyramidal tract. *Arch Neurol Psychiatry* 1938; **40**: 1049 [Abstract].

56. Klemme RM: Surgical treatment of dystonia, paralysis agitans, and athetosis. *Arch Neurol Psychiatry* 1940; **44**: 926 [Abstract].

57. Bucy PC, Case TJ: Tremor. Physiologic mechanism and abolition by surgical means. *Arch Neurol Psychiatry* 1939; **41**: 721–746.

58. Critchley M: Irving S. Cooper. pp. 43–54. In: *The Ventricle of Memory: Personal Recollections of Some Neurologists.* Raven Press: New York, 1990.

59. Keen WW: Intracranial lesions. *Med News (NY)* 1890; **57**: 439–446.

60. Beadles CF: Aneurisms of the larger cerebral arteries. *Brain* 1907; **30**: 285–336.

61. Horsley V: Remarks on the surgery of the central nervous system. *Br Med J* 1890; **2**: 1286–1292.

62. Horsley VAH: Diseases of the vertebral column, tumours, and compression palsies. pp. 854–871. In: Albutt TC (ed): *A System of Medicine, Volume 6*. Macmillan: London, 1899.

63. Keller T: Historical perspective. Victor Horsley's surgery for cervical caries and fracture: The centennial anniversary. *Spine* 1996; **21**: 398–401.

64. Horsley V: A clinical lecture on paraplegia as a result of spinal caries (compression myelitis) and its treatment. *Clin J* 1893; **1**: 321–328.

65. Horsley V: A clinical lecture on the diseases of the spinal cord requiring surgical treatment. *Clin J* 1897; **9**: 177–183.

66. Spiller WG, Musser JH, Martin E: A case of intradural spinal cyst, with operation and recovery. *Univ Penn Med Bull* 1903; **16**: 27–31.

67. Horsley V: A clinical lecture on chronic spinal meningitis: Its differential diagnosis and surgical treatment. *Br Med J* 1909; **1**: 513–517.

68. Elkington JStC: Meningitis serosa circumscripta spinalis (spinal arachnoiditis). *Brain* 1936; **59**: 181–203.

69. Shaw MDM, Russell JA, Grossart KW: The changing pattern of spinal arachnoiditis. *J Neurol Neurosurg Psychiatry* 1978; **41**: 97–107.

70. Long DM: Chronic adhesive spinal arachnoiditis: Pathogenesis, prognosis, and treatment. *Neurosurg Q* 1992; **2**: 296–319.

71. Horsley V, Taylor J, Colman WS: Remarks on the various surgical procedures devised for the relief or cure of trigeminal neuralgia (tic douloureux). *Br Med J* 1891; **2**: 1139–1143, 1191–1193, 1249–1252 (three parts).

72. Horsley V: An address on the surgical treatment of trigeminal neuralgia. *Practitioner* 1900; **65**: 251–263.

73. Stookey B, Ransohoff J: *Trigeminal Neuralgia: Its History and Treatment*. pp 169–180. Thomas: Springfield, IL, 1959.

74. Jefferson G: Sir Victor Horsley, 1867–1916. pp. 150–169. In: Jefferson G : *Selected Papers*. Pitman Medical: London, 1960.

75. Horsley V: On injuries to peripheral nerves. *Practitioner* 1899; **63**: 131–144.

Chapter 8

Measures of the Man

Unlike the conventional image of a successful doctor, Horsley was thin, pale, and restless, with piercing blue-gray eyes and a daunting manner.[1] He had a small lock of white hair just above his forehead (as did his brother Gerald), heavy eyebrows, and a rather bushy moustache. His clothing was comfortable – he preferred shirts with soft, loose collars – rather than fashionable, and he spurned the frock-coat, then the uniform of the medical establishment. He had a tremendous presence and an infectious laugh, attracting attention as soon as he entered a room, the impact of his personality immediately evident.

Horsley was intense and uncompromising, and he was always fighting something or someone.[1] Perhaps success had come too early, for he developed a fanatical conviction that his views were always correct, and he resented both opposing views and those who held them. His intellectual self-confidence and "inflexible antagonism"[2] to everything and everyone with whom he disagreed fed his ambitious and competitive nature. Early in his career, for example, he became involved in an angry exchange with Sherrington, a much-loved physiologist and future Nobel laureate, who had succeeded him as superintendent at the Brown Institution.

The Row with Sherrington

In 1893, Sherrington and Horsley independently began studying the termination of the corticospinal tract, the outpouring of nerve fibers from the cerebral cortex to the spinal cord, in non-human primates. This involved destroying a small region of the cerebral cortex and allowing the animal to survive for a period of time before sacrificing it, in order to trace the degenerating nerve fibers into the spinal cord. When Sherrington learned that Horsley and E. Lindon Mellus, an American working with him, were about to publish their findings, he sent a brief note to the *Lancet* with

his own account, which was published in early February, before those of his competitors.[3] Shortly thereafter, an irritated Horsley responded by pointing out that it was he who had suggested the original work to Sherrington and even planned the details of the study. In a private letter to Sherrington, he also implied that there was something sinister underlying the "as yet unaccounted for highly remarkable delay" in the publication of his own paper in the *Proceedings of the Royal Society*.

An acrimonious correspondence between Horsley and Sherrington followed in the *Lancet*, as well as privately. This culminated with Sherrington forwarding to the Royal Society the accusatory comments implied in Horsley's private letter to him.[4,5] Almost immediately, Rubert Boyce, who was then Horsley's assistant, wrote to the *Lancet* assuming responsibility for any misunderstanding that may have arisen. He had previously told Sherrington, at Horsley's request, of the work by Mellus; he thought that Sherrington had agreed to discontinue his own work on the subject, but conceded that he may have misinterpreted what was actually said. In any event, neither Horsley nor Mellus apparently had had any idea that they and Sherrington were working on the same topic.[6] Horsley suggested arbitration of the matter of primacy by a neutral committee of three persons, but Sherrington declined and thereafter made little public reference to the issue.

Nevertheless, the kindly Sherrington was quite upset by the whole affair. Some have suggested that he delayed publication of a seminal paper with Albert Leyton, a medical student,[7] on cerebral localization in non-human primates until 1917 to avoid any further argument with Horsley.[8] However, as Sherrington did not hesitate to publish preliminary accounts of the work,[9,10] this seems somewhat unlikely.[5] The paper's eventual publication was important – it not only characterized the extent of the motor

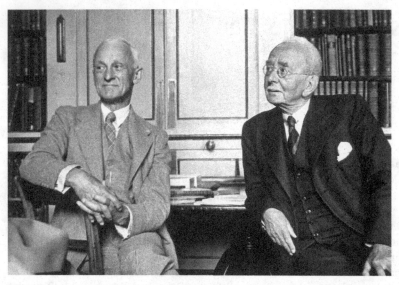

Figure 8.1 Harvey Cushing (*left*) came to Britain to study, but was disappointed by Horsley's surgical approach. He went on to become a world-famous neurosurgeon. Charles Sherrington (*right*), a much-loved physiologist and later Nobel laureate, succeeded Horsley as professor-superintendent at the Brown Institution. Their scientific interests overlapped, but they exchanged angry words over a question of scientific priority. (Photograph taken in 1938; from the Wellcome Collection, London.)

area of the brain but provided a detailed map of the primate motor cortex.[11]

Sensitivities, Insensitivities, and Idiosyncrasies

In later years, Horsley became involved in a second, more unseemly exchange that caused much controversy when he crossed swords with Karl Pearson – one of the founders of mathematical statistics – about the effects on children of parental alcoholism (discussed in Chapter 13). With Horsley, unfortunately, intellectual disagreement often became personal, and peaceful resolution was rarely an option, as exemplified by these exchanges. He regarded any opposition to his views as a personal challenge to be resolved not by discussion but by hostility and argument, sometimes bitter. To Horsley, things were black or white, right or wrong, and he favored a direct rather than a subtle approach to resolving any professional differences. There were other disagreements, especially related to medical and national politics, and these sometimes became quite vehement and vitriolic, reflecting rather poorly on Horsley. This became particularly apparent in his dealings with others while he served with the Medical Defence Union and the

General Medical Council, as discussed in Chapter 9.

To compound the problem, he did not always pick his battles wisely. On resigning from the chair of pathology at University College in 1896, for example, his unsuccessful canvassing for Vaughan Harley to succeed him both antagonized and personally offended Edward Schäfer, his teacher, friend, and former collaborator, and had a lasting effect on their relationship.

Although a perceived slight, whether intended or not, caused him to respond harshly, Horsley often offended others by his own words and actions without meaning to do so. He could be impatient and overbearing, imperiously disregarding those whom he judged to be foolish or insincere, and it is therefore no surprise that he tended to rub many people the wrong way. Nevertheless, despite the difficulties that occasionally surfaced in his interpersonal relations, Horsley had a liberal sense of fair play and took up many causes for the benefit of others. He spent much of his time in campaigning with vehemence for temperance and teetotalism, for women's suffrage, and for the welfare of children. He also helped, often with great passion, to establish and guide the Medical Defence Union, to reform both the General Medical Council and the British

Medical Association, and to develop nursing as a profession. These topics are considered in detail in later chapters.

Horsley judged others solely by their personal qualities. At a time when racial prejudice was common, he took as his private research assistant the dark-skinned James Risien Russell (1864–1939), an Edinburgh medical graduate of mixed ethnicity (Scottish and Guyanese), whose career he pushed to advance by urging Gowers and others to appoint him to the medical staff of leading London hospitals. The charismatic Russell eventually became professor of clinical medicine and full physician to both University College and the National Hospitals, charming all his patients even though he rarely examined them, and had an immense house in a fashionable part of London together with a chauffeur and Rolls Royce.

Some have alleged that Horsley's enthusiasm could go a little beyond the mark and verge on the scandalous. The American pathologist and neurosurgeon Percival Bailey (1892–1973) recalled that on one occasion an important diplomat, scouring the correspondence columns of *The Times*, found a scathing commentary against the antivivisectionists that made him chuckle until he found that he himself was named as its author. When challenged, Horsley confessed that he had written it, because "I've written so many, nobody pays any attention to me nowadays. I thought if I signed your name it might have some effect."[12] The story is almost certainly apocryphal, and in one preposterous version the name signed by Horsley was none other than that of the prime minister.

Many of Horsley's views became extreme with time, so that a colleague who dared to have an occasional drink came to be regarded by him as an alcoholic. However, his dry abrasive exterior actually shielded an innate kindness that was not always apparent, except in his dealings with those, such as patients or students, who needed his help. The American neurosurgeon Ernest Sachs (1879–1958) – grandson of the founder of the Goldman Sachs investment banking group – trained with Horsley and recalled years later how he "took me under his wing ... gave me every opportunity to learn his methods ... withheld nothing and gave me most generously of his time. He treated me like a son ... "[13] Another American surgeon, George Washington Crile (1864–1943) – who later co-founded the

Cleveland Clinic – worked in Horsley's laboratory as a young man and never forgot "the interest which Horsley showed in my problem, his courtesy and many kindnesses."[14]

In fact, Horsley was intensely loyal to those about him. Ernest Jones (1879–1958), his house surgeon at University College Hospital in 1902 and later a noted psychoanalyst and the biographer of Sigmund Freud, was particularly touched by Horsley's kindness. In 1906, Jones faced charges of inappropriate behavior with teenage girls; the girls' accounts were not believed in court and he was exonerated. Horsley went to the trouble of arranging a party at his house for the young physician, at which the president of the Royal College of Surgeons presented Jones with funds raised by professional colleagues to help defray his legal costs.[15] (An appeal for donations was then a common means of assisting prosecuted colleagues deemed to be innocent and subsequently acquitted by the courts, as discussed in Chapter 9.) Horsley himself contributed five guineas to the appeal. Jones later had a major role in negotiating Freud's escape to England from Hitler's Vienna in 1938.

Generosity was part of Horsley's character. He waived all charges to his professional colleagues, injured military personnel, and those who clearly could meet them only with difficulty, and he made no distinction between his private patients and the charity cases on which he consulted in hospital.

Surgeon and Scientist

During the last decade of the nineteenth century and the early part of the twentieth century, the only well-established clinical practice of neurosurgery in the world was that of Victor Horsley. As a surgeon, Horsley showed his patients nothing but kindness. He hated the idea of inflicting pain on them and would insist that they receive an anesthetic for even the most minor procedure.[16] He devised means of minimizing their discomfort postoperatively, when dressings were to be changed, and during their convalescence. His kindness to children was legendary. To spare a child who was dreading a second operation, he arranged for the boy to be sedated and put to bed at his usual hour, anesthetized him while he was asleep, and operated during the night despite the inconvenience to the other staff.[17]

Being naturally left-handed, Horsley had been forced to use his right hand for most tasks as a boy – as was then the custom – and he thus gained the operative advantage of being ambidextrous. Surgical procedures were performed with a rapidity and precision that were astounding and which visitors sometimes failed to comprehend. Ernest Jones recalled:

> The deftness and accuracy of his operating on the brain were something one could never forget, and he would coax a tumour from the thyroid as if by a gentle magic. His ambidexterity naturally helped him in this, and he seemed to expect the same gift in others. I remember when I fumbled over tying an artery with my left hand, my right hand being occupied with a Spencer Wells [forceps], he advised me to have my eyes tested for astigmatism.[18]

Robert Foster Kennedy (1884–1952), of Irish origin, studied at Queen's College, Belfast, and then went to London in search of neurological training, becoming the resident medical officer (a junior post) at the National Hospital in 1906, where he remained for four years. He kept his head when Horsley, as sometimes occurred, was in a bad mood and made life difficult for his juniors. As he wrote to his future wife in an undated letter soon after his arrival at the hospital:

> Tuesday morning was rather fierce and Horsley was in one of his bad humours. And I had the misfortune to have to give an anaesthetic to the fourth case. He was in a vile temper and slanged me and all the rest of the world – for a great man he is at times singularly petty – a vindictive fellow also, for yesterday I got a letter from him couched in indignant language because of trouble into which his optimism in operations had led him . . .[19]

Horsley could indeed be particularly short-tempered and irritable while operating, and expected his assistants to anticipate his needs and wishes. His "bad humours" probably reflected his anxiety. There was no junior surgeon to assist him for some years, and he had to turn to the two house physicians at the hospital for help. One commonly administered the anesthetic while the other provided more direct assistance.[20] The nursing staff had little experience of surgical techniques and would often hand him an unsuitable instrument, which he would unhesitatingly hurl across the room in a manner that was fairly common among surgeons until recently.

While at Queen Square, Foster Kennedy did not hesitate to air his views when they failed to conform to those of his seniors, but he did so inoffensively and with care. He occasionally disagreed with Horsley's tendency to operate early and on one occasion rather foolishly took the law into his own hands. As he again wrote to Isabel McCann, his fiancée:

> I was very anxious on Sat. night: a girl of fifteen was brought in – urgent. She had been playing cricket on Friday evening and was struck on the left temple by a fast ball.
>
> I felt sure she had fractured the base of the skull: she had complete paralysis of the right arm and leg. She was obviously improving, but was still critical. I was in rather a dilemma. If I rang up Gowers about the case, he'd say 'ask Sir Victor to see her' – and that meant opening the head, almost without thinking. On the other hand, if she were left alone and improved steadily, by Monday she'd be well enough probably to prevent the question of operation being raised. I decided – trembling – to hang on. I watched that child all Sat. night and through Sunday and today she's safe. If I'd have been wrong and she had died on Sat. night or yesterday, I'd have been in an ugly hole, but that's all right now! Circumventing staff men is an added excitement to life.[21]

In this latter instance, Kennedy's judgment can be faulted because hemorrhage in the suspected region can occur very rapidly and lead to a fatal outcome if not treated promptly. In the days before the availability of proper imaging techniques, early exploration would certainly have been justified, and Kennedy's courageous error might have cost the girl her life and him his career. And yet, on the occasions that he was proven correct, Horsley was big enough to give him the credit

A patient had been admitted for surgery of a right frontal lobe tumor of the brain, diagnosed by several senior physicians, but the young Kennedy decided it was an abscess. He arranged for the second stage of the operation (the brain dissection) to be the last of the day in case of sepsis, to Horsley's amused acceptance. The operation was difficult, as much of the brain was infiltrated with the unencapsulated lesion, with the typical appearance of a tumor. In the end, Horsley tied off its blood vessels and stuck the mass with a scalpel. There was, in Kennedy's words,

A gush of yellowish pus – I almost yelled with excitement in a silence absolutely deathlike, broken at last by Horsley with a great 'By God!' He let all the pus out, dissected out the membrane of the abscess cavity and then turned round to his gallery and said 'abscess had been Dr. Kennedy's diagnosis for the last fortnight' and afterwards he and a lot of other chaps came up and shook hands with me and gave me congratulations.[22]

On most other occasions, it must be said, Horsley was correct in his localization and identification of the pathological process, and Kennedy was wrong, as is only to be expected. Indeed, as Kennedy settled into his job, he came to realize the extent of Horsley's skill. "We were very busy yesterday. Horsley did five operations – I think any one of them would have been a sensation at home. ... They have all done splendidly."[23]

Foster Kennedy was a charming and excellent physician who nevertheless was unable to find a good permanent appointment in Britain despite the best efforts of Horsley and Gowers. He finally accepted an invitation to become chief of clinic at the new Neurological Institute in New York, then a place of promise but no reputation. It was to become a world-famous neurological center and one of the prides of American medicine. Kennedy served in World War I, first in the Royal Army Medical Corps and then with the Harvard Surgical Unit in General Hospital No. 22, of the British Expeditionary Force in Northern France (initially with a field ambulance unit and finally as a neurologist). On his return to New York, he moved to the large Bellevue Hospital, the oldest public hospital in the United States, where he became head of the neurology service, was appointed professor of neurology at Cornell, and eventually became president of the American Neurological Association. He was wise, much admired, and very influential. Among his later views were that shell shock was a form of "hysteria" and, more controversially, that eugenics was an important means of improving the health of the human race.

The American surgeon Harvey Cushing (1869–1939) spent fourteen months in Europe to further his medical career at the beginning of the twentieth century. He had intended to devote his time to men with particular surgical or neurological expertise, including Kocher in Berne, Sherrington in Liverpool, and Horsley in London. However,

He found Horsley living in seemingly great confusion: dictating letters during breakfast to a male secretary; patting dogs between letters; and operating like a wild man. H.C. [Cushing] gave him a reprint of his paper on the Gasserian ganglion, whereupon Horsley said he would show him how to do a case. They drove off the next morning in Horsley's cab ... to a well-appointed West End mansion. Horsley dashed upstairs, had his patient under ether in five minutes, and was operating fifteen minutes after he entered the house; made a great hole in the woman's head, pushed up the temporal lobe – blood everywhere, gauze packed into the middle fossa, the ganglion cut, the wound closed, and he was out of the house less than an hour after he had entered it. This experience settled H.C.'s decision to leave London; for he felt that the refinements of neurological surgery could not be learned from Horsley.[24]

This account by Cushing's biographer is surprising, for surely the young American was himself no stranger to multi-tasking; perhaps he mistook Horsley's operative speed for carelessness. In fact, Horsley's speed helped to reduce the duration of anesthesia, and he could show remarkable patience in the operating room when necessary.[16] In any event, Cushing was rather disparaging of all that he encountered in London and went elsewhere to advance his own career. He later seemed to become an admirer of Horsley and his work,[24] at one point even affectionately calling him "a daisy,"[25] despite considering him an impatient and somewhat impetuous surgeon.[26]

Cushing himself became an innovative neurosurgeon who trained many future specialists in this new field, a clinical investigator who stimulated others to greater depths of understanding, and a medical historian whose biography of Sir William Osler won him a Pulitzer Prize in 1926. He was a difficult person, driven and ambitious, critical of his assistants whom he often blamed for his own mistakes, a hot-tempered loser, unwilling to yield the limelight to any one, and respectful only of those who stood up to him. He resembled Horsley in his devotion to his own affairs regardless of others, and he had similar interests to Horsley regarding the brain and its responses to electrical stimulation, as well as in the pituitary gland and the gasserian ganglion.

Felix Semon, the laryngologist, worked with Horsley in the laboratory (see Chapter 4) and has described how he would have "flashes of genius by which quite suddenly he raised our experiments to higher ground."[27] In addition to their much valued friendship, Horsley had operated no fewer than four times on Semon's son for mastoiditis and provided much support when Semon's wife had a seizure and then lapsed into coma. "Nothing could have exceeded [his] kindness and zeal ... the generally gloomy prognosis was not shared by Horsley. He gave me hope, and, as on so many other occasions, he was right."[28] In 1911, Semon dedicated his two-volume *Forschungen und Erfahrungen* [Research and Experience] to his friend "in constant gratitude for his invaluable collaboration in the physiological portion of the work." Horsley responded that "you have done me far too much honour, and therefore [I] feel like some unworthy person who has just come into a large fortune! ... Personally I have never felt so delighted as with this addition to your innumerable kindnesses."[27]

There were, of course, many demands on Horsley's time, relating to his prominence as a surgeon. He was asked to see patients all over the country and he did his best to oblige, even if a special train was sometimes required to bring him to the patient and then return him to the capital.[29] He was also in demand as an expert witness in medicolegal cases, but his services did not come cheap – on one occasion in 1904, he charged one hundred guineas for giving evidence in a case at the Exeter Assizes, plus fifteen guineas daily for expenses.[30]

Horsley's co-workers generally loved the enthusiasm and energy with which he pursued any project,[2] but his colleagues, and especially his juniors, may well have felt overwhelmed by him at times. He reacted angrily if he felt excluded or was denied what he perceived to be his due, but was generous in the extreme to those who treated him in the manner that he expected. Thus, when presented with a manuscript reporting research carried out in his laboratory and bearing both his own name and that of his student as authors, Horsley crossed out his name with the remark "As long as it is customary, when two men publish a paper, to give credit to the one who is better known, I shall not allow my name to appear."[13] He

regarded his relationship with particular students not as that between teacher and pupil but as that of partners, for he learnt from them just as he also gave to them.[31]

Horsley has been described as a man "who used every ounce of his gifts – a very rare talent. ... He was never in a hurry and yet used every moment of his life actively. ... [He] would concentrate on the topic as if nothing else existed and no-one else mattered, as if time was of no importance: but, the business done, there was no delay."[32] He apparently believed that his needs and tasks were supremely important and automatically took precedence over any tasks of others. On arriving in Quebec for a visit to North America, he pointed out his luggage as if he were the only one in need of assistance and was swiftly put in his place by the busy porter: "And who the hell are you, anyway?"[32]

Comparative Anatomist

Many anecdotes about Horsley relate to his interest in comparative anatomy. Percival Bailey, a raconteur who was not above sacrificing accuracy for humor, recalled an escapade that may well be fictitious but is not difficult to believe. Horsley had a friend, Meyers, who developed an overarching interest in camels while professor of psychology in Cairo. On returning to his position at London University, Meyers brought with him a camel to which he was particularly attached. He built a heated barn for the animal in his garden, and imported dates and other special foods for the beast. No expense was spared. One day, while Meyers was delivering a lecture, Horsley rushed in, exclaiming that the camel had died. Meyers accused him of having operated on it. Horsley was not contrite: "Of course. Who could do it better?" Meyers was furious. "That's not the point, confound it," he said, "the point is that that was *my* camel." Horsley barely hesitated, "You wouldn't have let me if I'd asked you first, so I thought I'd operate first and tell you later. How was I to know the stupid brute would drink ether as if it were water? If he's dead, it's his own fault, not mine."[12]

The supposed appropriation of the camel was not the only instance of Horsley's interest in comparative anatomy and the evolution of the brain. On one better-substantiated occasion he was sent a huge barrel containing the head of an elephant packed in salt. The animal had been shot in India by a former student, who had then removed the head and injected it with formaldehyde brought along for that very purpose. Some photographs, sent separately, arrived at about the same time and showed the local natives watching open-mouthed as the decapitation proceeded.[33] Horsley was delighted and dropped everything else to remove the brain. Other specimens of particular interest also came his way in somewhat colorful circumstances. A certain Lieutenant Colonel Martin-Leake, medical officer to the Bengal-Nagpur railway, was a notable hunter as well as a skilled surgeon. In 1907, he was tracking a wounded rogue elephant that had killed a man and suddenly found himself confronted by the large and very angry animal. He shot it and subsequently spent nine hours removing the animal's brain, which he sent to Horsley in a stew-pan.[34] Martin-Leake had been a medical student at University College and was thus aware of Horsley's interests. He was also a man of remarkable courage and the first of only three men to twice win the Victoria Cross, the highest British medal for gallantry awarded to members of the armed forces in the face of the enemy. Horsley had operated on him in 1902 for a hand wound sustained in South Africa during the Boer war and – as was his custom – did so without charge to a fellow medical colleague.

Exotic animals were also available closer to home. On one occasion, Horsley rushed off to remove the brain of a walrus that had died at the London Zoo, justifying the inconvenience to his patients with the simple statement: "If people want me to learn, they must be willing to wait."[13,33] At the zoo, he found the unfortunate walrus laid out on a plank surrounded by a group of men. Horsley immediately took off his coat, removed the brain, and then turned the carcass over to the waiting men, each one of whom had come to collect the organs of special interest to himself.[33] The London press made much of the loneliness of the walrus' surviving companion.[35]

Scientific Awards and Other Honors

Horsley was the recipient of many honors, which are listed in Appendix 2, and only a few require additional emphasis or discussion here. In 1886, the same year as the invention of coca-cola, the building of the world's first gasoline-powered automobile (the Benz Patent-Motorwagen), the

dedication of the Statue of Liberty, and his appointment to the staff of the National Hospital, Horsley was elected to fellowship of the Royal Society of London. The society, founded in 1660, was the leading learned society for scientists in Britain. His proposers were Edward Emanuel Klein, the bacteriologist who came to personify the vivisectionists to an antagonistic segment of the public; George John Romanes, the physiologist and believer in evolution, after whom the Romanes lecture, given annually at Oxford University, is named; the neurologists J. Hughlings Jackson and David Ferrier; Edward Schäfer, his collaborator in studies of cerebral function; W. H. Gaskell, a cardiac physiologist; James Paget and John Marshall, leading surgeons of the day, the latter his former teacher at University College Hospital; and the physicist John Tyndall.

He gave the prestigious Croonian lecture at the Royal Society jointly with Francis Gotch, his brother-in-law, in 1891. They focused on their explorations of the mammalian nervous system and the manner and localization of its functions, as discussed in Chapter 4.[36] In 1894 Horsley received the Royal Medal of the society for his work on the physiology of the nervous system and on the thyroid gland. Established by King George IV in 1825, the medal was awarded annually for the two most important published contributions in the previous ten years to the advance of "natural knowledge" in the biological and physical sciences. The other medal for 1894 went to Joseph John Thompson for his contributions to physics; he went on to win the Nobel prize and is credited with identifying the electron. In that same year, Horsley received an honorary doctorate from the ancient University of Halle in Germany.

Among his other prizes, Horsley received the Cameron Prize for therapeutics from the University of Edinburgh in 1893, and, when accepting it, spoke on brain surgery and the thyroid gland. The Cameron Prize was a very prestigious award, the past recipients having been Pasteur (1889), Lister (1890), and Ferrier (1891), with no award made in 1892. Two years later, he won the Fothergill Gold Medal of the Medical Society of London for his work on the thyroid gland. The medal, created in 1787, was awarded every three years, and the recipient immediately preceding Horsley was Gowers, his neurological colleague and former teacher.

King Edward VII knighted both Horsley and his contemporary and fellow brain-surgeon, William Macewen, in 1902. They had pioneered a new specialty and advanced knowledge of the brain, and it was fitting that both were recognized for their individual contributions to this and many other fields of medicine. The announcement was published in the June Honours List that preceded the intended coronation of the new king.[37] The coronation itself, originally scheduled for late June, had to be postponed until August, however, after Edward developed appendicitis that necessitated surgery.

Horsley was invited to give the Linacre lecture at Cambridge University in 1909. The lectureship, at St. John's College, was founded in 1524 by Thomas Linacre, physician to King Henry VIII, and is the oldest medical endowment at Cambridge. Starting in 1908, the lectureship could be held for only a single year by "a man of mark" who was to give a single lecture for an honorarium of ten guineas. Horsley chose as his topic the motor area of the brain, his views on which were described in Chapter 4.

In 1911, Horsley became the first recipient of the international Lannelongue Prize, a gold medal and five thousand francs, awarded for the greatest contributions to the advance of surgery in the preceding decade. The prize was established by Odilon Lannelongue, a French surgeon, in memory of his wife Marie, and was to be awarded every five years by the French National Society of Surgery (now the National Academy of Surgery) on the recommendations of an international jury. In his acceptance speech, Horsley, still in his mid-fifties, complimented Professor Lannelongue and then spoke of the recent influence on British surgery of French physiologists, and especially of the late Claude Bernard who had provided a scientific underpinning to surgical practice much as he himself was attempting to do. Because of interruptions related to two world wars, there have been only a few winners of the prize since its creation. Among them are Wilder Penfield from Montreal who – like Horsley – treated epilepsy surgically and used electrical stimulation to map the functions of the human brain (see Chapter 4), and George Crile, one of Horsley's former research students, who went on to co-found the Cleveland Clinic.

Over the years Horsley was elected an honorary member of many foreign societies (listed in Appendix 2), including in 1912 the Royal Society of Sciences in Uppsala, which was founded in 1710 and is Sweden's oldest learned society, and to which he was appointed in succession to Lord Lister. He also was appointed to the General Medical Council, the Senate of the University of London, and to various positions in the British Medical Association, and he became president of the Neurological Society of London, the Medical Defence Union, and the British Temperance Society. He came to be regarded by his admirers as a fearless crusader for those unable to fend for themselves and by his enemies as a tiresome and inflammatory nuisance.

With the outbreak of the Great War, he joined the Army Medical Service as a volunteer, and in early 1916 was appointed companion of the Order of the Bath (CB), military division, by King George V for his distinguished service in the field as acting colonel (see Chapter 15). He died on active service just a few months later.

Domestic Life

Horsley's professional success reflected, at least in part, his domestic situation. He had become engaged to be wed in 1883 and – after four years and wearied of waiting – finally married Eldred Bramwell on October 4, 1887, in a quiet ceremony at the fashionable St. Margaret's, Westminster, on the grounds of Westminster Abbey. They honeymooned in Italy but – in Bologna – the bridegroom developed appendicitis and was briefly laid low. Fortunately his symptoms settled spontaneously, although they recurred periodically until, some twenty years later, he underwent an appendectomy by his friend Bilton Pollard, a former medical-school classmate and his colleague at University College Hospital.[38]

Eldred became a faithful, if somewhat earnest, companion. She was good at running the household and also acted very effectively as his secretary, managing his time, keeping his accounts, making his appointments, proofreading his publications, and writing his letters, which she occasionally even signed for him.[39] Returning home in the evening, he would simply "empty his pockets of the fees he had received during the day and pour them into her lap" and she would then take charge of matters.[39] Eldred was also an accomplished hostess, and became used to entertaining Horsley's friends or colleagues at any meal during the day or night, including breakfast, without any fuss. Things did not always go smoothly, however. On one occasion she hosted a dance for some of their friends and for Horsley's younger colleagues. Music was provided by a pianist and violinist, whose departure was to signal the end of the gathering, but some bright spark sat down at the piano and continued the entertainment. Eldred was furious and, eventually unable to contain herself, called out in a very unladylike display, "get out, the party is over!"[20]

Eldred had a strong, even dominating personality and came to have enormous influence over Horsley. She involved him in the cause of women's suffrage, helped him in his work against alcohol, and supported his political activities as a parliamentary candidate,[39] but the extent to which his views reflected her input is unclear. Although an ardent feminist, she held strong opinions on the behavior and decorum expected of women in public. If she encountered a lady smoking in public, for example, she had been known to dart forward and snatch the cigarette from the startled woman's mouth.[20]

The marriage was a good one, and Eldred relieved him of the many worries of daily life. In the charming words of Stephen Paget, "Heaven was so pleased with this marriage, that it made another, to go with it."[40] In December 1887, Horsley's sister Rosamund married Frank Gotch, his former classmate at medical school and subsequent partner in researches on the brain.

At home, Horsley was quite different from his public image as unbending and intolerant, showing instead a softer, affectionate, and genial side to his character. His tastes were simple. The Horsleys lived at Park Street until 1891 when they moved briefly to 33 Seymour Street, where their first son, Siward, was born on June 18, and then to 25 Cavendish Square, which they purchased as their permanent home. It was a fine house in a fashionable part of London, with a good-sized ground-floor consulting room that looked out onto the plane trees in the square. A large back room with a skylight served as Horsley's work area where he would perform dissections, cut sections for microscopy, and prepare visual aids

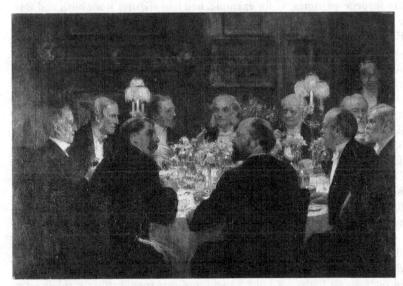

Figure 8.2 Dinner party hosted by Sir Henry Thompson to honor Ernest Hart, editor of the British Medical Journal, seated at back to the right of the mantelpiece. Horsley (third from left, foreground) is seated between Sir George Critchett, an ophthalmic surgeon, to his right, and Sir Richard Quain, an influential Irish physician, to his left. Thompson's dinner parties were known as "octaves" because eight courses accompanied by eight wines were served at eight o'clock to eight guests plus the guest of honor. (Oil painting by Solomon Joseph Solomon, circa 1897; image from the Wellcome Collection, London.)

such as lantern slides or photographs, which he would take and develop himself. On the shelves lining the walls were lecture notes, odd jottings, manuscripts, papers, and stacks of photographs, lantern slides, diagrams, and other paraphernalia.[41]

Curiously, the house had a remarkable neurological pedigree. It had been occupied by Charles Edouard Brown-Séquard (1817–1894), a founder-physician of the National Hospital and an improbable genius who contributed much to the understanding of the nervous and endocrine systems.[42] His successor at the National, Dr. Charles Radcliffe (1822–1889) also occupied the house. A man of refined taste but holding to eccentric scientific concepts, Radcliffe worked hard, contributed to the literature on epilepsy, and died the day after he retired without making real advances in the field.[43] And so the house became the home of the Horsleys. Unfortunately, the house and those adjacent to it exist no longer: a large department store has replaced them, and the calm of the square has succumbed to the rumble of London's traffic.

Horsley's second son, Oswald, was born on February 16, 1893, and his daughter Pamela Comfrey on April 19, 1895. He was close to the three children and one of his favorite pastimes was to take them to the zoo on a Sunday afternoon. The two boys went to Bedales, an expensive coeducational school that was founded in 1893 and had a less regimented approach than most other schools. The relationship between pupils and teaching staff was more level than hierarchical, and a direct hands-on and problem-solving experience was encouraged. The school had moved into purpose-built premises near Steep, a village in Hampshire, England, in 1900, and it was there that Siward and Oswald were sent. It was an excellent choice for the Horsley boys, and the school's non-denominational nature, emphasis on the individual, and progressive approach to education clearly coincided with Horsley's own beliefs. Students were issued with a hymn and psalm book, and the bias was Christian, but as a non-denominational school open to all faiths, children from non-conformist backgrounds were accepted at a time when most of the big public schools only accepted pupils from Church of England families.

Siward, a student there from 1903 to 1909, turned out to be a superb cricketer, and became editor of the school's *Chronicle*. Oswald, who followed his brother three years later, also excelled in sports, notably cricket and football, and became head boy. Both boys were members of the school orchestra. They seemed to enjoy their time at Bedales, and left their mark on the school (see p. 170).[44] Their cousin Oliver Henry Gotch, the only son of Francis Gotch and Rosamund, was also at the school from 1900 to 1907 and went on to become a consulting physician at St. Thomas' Hospital in London.[45]

It was a happy family and household until the teenage Siward had a seizure while at a concert at the Albert Hall. It is unclear whether he had experienced seizures previously but, in any event, further seizures occurred, epilepsy was diagnosed, and an operation was suggested. Horsley regarded himself as the most competent to perform it, and so he operated on his own son. There were no complications and all seemed to be well, but the seizures subsequently recurred. The epilepsy was a particular problem between 1910 and 1912, after which Siward spent a year fruit farming,[44] away from the stresses of city or academic life.

There were, of course, other surgical failures, often with tragic consequences, but at least these were less personal. Thirteen-year-old Ethel Wood, for example, had had seizures since birth and was examined by Horsley, but surgery failed to arrest her seizures, which increased in frequency despite medical treatment and the devoted care of her mother. Eventually the mother could stand it no longer, strangled the girl to "put her out of her misery" and turned herself in to the police.[46]

By the time of the 1911 census, only Pamela remained at home with her parents, for Siward was away studying chemistry and Oswald was still at Bedales, but they were well looked after by a butler, a cook, three housemaids, a kitchen maid, and a domestic nurse who helped Horsley in his private practice. In the summer months, Horsley generally rented a place in the East Anglia countryside for the shooting rights, and spent long weekends there. A morning of shooting would be followed by lunch and then work. Longer vacations were spent further afield, in later years in Scotland or the Orkneys, where he went sailing and fishing and supported local causes such as cattle and industrial shows.[47]

Horsley had an excellent memory, great powers of concentration, and – in order to be included in domestic life – often worked with his family and his

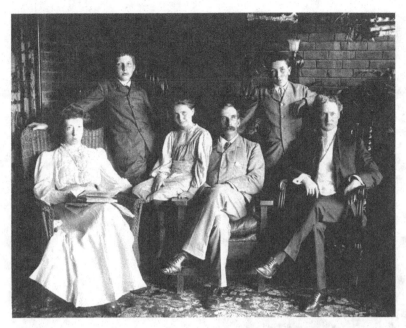

Figure 8.3 Victor Horsley at a conference in Toronto, Canada, in 1906 with, from left, his wife Eldred and children Oswald, Pamela, and Siward. The person on the extreme right is unidentified. (Image courtesy of the Queen Square Archives and Sir Victor Horsley's family.)

dogs around him. His favorite fox terrier liked to sit on his lap as he worked. He had the ability to retain his train of thought despite interruptions, and was able to join in family conversations while working on a manuscript or reviewing microscope slides, keeping for this purpose a microscope on a table in the middle of the drawing room. He was an excellent photographer, a skill that helped him in his academic work by adding to the quality of his medical publications and lectures. He also enjoyed drawing and would cleverly illustrate his letters or descriptive reports with little sketches. When writing to family members or friends, he often signed his name with a rebus, a prancing horse with a "V" for its saddle. In the evening, billiards or a variation of it brought excitement and relief from work. After a particularly busy day he might nap for a few minutes and, reinvigorated, would then be able to continue with his work or with other activities. He went to bed early and in his later years preferred not to go out to dinner.[48]

Other Interests

Horsley's retentive memory gave him the ability to scan a book and yet take in all its important details. He was fluent in French and German, and had no difficulty in keeping up with the foreign medical and scientific literature. He also was interested in history and was fascinated by the surgical endeavors of earlier times.

Trephining in the Neolithic period was of especial interest to him, and he spoke of it at the Anthropological Institute in London, discussing whether it involved boring, scraping, or sawing into the head. He believed, based on photographic appearances, that it most often involved sawing, occasionally supplemented by scraping, and observed that the openings in the skull tended to cluster over the motor region of the brain, a common site of origin for posttraumatic focal motor (Jacksonian) seizures.[49] Perhaps, Horsley reasoned, localized pain and tenderness from depressed skull fractures after head injury led first to removal of scar tissue and later of bone at the injured site, with fortuitous relief of focal seizures. He thus speculated that trephining sometimes came to be performed with the specific intention of relieving posttraumatic seizures, and in South America trephined skulls often do show evidence of preceding injury, such as fractures. In most instances, however, the motives for the

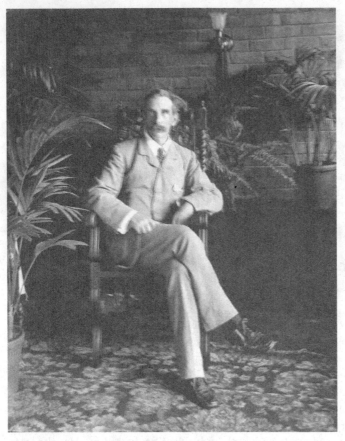

Figure 8.4 Victor Horsley in Toronto, Canada, in 1906. (Image courtesy of the Queen Square Archives and Sir Victor Horsley's family.)

procedure remain obscure – others have suggested that trephining allowed good or evil spirits to enter or leave the body, the head being selected as the operative site because even minor head injury sometimes leads to the appearance of death when consciousness is lost.[50]

In another talk, this time at the Middlesex Hospital Medical Society in March 1899, he discussed the medical profession and the state of surgery during Roman times, illustrating his talk with photographs of surgical instruments excavated from Pompeii and a small set taken from the pocket case of a Roman physician excavated in England at York. He also spoke of Galen and his work on the nervous system, deriving two principles from the study of his life: first, the need to avoid any deduction concerning the function of a tissue or organ based solely on observations of its structure and, second, the

importance of identifying and treating the cause of disease and not simply alleviating its symptoms.[51]

Horsley was interested in architecture and archaeology, on which he could speak with facility. In his house at Cavendish Square was a yellow-marble model of temple columns in the Roman Forum. When the opportunity arose during vacations in different parts of Britain, he was "always eager to explore some Pictish mound or barrow, some stone circle, cathedral, or monastery."[52] In 1899 he even lectured at the Royal Institution on the Roman defenses of south-east Britain against the attacks of the Scandinavian and Germanic tribes living on the shores of the North Sea, describing the walled camps in detail, including their structure and the arrangements within the walls.[53] On other occasions, he lectured to the public in museums or at various social gatherings,

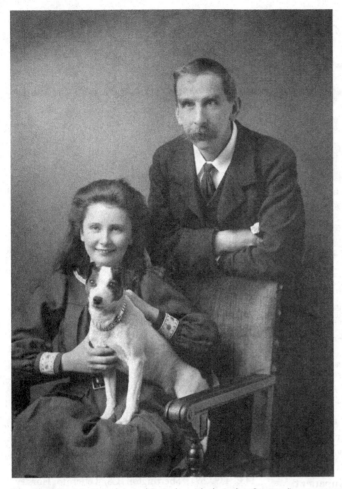

Figure 8.5 Victor Horsley and Pamela, with their dog Scamp. (Image courtesy of the Queen Square Archives and Sir Victor Horsley's family.)

speaking about various archaeological topics or on the history of surgery.[54] He was interested also in genealogy and spent much time in tracing his own lineage and the origin of his family name.[55]

Horsley was not a religious man. Although he considered himself an agnostic, he spoke on a number of occasions at the "pleasant Sunday afternoon" (PSA) meetings of the Brotherhood Movement of the Free Churches. These meetings, neither political nor sectarian, had become popular with the working classes in the early years of the twentieth century. They encouraged responsible, ethical behavior in a Christian context, and Horsley spoke on a variety of topics ranging from citizenship, charity, morality, self-sacrifice, public affairs, and the status of women, to disease. He spoke on abstract topics or in support of

a particular institution or charity. His talks, as judged by his notes, had an air of spirituality without divinity.[56]

Mechanical activities that could be performed without much thought – on automatic pilot, so to speak – helped him to put aside the cares of the day. He thus was able to relax when using a microtome to prepare tissue sections for microscopy, often humming or whistling tunes from a Gilbert and Sullivan opera or chatting about one thing or another.[41] He remained physically active. He had enjoyed playing tennis as a student and young doctor. As an established London surgeon, he enjoyed bicycling about the city to see his patients, to the startled consternation of some of his neighbors, including Christopher Heath, his senior colleague at University College Hospital, who found such behavior unseemly.

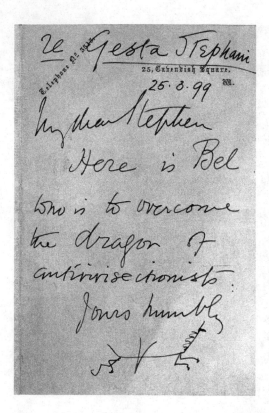

Figure 8.6 Letter from Horsley to Stephen Paget dated 25 March 1899, referring to antivivisection and signed with his special rebus, a prancing horse with a "V" for a saddle. (Image from the Wellcome Collection, London.)

Horsley loved motoring, preferring to drive himself in his forty-five horsepower, four-cylinder Daimler[57] rather than be driven, and this, too, took his mind off his work or his various obligations. He would become quite impatient while being driven slowly and indecisively by a colleague. Driving along country roads, he was able to relax as London receded into the distance. He would sometimes drive sixty miles or more to see a patient at a local hospital and then operate without any sign of fatigue from the journey.[39] Perhaps of necessity, he also became quite a mechanic – if anything went wrong with the car, he would take off his jacket, roll up his shirt sleeves, lift up the bonnet of the car, and set to work to find the problem, usually to the merriment of his children.

Notes

1. Abraham JJ: *Surgeon's Journey*. p. 390. Heinemann: London, 1957.

2. Sharpey Schafer E: The Victor Horsley Memorial Lecture on the relations of surgery and physiology. *Br Med J* 1923; **2**: 739–744.

3. Sherrington CS: Note on experimental degeneration of the pyramidal tract. *Lancet* 1894; **143**: 266.

4. Correspondence. Sherrington CS: Experimental degeneration of the pyramidal tract. *Lancet* 1894; **143**: 439, 571; Sherrington CS, Letter to Horsley dated February 17, 1894. Section E4/19, Horsley Papers, Special Collections, UCL Library Services (London, UK); Horsley V: *Lancet* 1894; **143**: 370–371, 571.

5. Vilensky JA, Stone JL, Gilman S: Feud and fable: The Sherrington-Horsley polemic and the delayed publication. *J Hist Neurosci* 2003; **12**: 368–375.

6. Boyce R: Experimental degeneration of the pyramidal tract. (Letter to the editor.) *Lancet* 1894; **143**: 501.

7. Leyton ASF, Sherrington CS: Observations of the excitable cortex of the chimpanzee, orang-utan and gorilla. *Q J Exp Physiol* 1917; **11**: 135–222. (The co-author of the preliminary accounts of this work was named "Grünbaum," which was Leyton's original surname. He changed it by deed-poll during World War I because of anti-German sentiment.)

8. Fulton JF: Sir Charles Scott Sherrington, O.M. (1857–1952). *J Neurophysiol* 1952; **15**: 167–176.

9. Grünbaum ASF, Sherrington CS: Observations on the physiology of the cerebral cortex of some of the higher apes. *Proc R Soc Lond* 1901; **69**: 206–209.

10. Grünbaum ASF, Sherrington CS: Observations on the physiology of the cerebral cortex of the anthropoid apes. *Proc R Soc Lond* 1903; **72**: 152–155.

11. Lemon RN: An enduring map of the motor cortex. *Exp Physiol* 2008; **93**: 798–802.

12. Bailey P: Historical vignette: Anecdotes from the history of trephining. *Surg Neurol* 1994; **42**: 83–90.

13. Sachs E: Reminiscences of an American student. *Br Med J* 1957; **1**: 916–917.

14. Crile G: *George Crile: An Autobiography*. p. 69. Lippincott: Philadelphia, PA, 1947.

15. Subotsky F: With the benefit of hindsight: Lessons from history. p. 46. In: Subotsky F, Bewley S, Crowe M (eds): *Abuse of· the Doctor-Patient Relationship*. p. 46. Royal College of Psychiatrists: London, 2010.

16. Trotter W: Obituary. Sir Victor Horsley, C.B., F.R.S., M.B., F.R.C.S. Surgical work. *Br Med J* 1916; **2**: 162–163.

17. Paget S: *Sir Victor Horsley: A Study of His Life and Work*. pp. 270–271. Constable: London, 1919.

18. Jones E: Sir Victor Horsley. [Letter to the editor.] *Br Med J* 1957; **1**: 1065.

19. Butterfield IK: Letter 3, p. 20 (undated). In: *The Making of a Neurologist: The letters of Foster Kennedy M.D., F.R.S.Edin. 1884-1952 to his wife*. Stellar Press: Hatfield, Hertfordshire, 1981.

20. Walshe FMR: Personal communication, July 15, 1966.

21. Butterfield IK: Letter 9, p. 25 (undated). In: *The Making of a Neurologist: The letters of Foster Kennedy M.D., F.R.S.Edin. 1884-1952 to his wife*. Stellar Press: Hatfield, Hertfordshire, 1981.

22. Butterfield IK: Letter 10, pp. 26–27 (undated). In: *The Making of a Neurologist: The letters of Foster Kennedy M.D., F.R.S.Edin. 1884-1952 to his wife*. Stellar Press: Hatfield, Hertfordshire, 1981.

23. Butterfield IK: Letter 11, pp. 27–28 (undated). In: *The Making of a Neurologist: The letters of Foster Kennedy M.D., F.R.S.Edin. 1884-1952 to his wife*. Stellar Press: Hatfield, Hertfordshire, 1981.

24. Fulton JF: *Harvey Cushing: A Biography*. pp. 163–168. Thomas: Springfield, IL, 1946.

25. Fulton JF: *Harvey Cushing: A Biography*. p. 236. Thomas: Springfield, IL, 1946.

26. Fulton JF: *Harvey Cushing: A Biography*. p. 257. Thomas: Springfield, IL, 1946.

27. Semon HC, McIntyre TA (eds): *The Autobiography of Sir Felix Semon K.C.V.O., M.D., F.R.C.P.* pp. 320–321. Jarrolds: London, 1926.

28. Semon HC, McIntyre TA (eds): *The Autobiography of Sir Felix Semon K.C.V.O., M.D., F.R.C.P.* pp. 224–225. Jarrolds: London, 1926.

29. Anon: Surgeon's special train. Sir Victor Horsley summoned by wire. *Daily Mail (Lond)* April 20, 1909, p. 3

30. Anon: Medical witnesses' fees. *Daily Mail (Lond)* June 23, 1904, p. 3.

31. Horsley V: Letter to Dr. Bernard Sachs, New York, dated August 29, 1908. (Reproduced typed copy.) In Sachs MK : *A Saga of Forty-Five Flawless Years*. Unpublished material held at the Bernard Becker Medical Library, Washington University School of Medicine, St Louis, Missouri

32. Jones E: *Free Associations: Memories of a Psycho-Analyst*. pp. 87–89. Basic Books: New York, 1959.

33. Sachs E: *Fifty Years of Neurosurgery: A Personal Story*. pp. 39–40. Vantage: New York, 1958.

34. Barnsley RE: Sir Victor Horsley. [Letter to the editor.] *Br Med J* 1957; **1**: 1065.

35. L.G.M.: Lonely "zoo" walrus. *Daily Mail (Lond)* December 1, 1908, p. 5

36. Gotch F, Horsley V: Croonian Lecture: On the mammalian nervous system, its functions, and their localisation determined by an electrical method. *Philos Trans R Soc Lond B* 1891; **182**: 267–526.

37. Anon: Coronation Honours. *Br Med J* 1902; **2**: 75–76.

38. Pollard B: Correspondence. Section E4/16, Horsley Papers, Special Collections, UCL Library Services (London, UK).

39. MacNalty A: Reminiscences of Sir Victor Horsley. *Ann R Coll Surg Engl* 1962; **31**: 120–126.

40. Paget S: *Sir Victor Horsley: A Study of His Life and Work*. p. 129. Constable: London, 1919.

41. MacNalty A: Sir Victor Horsley: his life and work. *Br Med J* 1957; **1**: 910–916.

42. Aminoff MJ: *Brown-Séquard: An Improbable Genius Who Transformed Medicine*. Oxford University Press: New York, 2011.

43. Eadie MJ: *Rigor mortis* and the epileptology of Charles Bland Radcliffe (1822–1889). *J Clin Neurosci* 2007; **14**: 201–207.

44. Gimson BL (ed): Horsley, Oswald and Horsley, Siward Miles. In: *The Bedales School Roll 1952*. p. 137. Bedales Society: Steep, Hampshire, UK, 1952.

45. Gimson BL (ed): Gotch, Oliver Horsley. In: *The Bedales School Roll 1952*. p. 111 Bedales Society: Steep, Hampshire, UK, 1952.

46. Anon: Mother's confession: A pitiful tale. *Daily Mail (Lond)* January 8, 1913, p. 6.

47. Papers relating to Orkney. Section D4, Horsley Papers, Special Collections, UCL Library Services (London, UK).

48. Cairns H: Diary entry, January 13, 1934. Cited by Fraenkel GJ : *Hugh Cairns: First Nuffield Professor of Surgery University of Oxford.* p. 93. Oxford University Press: Oxford, 1991.

49. Horsley V: Trephining in the Neolithic period. *J Anthropolol Inst Gr Br Ire* 1888; **17**: 100–106.

50. Prioreschi P: Possible reasons for Neolithic skull trephining. *Perspect Biol Med* 1991; **34**: 296–303.

51. Horsley V: Galen. *Middlesex Hosp J* 1899; **3**: 37–52.

52. Bond CJ: *Recollections of Student Life and Later Days.* Lewis: London, 1939.

53. Horsley V: Roman defences of south-east Britain. *Not Proc R Inst Gr Br* 1899; **16**: 35–44.

54. Papers relating to archaeology. Section D3, Horsley Papers, Special Collections, UCL Library Services (London, UK).

55. Papers and correspondence relating to genealogy, including documents relating to William Horsley. Section D6, Horsley Papers, Special Collections, UCL Library Services (London, UK).

56. Horsley V: Notes for lectures to the Brotherhood Movement. Section C8, Horsley Papers, Special Collections, UCL Library Services (London, UK).

57. Anon: Orders placed. *Automotor J* 1907; **12**: 413.

The Politics of Protection

Horsley was not one to win friends with an easy smile, gentle asides, and whispered confidences, and he certainly did not always bother with subtleties or even genteel niceties in expressing his views. Some have wondered what drove an outspoken and confrontational man like Horsley into the "muddy pool of politics."[1] He became involved early in a number of social issues in which he had a personal stake, such as opposing the clamor and charges of the antivivisectionists and speaking in support of the temperance movement, as discussed in other chapters. The challenges, verbal sparring, and camaraderie were to his liking and he gained increasing national prominence by his stands. This led him to become more engaged in the cut and thrust of medical and then national politics, enjoying the support of many of his contemporaries in doing so. It was as if he needed something with which to challenge himself, something to fight about. The experience of having to deal with his son's epilepsy and his own failure to cure it by surgery may well have caused Horsley to turn further from clinical work and become even more immersed in social and political activities.[2]

Horsley's aims became increasingly to protect the reputation and livelihood of members of the medical profession from assault by an uninformed or misinformed lay public and, equally, to protect the public from medical negligence, incompetence, and charlatans. This soon extended to protecting the public from blundering or untrained nurses and midwives, and then to measures for providing health insurance for much of the working public. In these various goals, Horsley – gifted and driven – was clearly ahead of his times, but he became isolated by his celebrity status and a belief in his own infallibility, unwilling to listen to the opinions of others and often becoming hostile both to them and their views. Indeed, he became increasingly quarrelsome, and – ignoring the usual constraints that

guide social interactions – did not hesitate to express himself with a brutal honesty that could be corrosive, unsettling, and sometimes humiliating. Although he came to champion many worthwhile causes, his manner of doing so sometimes detracted from his achievements and made him no friends.

The Medical Defence Union

In the summer of 1884, a general practitioner in Chesterfield, England, was accused of raping Eliza Swetmore, the wife of a coal miner, in his surgery. The patient, who was an epileptic, had begun having an epileptic seizure, and the doctor – David Bradley – after holding a bottle of *sal volatile* ("smelling salts") to her nose to revive her, hurried to an adjoining room to get help. He returned to find that she had run to a neighbor's house claiming to have been raped. No-one had heard her call out and there were no obvious signs of a struggle. Nevertheless, at his trial at the Leicester Assizes before Lord Chief Justice Coleridge, the unfortunate Bradley, who could not afford legal representation, was found not guilty of rape but guilty of attempted rape (with which he had not actually been charged) and sentenced to imprisonment for two years, with hard labor. No expert witnesses were called on his behalf.[3]

An outcry by the medical profession followed the conviction, for the evidence seemed not to support the charge and the supposed victim was held to be delusional by virtue of her epilepsy. The medical press and many leading members of the profession campaigned for an enquiry, but the responsible government minister – the home secretary, Sir William Harcourt – refused to intervene. Following a change in government, however, the case finally was reviewed and in July 1885 Bradley was released after having been imprisoned for eight months. Innocence was not proved, but the doubt surrounding the case was felt not to justify further detention.[4]

Bradley's case received a lot of publicity but was not exceptional. As was also true of other doctors in similar circumstances, he faced loss of his reputation and livelihood simply by having been charged, regardless of the final judgment of the court. Doctors who were slandered or libeled generally had to arrange and pay for their own defence to prevent professional ruin. Medical malpractice insurance did not exist. Senior physicians and surgeons often came to the financial aid of colleagues acquitted by the courts, and Bradley received a purse of four hundred guineas by subscription of the medical profession. Sir William Jenner was foremost among the contributors and the lead author of a letter published in the *Lancet* and in the *Medical Press and Circular*, which stated

> We raise our emphatic and indignant protest against the ready credence which the law has given, in his case, to a form of accusation very easy to make, but not always easy to disprove. We do this for our own sakes, because medical men in the daily discharge of their duties, which are often of a delicate character, are exposed, more than other men, to have such charges brought against them. We protest also on public grounds, since it is detrimental to the interests of society that such duties should be rendered more difficult than they naturally are, and because it is even more deplorable that the innocent should suffer than that the guilty should escape. We are fully aware that the tardy and inadequate measure of justice which has at length been dealt out to Dr. Bradley can in no way atone for the cruel wrong which has been done to him, and we are sensible that no action on our part can make amends to him for the suffering and loss he has had to bear.[5]

The sorry plight of David Bradley and others similarly affected brought home the need to protect the good name and livelihood of doctors charged with an offence of which they might well be innocent. The Medical Act of 1858 had defined the profession by setting the educational standards required of anyone practicing medicine in the United Kingdom and established the General Council of Medical Education and Registration (the "General Medical Council") to oversee such standards and maintain a medical register of qualified practitioners for the protection of the public.

Nevertheless, unqualified practitioners continued to flourish and dissatisfied patients increasingly brought frivolous or malicious lawsuits against their doctors, underscoring the need for some mutual defensive strategy to protect doctors in such circumstances. The existing professional associations offered no help in this regard.

Robert Lawson Tait, an innovative surgeon and gynecologist and one of the earliest to use modern aseptic operative techniques, led the profession in calling for the establishment of an organization to provide legal assistance to doctors.[6] In 1885, the Medical Defence Union was founded to promote and support the character and interests of its members, and to advise and defend them in cases involving professional matters. Charles F. Rideal, a writer and lecturer on the works of Charles Dickens, was instrumental in establishing it and served as the founding secretary of an organization that became the first of its kind in the world.[7] An annual subscription of ten shillings covered advice and legal fees, but not the costs or damages awarded to plaintiffs.

The new organization had a mixed reception. Although some four hundred doctors joined within the first four months, others hesitated, concerned that its objectives were not solely to provide legal protection but also to prosecute unauthorized practitioners at an uncertain cost. Moreover, financial irregularities almost bankrupted the organization shortly after its inception. It was restructured: doctors replaced the original signatories for the company, and officers were elected.[8] The articulate and energetic Lawson Tait became the first president early in 1887, and the membership and funds of the organization then began to grow. During 1892, however, it faced several new crises. First, a number of the members resigned to form a new mutual organization, the London and Counties Medical Protection Society, following dissatisfaction with changes to its constitution. Then its president himself became the defendant in a lawsuit for libel (Denholm v. Tait).

In brief, a Dr. Denholm referred a patient with fibroids to specialists, who treated her unsuccessfully by electrolysis, then an accepted approach. Tait was eventually consulted, recommended surgery, and removed a massive tumor. The patient died within forty-eight hours, supposedly from hemorrhage that Tait, in a letter to her husband, ascribed to sloughing from the electrical treatment: "Had she never been submitted to that treatment the case would have been a straightforward one, and her recovery almost certain."[9] Denholm took this letter as a reflection on his management and started legal proceedings against Tait, whom the Medical Defence Union defended. A postmortem examination, in Tait's absence, showed death to have resulted not from hemorrhage but from peritonitis. The autopsy, however, was performed by gaslight and in the coffin; a collection of blood in the broad ligament was overlooked; and the evidence of peritonitis was slight,[9] so that the findings, in reality, were inconclusive. It was generally agreed, moreover, that Tait was entitled to report truthfully to the patient's husband the facts of the case and causes of failure as he saw them, and that such a letter was a privileged communication. At trial the involved parties eventually agreed to withdraw the case and any related accusations[9,10] and Tait accepted this settlement without his costs being covered. This left the organization in debt, for Tait was reluctant to cover the expense himself, although he had originally agreed to do so. An acrimonious dispute followed – some maintained that Tait's costs should not be paid, others that Denholm's also should be covered, and yet others that the organization should not have taken sides. Indeed, one outcome of the sorry affair was that the society resolved not to support or defend in the future a case in which both parties were doctors. Another was that early in 1893, Tait resigned the presidency.

Horsley, who had been elected a member of the governing council in 1892, was now elected president, and he held office from 1893 until 1897, when he was elected to the General Medical Council as a representative of the profession. It was a difficult time, with a competing organization and transfer of the main office from the provincial city of Birmingham to the capital, London.

Another legal intervention, the Bloxham case, brought its own problems in 1894. A certain Dr. Collie sought to restrain Dr. Bloxham from practicing within three miles of his own practice, based on an agreement signed by Bloxham when he became Collie's assistant. Collie wanted also to recover a penalty plus damages from Bloxham for breaking their agreement. Bloxham, in turn, sought damages from Collie for breach of a verbal agreement in which he would have become Collie's partner and received one quarter of the net profits of the practice. In a settlement agreed by the court, all accusations of professional misconduct were withdrawn, Bloxham agreed not to practice within three miles of Collie's residence for ten years, Collie's other claims were abandoned, and no costs were levied on either side.[11]

Both Bloxham and Collie were members of the Medical Defence Union. Although Bloxham was denied the union's assistance because his case was deemed a business dispute, Collie – a vice president of the organization – received its help for his defence "as a distinctly exceptional case."[12] Bloxham then sued to prevent the organization's involvement, claiming that this was beyond the normal scope of its activities. The governing council eventually agreed not to use its funds in the litigation between Bloxham and Collie, but critics were greatly angered by its attempted involvement in the case and called for a special general meeting, which was held on May 8, 1894, chaired by Horsley. It was stormy. Horsley announced, but Bloxham denied, that both Collie and the union had offered arbitration to Bloxham. It was questioned why the organization had got involved at all since it had been agreed just a year earlier that it should not take sides in cases between doctors. Horsley allowed a free-ranging discussion, agreed that the articles of association required review and possible revision, and announced that the governing council would set up a special committee to examine the issues.[13,14] Bloxham subsequently brought suit against Horsley for slander and also against the union, but both cases were dismissed.[12]

Horsley and the other officials were able to retain or regain the confidence of the membership despite the notoriety and concerns brought out by the Bloxham litigation. In fact, under Horsley's leadership the membership increased by almost twenty percent, and the principle of mutual legal defence was safely established. The organization was not an insurance company, however, and the benefits of membership consisted of discretionary medical indemnity, subject to the memorandum and articles of association.

Doctors in other countries were also grappling with their vulnerability to legal threats, and the financial and professional consequences of litigation, and they took note of the mutual organization of the Medical Defence Union. In the United States, for example, various legislative remedies were proposed[15,16] but were not well received,[17] and the concept of mutual defence thus gained ground. In 1887, a report in the *Boston Medical and Surgical Journal* (later the *New England Journal of Medicine*) urged physicians to combine to protect themselves,[18] and by the early years of the twentieth century several local medical societies and professional organizations were sponsoring legal defence organizations and medical malpractice insurance.[19] Private malpractice insurance did not take hold in America until well after the turn of the century.[17] Back in Britain, attempts by the two medical defence organizations to combine foundered on several issues, including the choice of name for an amalgamated organization.[20]

By 1903 the membership of the Medical Defence Union had reached six thousand, some nine hundred doctors having joined in the previous year. When the British Medical Association then proposed – not for the first time – to develop its own medical defence department and thereby absorb the existing defence societies, Horsley – now one of the association's leaders – supported the plan enthusiastically. The existing societies, however, chose to remain separate'[21,22] in part because those of their subscribers not belonging to the association would be compelled to join it – at an added expense – to retain their protection.[23] Thus the move foundered.

During Horsley's presidency, the union prosecuted a number of persons who had engaged in the practice of medicine or used the title of "physician" or "M.D." despite lacking the necessary qualifications. The results were often baffling, frustrating, or otherwise unsatisfactory. For example, an unqualified person named Matthews was regarded as a medical practitioner by the local citizens of Norwich. As Horsley described it, the issue was taken to a "bench of magistrates who determined in their wisdom that it was exceedingly wrong of Mr. Matthews to 'inadvertently' . . . use the word 'surgeon' in one of his advertisements, but he was perfectly entitled to use the word 'doctor.'"[24] In fact, provided there is no intent to deceive, the use of the title of "doctor" – as opposed to "doctor of medicine" – is permissible, for there are doctorates in disciplines other than medicine. In any event, it was soon realized that actions against unqualified medical practitioners were difficult and often unsuccessful, and

their prosecution was therefore left to the General Medical Council, which had greater resources at its disposal.

Horsley left the Medical Defence Union in much better shape than when he had assumed office. He had helped it through painful times. It has thrived since then, as has its offshoot, the Medical Protection Society. Both exist today but the scope of their activities has changed to meet new challenges. In looking back in 1898 to his service with it, Horsley confessed that he had particularly enjoyed and benefited from his time on its governing council. He had "learnt from them what politics might be; he learnt from them what the business of medical politics should be, and he also learnt what was going on in the General Medical Council."[24]

The General Medical Council

The original purpose of the General Medical Council was to help the public in distinguishing between qualified and unqualified practitioners, a distinction that previously had been difficult given the more than twenty different standards used to certify medical competence. It was not intended to promote the welfare of the medical profession or even to crack down on "quackery." The council developed recommendations on minimum requirements for general and professional education and examinations, and compiled and published annually a *Medical Register* of those who were qualified to practice because they met these requirements. It also had a disciplinary function, being required to erase from the register the name of any practitioner convicted of a criminal offence or otherwise "judged after due inquiry to have been guilty of infamous conduct in any professional respect."

Unfortunately, the Medical Act of 1858 had resulted in the related law being somewhat murky and allowed registration based on a single qualification in medicine *or* surgery.[25] A second Medical Act, passed in 1886, tightened up various procedures and established, among other things, that applicants for registration needed to have passed qualifying examinations in each of medicine, surgery, *and* midwifery – a simple certificate of attendance at a course of lectures in, for example, surgery was no longer sufficient for a would-be physician.[26] It also introduced direct representation of the profession, authorizing the election of five medical practitioners to the council by the postal votes of the whole profession.

The Medical Acts did not stop the public from seeking aid from unqualified practitioners if they wished, and unqualified practitioners remained free to work and to profit thereby as long as they did not claim to be practicing medicine. The Acts did, however, restrict them from using a title, such as "physician," that implied qualification.[27] Unfortunately, lawsuits frequently ended in seemingly nonsensical quibbling, verbal gymnastics, or misunderstandings. As recorded by Horsley:

> In the proceedings of the Appeal Court ... one judge was under the impression that the College of Physicians was a body which granted university degrees! and the other judge not only said that a physician was a person who practised surgery (!), but also that though a modern (that is, 1886) L.S.A. [Licentiate of the Society of Apothecaries[28]] could not call himself "a surgeon," he *could* call himself "a surgeon specially licensed to practise surgery," and said further "surgeon may be a general word and physician may be a specific word."[29]

The situation was even more complicated because qualifications were sometimes used in a manner that suggested an attempt to mislead, and the courts were not consistent in how they viewed such cases. Thus, the use of such postnominals as "M.D., U.S.A." could have suggested deceptively that the holder was qualified to practice in Britain, but the magistrate dealing with one such case in 1896 accepted that the addition of "U.S.A." implied that the holder knew he was not, and therefore there was no false pretense within the meaning of the Act. By contrast, similar cases had led to convictions.[25]

Encouraged by Horsley, from the late 1890s the General Medical Council began to take on an increasing number of cases involving misrepresentation. Its composition was changing, as were its priorities. Each of the universities and professional organizations conferring medical degrees or diplomas in the United Kingdom was allowed to appoint one member. Five additional members were appointed directly by the government, and another five were elected by the registered practitioners, thereby ensuring that the profession had a voice in the council's affairs. The total number of members was thirty-four in 1906.[27]

Victor Horsley was elected to it in October 1897 as a direct representative of the profession for England and Wales, gaining six thousand nine hundred and forty-six votes, a majority of more than eight hundred votes over his nearest rival, the physician Sir Walter Foster.[30] His supporters hoped he would advocate fearlessly for a less apathetic policy and a less autocratic governance. They were not to be disappointed. In part at Horsley's urging, the council became increasingly active in safeguarding the interests of doctors and cracking down on those perceived to be "quacks." Horsley was re-elected in 1902 for a second term but stood down in 1907, feeling that he had achieved his aims.

In addressing a dinner meeting at the Café Royal in London on October 28, 1898, soon after starting on the council, Horsley discussed some of the anomalies and problems that he had encountered. He had always assumed that those entered on the *Medical Register* were entitled to certain privileges not enjoyed by others, namely, the title of doctor or surgeon and the sole right to practice medicine. (The ambiguity regarding the prefix of "doctor," mentioned earlier, seemed to have escaped him.) He found it curious that not all the members of the council felt the same way and was dismayed by the council's reluctance to challenge in court those unqualified to practice medicine. He was also disturbed that the courts responded in an apparently arbitrary and inconsistent manner to such challenges. As he pointed out, one magistrate might interpret the law to mean one thing, whereas a second might conclude the exact opposite on precisely the same point. Comparing his experience with that gained through the Medical Defence Union, Horsley noted that the "General Medical Council had only quite lately seen that it owed a duty to the profession. It had been taking the money of the profession for years and years, but ... refused to recognise that it owed any duties towards that profession. On the contrary, it was always very ready to receive complaints against members of the medical profession for the enforcement of discipline in the profession itself, but it would not touch the question of protecting the profession."[24]

He had other concerns. For example, in 1896 he had referred to the dangerously arbitrary powers possessed by the council's president, who could impede the business of the council, especially in its prosecution of certain offenders against the Medical Act.[31] The penal procedures were subsequently revised to transfer power from the president to a committee, but the president – Horsley alleged – could still impede the committee's meetings.[32] On being told that the president was ill, he retorted unsympathetically that it may "be necessary for the President to resign an office the duties of which he could not fulfil."[33] The president died barely a week later.

Horsley went on to complain that the new president had made it difficult for him to gain access to the council's documents,[34] perhaps in part because these were so few. In late December 1898, in a published address, he protested that, apart from the little that appeared in the medical journals, no record was kept of what was said in council, not even a shorthand note of public or private meetings. He also objected to the secrecy surrounding the council's activities, which were funded by public money.[35] More constructively, he urged the development of a "one-portal" system for entry to the *Medical Register* and thus to the medical profession in place of the existing system, with its different standards for qualification by different bodies (that is, the universities, professional colleges, and Society of Apothecaries).

His comments and criticisms of the council were thoughtful in substance but lacked much in style. In 1896, the *Lancet* published a letter from him, with an editorial footnote: "We have thought it best to omit from Mr. Horsley's letter a paragraph contained in the manuscript which referred to the President of the General Medical Council in an unnecessarily personal manner."[36]

He quarreled with Brudenell Carter, an ophthalmological surgeon at Horsley's hospital in Queen Square, who was also on the council. Horsley noted that:

> "Mr Carter . . . is not elected by medical men at all as their representative on the General Medical Council but by a few druggists and other persons who style themselves the master and wardens of the Society of Apothecaries and who know no more about medicine than about bootmaking. . . . he does not really represent a licensing body at all but that he represents a handful of tradesmen who, though not having any medical education, notoriously prescribe over the counter in the druggist's shop of the ground floor of the Apothecaries' Hall."[37]

And a few weeks later,

> "In the case of Mr Brudenell Carter who represents the Apothecaries' Society we have the unedifying spectacle of a seat on the General Medical Council being occupied by a man who is sent there by a handful of city grocers who have not a particle of medical education."[38]

Such offensive comments by Horsley against Carter were not new. They did lead eventually to an apology, rather grudging, when finally he was called to task on it.[37] His barbed comments illustrate a perfectly valid point, however, namely that the various corporations (that is, the colleges, universities, and Society of Apothecaries) that appointed a representative to the council did so by vote of the members of their own governing councils rather than their entire membership. In consequence, their nominee "represents only the little coterie who elected him" and this, Horsley contended, led to the "utmost indifference on the part of the so-called representatives of the corporations to the interests of those whom they nominally represent."[38]

Horsley's sharp tongue and injudicious manner are also well illustrated by his interactions with Edwin Alabone, who had studied at Guy's Hospital, became a member of the Royal College of Surgeons (MRCS) in 1870, and was placed on the *Medical Register* by the General Medical Council. Alabone subsequently authored a book, *The Cure of Consumption*,[39] in which he referred to a secret remedy, thereby bringing on himself the ire of the surgeons, especially when it also transpired that he was the subject of a laudatory article in a weekly periodical and that advertisements for his treatment had appeared in various magazines.[40] He was expelled from the college for advertising and his name therefore had to be erased from the register as having no accepted qualifications, but not for any other reason. He nevertheless continued in his flourishing practice, treating tuberculous and other patients by inhalation of a tincture of lachnanthes – a plant native to parts of North America – until the law caught up with him. In 1900, he was prosecuted by the General Medical Council for pretending to be a medical practitioner and using various postnominals to support this pretense. In actual fact, the postnominals were "M.D. Phil.," which indeed he had earned in Philadelphia, and "ex-MRCS," which was correct. The magistrate therefore found in favor of Alabone and dismissed the charges against him, not realizing that the American institutions from which Alabone had obtained a qualification were bogus.[40,41]

There followed a flurry of letters in the medical journals. Horsley criticized the incompetence of the council's attorneys and claimed that Alabone had been struck off the register for "infamous conduct."[42] Alabone's attorneys then rightly pointed out that there had been no implication of infamous conduct in his erasure from the register,[43] to which Horsley responded that an offence against professional ethics leading to expulsion from a college was tantamount to infamous conduct, a point that the editorial staff of the *Lancet* found misleading.[44] Alabone and his supporters were outraged and wrote to Horsley,[45] who now kept uncharacteristically silent. Alabone accordingly published a book, twenty-nine pages long, *Infamous Conduct: Edwin W. Alabone versus Victor Horsley*, in which he took Horsley to task for failing to either withdraw or explain himself.[46] It was a bad time for Horsley – he had been publicly corrected by the editorial staff of the *Lancet*, had questioned unwisely the competence of both the council's legal advisers and the magistrate, and had misstated facts in a seemingly malicious manner concerning a colleague.

Horsley's time on the General Medical Council was stormy but he helped to bring about much needed reforms by publishing a series of reports to the registered practitioners of England and Wales in which he showed the need for change. He was by turn appealing, outrageous, reasoning, and insulting in making points to win his arguments for, as he judged it, the benefit of the profession and public. Nevertheless, his pleas to make the council more representative of its constituents fell on deaf ears. Nudged by Horsley, however, the council's focus changed, and – in addition to its educational mission – it moved more actively to limit the practice of medicine by unqualified persons and to prevent the use of advertising or canvassing by medical practitioners to procure patients. Horsley himself chaired a committee to focus on the very real problem of fraudulent personation of dead or distant practitioners by the unqualified, and recommended specific measures to prevent this, including the use of handwriting to identify applicants for registration.[47,48] The procedures and practices of the council in reaching its various

objectives also became less forbidding and more transparent, in no small measure due to Horsley's influence.

Since Horsley's time, the composition and governance of the council has changed. Its role has expanded, but it continues to set professional, educational, and ethical standards for doctors in Britain; oversees the undergraduate and postgraduate training of doctors; provides guidance on best medical practice and related learning materials; maintains the *Medical Register*; and helps to protect patients and promote public confidence in the medical profession.

Midwives and Nurses

The Registration of Midwives

One of Horsley's campaigns was concerned with the regulation of midwives, many of whom had no training whatsoever. Their ignorance and incompetence sometimes led to unnecessary suffering, the spread of infection, or death in childbirth. Some of them worked even when intoxicated with alcohol or drugs, or took it upon themselves to perform operations or prescribe medication despite a lack of experience or qualifications. The fact that they could charge for their misguided management added insult to injury. Horsley had corresponded on the topic in the medical journals for several years, going back to 1895 (see Appendix 3) and continuing thereafter as drafts of a proposed parliamentary bill were discussed, aiming to protect the health and safety of the public, the professional standing of midwives, and the privileges of the medical profession.

The Midwives Act was passed in 1902 and came into force in 1903, establishing a Central Midwives Board to oversee the training and examination of midwives. A *Midwives Roll* was set up to list those claiming to be midwives, initially regardless of whether they had undergone any special training. After a transitional grace period, unlisted persons were not permitted to call themselves or function as midwives or to charge for their services without completing specific training that qualified them to be listed on the roll. Supervisory bodies were established to investigate cases of malpractice or professional misconduct.

The General Medical Council took no part in the formation and administration of the new board, its duty being restricted to advising on the rules framed by the board before the government approved them.[49] Horsley, with his understanding of the working of the Medical Acts and his familiarity with proposals for reform in medical legislation, was an influential member of the Midwives' Committee of the council. As always, one of his particular concerns was to ensure that trainees in midwifery received adequate instruction so that they could provide competent care.[50] At the same time, he emphasized the need to define their responsibilities so that they did not subsume those of doctors but limited their activities to the conduct of normal labor.[51,52] Some of his colleagues on the General Medical Council failed to appreciate the importance of this last point until Horsley exercised his formidable powers of persuasion.[53]

The Central Midwives Board continued for some years but was replaced in 1983 by a separate council for nurses, midwives, and health visitors, and then – twenty years later – by a Nursing and Midwifery Council that has similar functions to those of the General Medical Council.

The Registration of Nurses

The nurses lagged behind the midwives. The British Medical Association had expressed its belief in 1895 that parliament should act to provide for the registration of nurses. In the following year, its representatives met with those of the nursing profession for further discussion, but there was little progress.[54] In 1905, a select committee of the House of Commons recommended that a register of nurses be maintained by a central body appointed by the state, and the title of "Registered Nurse" restricted to those on the list. Horsley appeared before the committee on May 18, 1905, arguing that state registration would indeed be valuable: "If an individual has gone through a long course of professional training to acquire expert knowledge, that individual is justified in requiring from the State the registration of the fact, and unless the individual misbehaves in any way, that registration remains good."[55] Others disagreed, and bills for the registration of nurses were put forward annually from 1903 until the outbreak of World War I, without gathering general support.

In May 1909, Horsley represented the British Medical Association in a delegation to Mr. Asquith, the prime minister, in support of the state registration of nurses.[56] He attempted to convince the premier that the views he expressed were those of the profession as a whole, but the canny Asquith pointed to a number of persons who had voiced objections.[57] In 1914, when another parliamentary bill was being considered, Horsley published a long letter in the *British Medical Journal* about the state registration of nurses, criticizing the influential Lord Knutsford (chairman of the London Hospital House Committee), for quoting the contrary opinions of private individuals on a circular containing several incorrect assertions.[58] Knutsford, who opposed the bill, had written to matrons and nursing superintendents, asking those against the bill to sign a letter to that effect rather than requesting signatures both for and against the measure; he had then circulated misleading information about the composition of the proposed nursing council.[59] Horsley cited in his letter the support of the British Medical Association and its various committees and representative meetings, as well as that of the nurses' associations in England, Scotland, and Ireland, all of which endorsed the bill before parliament. His comments in 1914 were the same as he had addressed to Mr. Asquith five years earlier. Horsley subsequently pointed out that he had visited several of the matrons (including the matron of his own hospital) who allegedly supported Knutsford but whom he knew to be in favor of registration, finding that their letters of support were ten years old – "people did not go on living without learning."[60]

Following the outbreak of war in 1914, many untrained women volunteered to serve as nurses. Earlier proposals to form a reserve of military nurses had met with opposition on many fronts, including from Knutsford, who felt that nurses could always be found to serve with the military if needed, but to allow them to volunteer for a military reserve might pose problems for civilian hospitals in wartime. The lack of organization of the various authorities responsible for training nurses and of the nurses themselves now dismayed Arthur Stanley, a member of parliament who chaired the Joint War Committee of the British Red Cross Society and the Order of St. John of Jerusalem in England. In late 1915, he proposed the creation of a College of Nursing, and with the support of Sarah Swift, matron-in-chief of the British Red Cross, the new body finally came into existence on March 27, 1916, initially as a limited-liability company known as the College of Nursing Ltd., with just thirty-four members. Its aims were to improve the training of nurses through a uniform curriculum at approved nursing schools, to maintain a register of trained nurses, and generally to advance nursing as a profession.

Horsley was appalled, disappointed because of the private nature of what he regarded as a sham institution rather than a truly educational body, fearful that the drive for a state-regulated system would falter, angry that a private entity had hijacked the concept for profit. He wrote anxiously to his friend Alfred Cox, then medical secretary of the British Medical Association, impatient at being unable to help while serving "on a burning mud flat in the midst of cholera, dysentery, diarrhea, etc." with the military forces overseas.[61] He did not live to see the new organization flourish. It was to become the Royal College of Nursing in 1939, and now has almost a half-million members.

The registration of nurses – and the educational and other requirements for registration – were taken over by the General Nursing Council for England and Wales when established by parliament in 1919, and are now the responsibility of the Nursing and Midwifery Council that was established in 2002.

The Coroner and The Doctors

Coroners are responsible for establishing and certifying the cause of death when this has occurred in unexpected or suspicious circumstances or for unclear reasons. In the late nineteenth century, coroners in England and Wales were appointed by the local authorities but were themselves directly accountable to the lord chancellor for their activities, and their conduct was codified by law. The effectiveness of the system depended on the abilities of those working within it.

In 1902, the London County Council appointed a lawyer, Mr. John Troutbeck, coroner to the southwest district of London. It also recommended that the coroner should be notified of every death occurring after a surgical intervention so that a preliminary inquiry and, if necessary, an inquest could be held, and further required that postmortem examinations be performed by a skilled pathologist unless the involved doctor was competent to do so.[62] For unclear reasons, Troutbeck did not bother with the evidence of doctors present at the time of death or with prior knowledge of individual cases, and he selected a Dr. Ludwig Freyberger, a self-declared expert with no special qualifications, to perform all his autopsies. The local doctors soon complained about loss of the income previously derived from performing autopsies or attending inquests. A deputation representing the medical profession complained to the lord chancellor in May 1903, among them Horsley on behalf of the British Medical Association. When Troutbeck rebutted their claims, Horsley listed a series of inquests in which incorrect verdicts were recorded because Troutbeck withheld the evidence of doctors involved in the cases.[63,64] As an example, Horsley cited the case of a child with measles, who was seen by a doctor just after death. Troutbeck did not call the doctor to testify, and some days later, after the rash had disappeared, an autopsy was performed by Dr. Freyberger, who had no prior knowledge of the case. Blood poisoning was given as the cause of death and, as this was the only evidence taken by the coroner, an erroneous verdict was returned by the misdirected jury.[63,64]

The lord chancellor simply sent Troutbeck's response to these complaints on to the British Medical Association without comment or further reply until, after waiting for many months, the association appealed to Arthur Balfour, the premier. Balfour felt unable to intercede, leading Horsley to publish the exchange of letters.[65] Within a few days, the lord chancellor's office found the time to respond: while dismayed by the coroner's practice, his lordship did not feel that it justified Troutbeck's removal from office and had no other recourse.[66]

In June 1908, the situation deteriorated. Despite the advice of the Coroners' Society that an inquest was unnecessary in circumstances in which surgery may simply have hastened death, Troutbeck held an inquest into the death of Gertrude Muirhead, a music teacher. She had died shortly after Horsley had removed a brain tumor that had threatened her with total blindness, severe headaches, and an inevitable death within the next few months. Horsley was called as a witness and declared that he could not see the need for the inquest. Troutbeck explained that death hastened by an operation could not possibly be considered natural and accordingly justified the inquest, generating an angry retort from Horsley. In any event, the jury returned a verdict of "accidental death" at the coroner's direction, satisfied that the operation was reasonable and proper care had been taken.[67,68] Horsley, still angry, wrote to *The Times*, declaring that the cause of death (heart failure) was never in doubt and that Troutbeck's claim regarding coroners' jurisdiction in general "would put an end to the practice of medicine as well as surgery, besides involving ratepayers in an enormous cost in coroners' fees," because the giving of medications or any surgical intervention was always an "unnatural event."[63] Further, as neither the coroner nor the jury possessed medical expertise, "this new claim by Mr. Troutbeck of judicial omniscience must appear to every reasonable man to be preposterous."[63]

A lively correspondence followed in the broadsheet. Some considered Troutbeck's actions were personally motivated because of Horsley's earlier complaints against him.[69] Others wrote of the background of the case and of Troutbeck's seeming incompetence.[70,71] Troutbeck himself complained that Horsley had misled the public, missed a second brain tumor, and misquoted him, and went on to imply that Horsley had operated unnecessarily.[72] Horsley came back, tartly observing that the second "tumor" was actually a "false capsule" that he had deliberately left behind because removing it was too risky and that if a second tumor had actually been left behind, Troutbeck's direction to the jury made no sense. Further, he resented Troutbeck's unwarranted assertion as to his clinical judgment,[73] for the patient had been fully informed and consented voluntarily to the surgery.[70] The editor of *The Times* now concluded that Troutbeck's behavior was ill-advised and intolerable, and that it was "high time for the Lord Chancellor to intervene,"[74] a position that the president of the British Medical Association (representing some twenty thousand doctors) endorsed with alacrity,[75] for a principle was involved that related to the entire profession, not just to Horsley.[76]

What had begun as a dispute regarding professional income related to working with the coronial system had evolved into a broader dispute regarding the accountability and independence of doctors. The dispute seemed to settle down but similar issues came up again over the next few years, not directly involving Horsley. New acts were introduced to parliament, but only in 1926 was the law finally revised such that it required a coroner in England and Wales to be a qualified lawyer or medical practitioner, with a minimum of five years' working experience; recognized as an expert a legally qualified medical practitioner; and permitted coroners to request an autopsy without necessarily having to proceed to an inquest (that is, a fact-finding inquiry), depending on the circumstances. It also contained various advisory rules. The functions and duties of coroners have been affected by subsequent acts of parliament, but these do not need to be discussed here.

Horsley's challenge to the system may have been ill advised, but he played an important even if incidental part in redefining the coroners' role and scope of activities. The famous inquest that so offended him made doctors more accountable to the public and raised important issues such as that of informed consent.[62] It also underlined the independence of the coronial system, where the aim is not to apportion blame or determine criminality but simply to determine how and when death occurred. In Britain and many other countries, death that occurs during, immediately after, or as a consequence of an operation must indeed be reported to the coroner, as must death related to a medical or nursing procedure, regardless of whether the procedure was justified or properly performed.

Notes

1. Osler W: Obituary of Sir Victor Horsley, C.B., F.R.S., M.B., F.R.C.S. Personal appreciation. *Br Med J* 1916; **2**: 165.

2. Robinson P [Victor Horsley's daughter]: Letter to Sir Geoffrey Jefferson dated August 9, 1957. Archives, John Rylands Library (University of Manchester). Sir Geoffrey Jefferson Papers. JEF/1/2/4/2/2/18. Available at: http://archiveshub.ac.uk/data/gb133-jef.xml [last accessed June 22, 2021].

3. Anon: A miscarriage of justice. *Med Press Circ* 1885; **90**: 13–14.

4. Anon: Medical notes in parliament. The case of Dr. David Bradley. *Lancet* 1885; **126**: 136 and 185.

5. Anon: The case of Dr. Bradley: Presentation by the medical profession. *Lancet* 1885; **126**: 1162; The case of Dr. Bradley: Dinner and presentation at Sheffield. *Med Press Circ* 1885; **91**: 580–581.

6. Anon: Proposed Medical Defence Union. *Br Med J* 1886; **1**: 943–944.

7. Rideal CF: The Medical Defence Union. [Letter to the editor.] *Br Med J* 1885; **2**: 936; *Lancet* 1885; **126**: 924.

8. Anon: The Medical Defence Union. *Br Med J* 1887; **2**: 1227.

9. Anon: Medico-legal and medico-ethical. Denholm v. Tait. *Br Med J* 1892; **1**: 739.

10. Anon: Denholm v. Tait. *Lancet* 1892; **139**: 761–762.

11. Hempson, Elgar: Collie v. Bloxham: Bloxham v. Collie. [Letter to the editor.] *Lancet* 1894; **143**: 1591.

12. Forbes R: *Sixty Years of Medical Defence.* pp. 15–30. Medical Defence Union: London, 1948.

13. Anon: Medical Defence Union. *Br Med J* 1894; **2**: 780–781.

14. Anon: Medical Defence Union. *Med Press Circ* 1894; **108**: 529.

15. Sanger EF: Report on malpractice. *Boston Med Surg J* 1879; **100**: 41–50.

16. Powel AM: Surgical malpractice. *St Louis Med Surg J* 1882; **42**: 231–236.

17. De Ville KA: *Medical Malpractice in Nineteenth-Century America.* pp. 204–206. New York University Press: New York, 1990.

18. Anon: Stogdale vs. Baker. *Boston Med Surg J* 1887; **117**: 610–611.

19. Anon: Organized medical defense. *JAMA* 1902; **38**: 37 and 43.

20. Horsley V: The Medical Defence Union, Limited, and the London and Counties Medical Protection Society, Limited. [Letter to the editor.] *Lancet* 1896; **147**: 735.

21. Anon: British Medical Association and medical defence. *Lancet* 1904; **163**: 1452–1454.

22. Anon: Medical defence. *Lancet* 1904; **163**: 1439–1440.

23. Anon: Notes and news. *W Lond Med J* 1904; **9**: 155–156.

24. Anon: Mr. Victor Horsley and medical reform. "Medical politics." *Br Med J* 1898; **2**: 1437–1439.

25. Anon: Reform of the Medical Act, 1858. *Br Med J* 1896; **1**: 1401–1403.

26. Finch E: The centenary of the General Council of Medical Education and Registration of the United Kingdom (The General Medical Council) 1858–1958 in relation to medical education. *Ann R Coll Surg Engl* 1958; **23**: 321–331.

27. MacAlister D: Introductory address on the General Medical Council: Its powers and its work. *Br Med J* 1906; **2**: 817–823.

28. The Worshipful Society of Apothecaries, founded by Royal Charter in 1617, served from 1815 as an examining authority for the medical profession, licensing and regulating medical practitioners in England and Wales until the end of the twentieth century. Its licentiates initially used the postnominal LSA but, later, LMSSA was used to reflect qualification in both medicine and surgery. Among the society's licentiates were John Keats, the poet; Elizabeth Garrett Anderson, the first women in Britain to gain a medical qualification; and Sir Ronald Ross, the first British Nobel laureate.

29. Horsley V: The General Medical Council and the Hunter case. [Letter to the editor.] *Br Med J* 1899; **1**: 374–375.

30. Anon: The election of a direct representative on the General Medical Council. *Lancet* 1897; **150**: 1072.

31. Horsley V: On certain undesirable powers possessed by the president of the General Medical Council. *Br Med J* 1896; **2**: 499–502, 699.

32. Anon: The penal powers of the General Medical Council: A report to the registered practitioners of England and Wales. *Lancet* 1898; **151**: 253–254.

33. Horsley V: The duties of the president of the General Medical Council. [Letter to the editor.] *Lancet* 1898; **151**: 676.

34. Horsley V: The General Medical Council: Inspection of documents. [Letter to the editor.] *Br Med J* 1899; **1**: 52–53.

35. Horsley V: The Manchester Medico-Ethical Association. Address by Mr. Victor Horsley on the procedure of the General Medical Council and the reform of the Medical Acts. *Br Med J* 1898; **2**: 1883–1887; Horsley V: Abstract of an address on the work of the General Medical Council. *Lancet* 1898; **152**: 1692–1695.

36. Horsley V: The General Medical Council: critics and candidates. [Letter to the editor.] *Lancet* 1896; **148**: 907–908.

37. Carter B, Horsley V: The Society of Apothecaries of London. Statement by Mr. Brudenell Carter – reply by Mr. Horsley. *Lancet* 1899; **154**: 1560–1562.

38. Horsley V: The direct representatives' meeting at Newcastle. Mr. Victor Horsley's address. *Br Med J* 1899; **2**: 1501–1504; *Lancet* 1899; **154**: 1474–1477.

39. Alabone EW: *The Cure of Consumption, Asthma, Bronchitis, and Other Diseases of the Chest; With Chapters on Laryngitis, Tabes Mesenterica, Post-Nasal Catarrh, and Hay Fever. Illustrated by Numerous*

Cases Pronounced Incurable by the Most Eminent Physicians. 37th edition. Kemp: London, 1903.

40. Vaile M, Gilbert S: The curious case of Dr Alabone – heterodoxy in 19th century medicine. *J R Soc Med* 2005; **98**: 281–286.

41. Anon: The General Medical Council v. Alabone. *Lancet* 1900; **155**: 715.

42. Horsley V: Conference on medical organisation at Manchester. The Medical Acts. *Lancet* 1900; **155**: 1302–1303.

43. Cheverton BA: Mr. Victor Horsley and the Medical Acts. [Letter to the editor.] *Lancet* 1900; **155**: 1533.

44. Horsley V and the Editors of the *Lancet*: Mr. Victor Horsley and the Medical Acts. [Letter to the editor.] *Lancet* 1900; **155**: 1605.

45. Alabone EW: Letter to Victor Horsley dated March 10, 1901. Section E4/1, Horsley Papers, Special Collections, UCL Library Services (London, UK).

46. Alabone EW: *Infamous Conduct: Edwin W. Alabone versus Victor Horsley*. Powage Press: Aspley Guise, Beds., UK, 1901.

47. Anon: The General Council of Medical Education and Registration. *Lancet* 1900; **155**: 1555–1562.

48. Anon: The General Council of Medical Education and Registration. Report of proceedings. The prevention of personation. *Br Med J* 1902; **1**: 1416–1417.

49. Anon: The General Council of Medical Education and Registration. *Lancet* 1902; **160**: 1494 and *Br Med J* 1902; **2**: 1718–1719.

50. Anon: General Medical Council. *Med Times Hosp Gaz* 1903; **31**: 429–432.

51. Horsley V: The midwives registration bill. [Letter to the editor.] *Br Med J* 1898; **1**: 915.

52. Horsley V: The midwives bill. [Letter to the editor.] *Br Med J* 1899; **2**: 313.

53. Horsley V: The proposed registration of midwives. *Lancet* 1899; **153**: 1732–1734.

54. White R: Some political influences surrounding the Nurses Registration Act 1919 in the United Kingdom. *J Adv Nurs* 1976; **1**: 209–217.

55. Horsley V: Witness testimony, May 18, 1905. pp. 61–73. In *Report from the Select Committee on Registration of Nurses; Together with the Proceedings of the Committee, Minutes of Evidence, and Appendix*. His Majesty's Stationary Office: London, 1905.

56. Anon: State registration of nurses. Deputation to the premier. *Br Med J* 1908; **1**: 1247–1250.

57. Anon: Registration of nurses. *Daily Mail (Lond)*, May 14, 1909, p. 3.

58. Horsley V: State registration of nurses. [Letter to the editor.] *Br Med J* 1914; **2**: 315–316.

59. Anon: Anti-registration tactics. *Br J Nurs* 1914; **53**: 6–7.

60. Anon: The nursing and midwifery conference. *Br J Nurs* 1914; **52**: 394–396.

61. Cox A: Obituary of Sir Victor Horsley, C.B., F.R.S., M.B., F.R.C.S. Work for the British Medical Association. *Br Med J* 1916; **2**: 164–165.

62. Zuck D: Mr Troutbeck as the surgeon's friend: The coroner and the doctors – an Edwardian comedy. *Med Hist* 1995; **39**: 259–287.

63. Horsley V: A coroner on operations. [Letter to the editor.] *The Times (Lond)*, June 6, 1908, p. 12.

64. Anon: The relation of coroners to the medical profession. Conferences as to the action of the coroner for south-west London. *Br Med J* 1904; **2** (Suppl. 26): 52–61.

65. Horsley V: Report on the procedure of the coroner for south-west London and the inaction of the government in relation thereto. *Br Med J* 1905; **2** (Suppl. 68): 146–148.

66. Anon: The government and the profession. *Br Med J* 1905; **2**: 291–292.

67. Anon: A coroner on operations. *The Times (Lond)*, June 4, 1908, p. 14.

68. Anon: 1,000 operations daily. Coroner on the need for inquiry. *Daily Mail (Lond)*, June 4, 1908, p. 3.

69. Shearer DF: A coroner on operations. [Letter to the editor.] *The Times (Lond)*, June 9, 1908, p. 6.

70. Biggs MG: A coroner on operations. [*Letter to the editor.*] *The Times (Lond)*, June 10, 1908, p. 8.

71. McManus LS: A coroner on operations. [Letter to the editor.] *The Times (Lond)*, June 12, 1908, p. 20.

72. Troutbeck J: A coroner on operations. [Letter to the editor.] *The Times (Lond)*, June 10, 1908, p. 8.

73. Horsley V: A coroner on operations. [Letter to the editor.] *The Times (Lond)*, June 12, 1908, p. 20.

74. Anon: A coroner on operations. *The Times (Lond)*, June 12, 1908, p. 13.

75. Davy H: A coroner on operations. [Letter to the editor.] *The Times (Lond)*, June 19, 1908, p. 14.

76. Anon: Death after operation: Surgical opinion. *Daily Telegraph (Lond)*, June 16, 1908, p. 4.

Chapter 10

Not So Trivial Pursuits: The Slide into Politics

In addition to the leading role he played in various professional organizations that served to protect doctors and the general public, each from the other, Horsley attempted unsuccessfully to reform certain aspects of the Royal College of Surgeons and then assumed an important role in reforming and leading the British Medical Association, ensuring that it became more representative of the profession and more concerned with the welfare of its members. He enjoyed being in the public eye, having his views heard, and influencing the course of events in accord with his liberal principles. He used his position in the association to support legislation to improve the health and welfare of children and then became an ardent advocate of the National Insurance Bill, which caused him to be cast aside by many of his friends. An idealistic man of strong opinions who was always ready to help those less fortunate than himself, his support of social legislation was not for personal gain. Indeed, it cost him dear, for his private practice withered as colleagues stopped referring patients to him, either in anger or in the belief that he was turning from a clinical to a political career. In turn, he became a parliamentary candidate, hoping to promote other legislation to advance social welfare, but the outbreak of war interrupted these hopes and aspirations.

Royal College of Surgeons of England

Although Horsley was both a fellow and a member of the Royal College of Surgeons of England, he had little involvement with its policies and practices, preferring instead to work more inclusively. He opposed, however, the college's policy that prevented its members – as opposed to its fellows – from serving on the governing council or even voting in elections to the council, believing this to be undemocratic. Membership by examination was a means of entering clinical practice, whereas

fellowship status rewarded those who had passed more advanced examinations to practice as surgeon-specialists. The lack of direct representation of members bothered Horsley, who in 1912 and 1914 moved resolutions for change at the annual meetings of the college, but his efforts were unsuccessful, as were protests by the membership as a whole.[1] The council, led by its president, Rickman Godlee, felt that its focus and obligations were better met by its existing constitution and that the inclusion of members was unnecessary as their professional issues could be referred to the British Medical Association. It was only after many years and two world wars that the issue was resolved and members gained some representation on the council.

British Medical Association

The British Medical Association was founded as a provincial association in 1832, expanded to become national in name and reach in 1855, and then extended into the British Empire, with branches being established in different parts of India, Ceylon, Asia, Africa, Australia, New Zealand, Canada, and the West Indies before the turn of the century. Despite its early focus on general practitioners, it became apparent by the end of the nineteenth century that the organization was not meeting their expectations. Many doctors therefore wondered about establishing a new association to advance medico-political reforms in Britain.

At a conference on medical politics held in November 1899, Horsley opposed the idea, believing instead that the existing organization should take on such reforms. It had involved itself previously in contemporary medical controversies and political issues, but it needed to align itself more fully with the needs of its members and of the profession as a whole. He also had a number of personal concerns, among them that many of the association's officers felt their positions were honorific and required no actual work. Some of the officers, he believed, felt that urges favoring medical reforms were "only the production of a small, insignificant coterie of discontented men 'agin the Government' who are always disposed to get up a row for the sake of a little notoriety." These officers needed to understand that their constant obstructiveness was "due to a combination of a want of knowledge and of sympathy."[2]

In May 1900, delegates from different local medical societies met to consider common concerns, clarify the needs of general practitioners, and determine how to improve the organization of medicine.[3,4] Although a specialist, Horsley was asked to speak first because of his knowledge of the Medical Acts and his views on medical reform.[4] Forceful, tireless, and radical in his beliefs, he became "the great driving force" in pointing to the need for change, and others joined him in channeling these reforms so that – rather than leading to a new organization – they occurred through the existing association. However, the changes initially proposed did not allay all the concerns of Horsley and his followers, who consequently rejected them.[3,5]

At the following annual meeting, Horsley proposed that a committee be appointed to revise the constitution, and this was carried unanimously.[6] It was subsequently resolved that the organization should function in such a manner that every member had a reasonable opportunity to attend every important meeting. The association was divided into local divisions (or medical societies) to which all the members living in the area belonged, with divisions grouped together as branches for administrative purposes. The annual meeting became the annual meeting of the representatives of divisions from all over Britain and the empire, and was designated the representative meeting, sometimes referred to as the "medical parliament." It became the forum where – as Horsley wished – policy was to be decided. Horsley was elected the first chairman of the representative body, holding office from 1903 to 1906, and remained a member of the representative meeting until 1912. As pointed out some years later, "The revivified Association can never forget the debt which it owes to Sir Victor Horsley, whose dominating personality, intense enthusiasm, and indefatigable efforts did so much to put life into dead bones and make our Association the living power which it is today."[7]

Horsley was a member of the council of the association from 1900 to 1912, chaired many committees, and helped to develop the articles and byelaws that made the association more democratic. He took a leading role in developing policies regarding reform of the regulations concerning coroners, the state registration of midwives and nurses, and the suppression of medical practice by the unqualified and by charlatans (see Chapter 9), as well as the medical inspection and treatment of schoolchildren (see later).[8] Unlike most of his medical contemporaries, however, he also supported plans for national insurance.

He did not always get his way and, when frustrated, could be quite vindictive. In 1900, during discussions at the annual meeting about the *British Medical Journal*, he proposed a cut in the salary of its editor – his former medical school classmate, Dawson Williams – for supposedly failing to promote the interests of the profession as Horsley saw them.[9] After protests and an explanatory statement by Williams,[10] Horsley only reluctantly withdrew his proposal.

Horsley served the association well, and when he completed his term as chair of the representative meeting, his colleagues purchased some expensive silver-plate for him. He declined any formal presentation, however, believing that personal presentations should not be made for public service, except by the state.

Social Legislation: In Defence of Children

At the beginning of the twentieth century, children from impoverished families often worked in factories or domestic service, on farms or in the mines, at home or on the streets. They were required to attend elementary school until the age of ten, but truancy was common and many children were illiterate. Street urchins were dirty, ill-clothed, and undernourished; they smoked tobacco, drank alcohol, begged, stole, and sold themselves. Many were ill, disabled, or deformed. Trouble brought them harsh penalties: they could be whipped or sent to adult prisons for even minor infractions. They were a constant thorn in the social conscience and a rich source of recruits to the criminal underworld. The 1908 Children's Act helped to alleviate some of the issues: it established juvenile courts and detention centers, gave local authorities the powers to protect children from extreme abuse and cruelty, made it an offence for parents to neglect a child's health, and made it more difficult for children to obtain cigarettes or alcohol. Nevertheless, much remained to be done.

During the Boer War (1899–1902) the recruiting statistics were such that of eleven thousand volunteers for military service from Manchester, it was said that eight thousand had to be turned away as physically unfit. These numbers may be questioned,[11] but there is no doubt that many would-be military recruits were not fit enough physically to serve sovereign or empire. This underscored the need to develop a system for inspecting schoolchildren medically at periodic intervals and for ensuring their adequate nutrition and health. Such care would also ensure that every child was better able to benefit from the elementary education provided by the state following enactment of the Education Bill of 1902,[12] which had placed all elementary schools under the control of local education authorities in England and Wales, thereby providing for a national educational system. A selective system of secondary (that is, post-elementary) schools was also established, consisting of state-supported grammar schools (in addition to the elite, fee-charging public schools).[13] In 1903, a royal commission made various recommendations concerning physical education in schools,[14,15] and in the following year an interdepartmental committee, enquiring into allegations of physical deterioration based on the recruitment figures mentioned earlier, also made recommendations with both the national interest and the welfare of individual children in mind.[16] There was general agreement that alcohol consumption, an inadequate diet, and a lack of exercise were important contributory factors, and that educational reform and the schools themselves would be important in countering these factors.

Compulsory elementary education had begun in Britain in 1880. By 1906, it was clear that children from very poor families needed assistance to prevent malnutrition and to allow them to benefit fully from the education provided. Parliament accordingly passed legislation requiring school meals, paid for by local taxation ("rates"), to be supplied free of charge to children whose parents could not afford them.

Another parliamentary act, in 1907, required local education authorities to provide for school medical inspections of all children and "to make such arrangements as may be sanctioned by the Board of Education for attending to the health and physical condition of the children." The aims were to adapt the educational system to the needs and abilities of the child, to detect unsuspected medical disorders, and to gain information about physical and mental development during childhood. These measures, combined with teaching the elements of personal hygiene and ensuring that classrooms were clean and well ventilated, would – it was hoped – diminish the incidence of various common diseases, check the spread of infectious diseases, and improve physical fitness nationally.

The school inspections were to be performed in conjunction with the existing public health authorities, supervised by the local medical officer of health. However, a newly established medical department at the board of education was to be in overall charge rather than any local government agency, in order to ensure close cooperation between education and public health officials. The doctors in general and, more especially, the administrators of the London County Council (established in 1888 as the local government agency of the metropolis) were concerned about the costs and time involved, reimbursement issues, the number of children to be inspected, the nature of the care to be provided, and staffing requirements. Further, the London officials were opposed to a national approach, preferring their own education committee and its chief medical officer to be responsible.

For a while there was little movement. Then in March 1911, Horsley presided at a discussion held at Clifford's Inn, a former inn of chancery, and pointed out that the system of medical inspections carried out in the metropolis – where inspections were still restricted to a few of the children entering certain selected schools – did not meet the statutory requirement. He characterized the action in London as "a breach of faith with the nation" and went on to advocate for the establishment of school clinics, which he believed was the only way to provide adequate medical care to school-age children.[17] (Such a clinic had been opened in Bow, a poor section of London, by the reformers Margaret and Rachel McMillan.) The issues raised by Horsley were brought up in parliament, where Walter Runciman, president of the board of education and the wealthy son of a shipping magnate, responded: "I have a great deal of respect for this distinguished surgeon's opinion upon the subjects on which he speaks with special authority, but I am not sure that the organization of the medical inspection of school children is one of them."[18]

Nevertheless, shortly thereafter, Runciman and his officials received a large group of doctors led by Horsley, who complained about the methods adopted in the capital. They demanded that the local authorities should be required to carry out their duties in accordance with the 1907 Act and should adopt the school clinic system advocated by Horsley and the British Medical Association.[19] The officials at the board of education claimed to be in full agreement. They pointed out that they had previously expressed to the leaders of the London County Council, but "in milder language," the proposals of Horsley and his colleagues and had received promises that things would improve.

Eventually, London did come into conformity with the rest of the country regarding medical inspections, although it followed a rocky road to compliance. At first, "inspections" consisted merely of a "march past" of those entering school rather than a medical inspection as normally understood, but by 1912 things had changed for the better despite the enormous resources required because of the numbers involved.[20] For example, in London during the year 1911, more than two hundred thousand children underwent medical inspection, and more than half of them showed "defects." One third had enlarged tonsils and adenoids; four fifths had rotten teeth; between two and three thousand had ringworm; and almost fifteen thousand children were found to be "verminous" and had to be sent to one of the nine cleansing stations established for verminous children.[21]

Horsley led another deputation from the British Medical Association to the board of education in May 1912, this time with regard to the medical treatment of children. This was a particularly thorny problem for the association because, in addition to resolving the social issues, it had to safeguard doctors' salaries in its proposals. Working-class children requiring medical care had received treatment previously either as charity cases at one of the voluntary hospitals or through poor-law doctors. These options, if continued, risked drawing patients away from private medicine, and the association was therefore against them. The better options – providing good care plus an income for doctors – involved establishing clinics within schools or encouraging the private treatment of children by their family

doctor.[22] The school clinics seemed the only universally applicable option.[23]

The association believed that all schools in the metropolis should be grouped and that for each group there should be a school clinic staffed by paid local practitioners. Instead, London was using local hospitals, which involved "waste, confusion, and administrative chaos."[20] Only eight hospitals, all within a small region of the metropolis, were being paid to participate. The system was unworkable because of difficulties with geographic access, the inappropriateness of hospital treatment for many childhood ailments, and the difficulty of caring for the needs of children in hospitals.

The new president of the board of education (Jack Pease, later Lord Gainford) agreed that the existing system in London was not ideal, was anxious that involvement of the hospitals should not become permanent, and wanted the system to evolve along the lines discussed, with the establishment of school clinics. Discussions were in progress with local education authorities and grants were being made to help fund the cost of medical treatment of children attending public elementary schools and of those with tuberculosis or other medical disorders for which open-air treatment was beneficial.[24]

Horsley's embrace of the principle that schoolchildren should undergo regular medical inspections and – if necessary – treatment, and that school meals should be provided at no charge for the needy, reflected his growing interest and active involvement in social welfare and related legislation. The first decade of the twentieth century saw the increasing acceptance in Britain of the concept that the state should provide certain basic benefits unconditionally to its citizens, and that some were less able than others to provide for themselves through no personal failing. This increasing social awareness led to the development of the National Insurance Act of 1911.

The National Insurance Act

In the early part of the twentieth century, many general practitioners worked in "contract practice." They charged a small weekly sum for providing medical care as needed to subscribers or received an agreed salary to care for the members of a local works club, medical aid society, or friendly society.[25] Such schemes enabled the working classes to receive at least some sort of health care, limited though it might be, and helped to augment the earnings of medical men who nevertheless often looked with distaste at contract practice and the patients it brought to them.[26] Many doctors regarded the work as unseemly or ill-paid. Some felt uneasy about taking money when there had been no call on their services, others that calls were excessive or that patients in the scheme could well afford to pay full rates for service.

In fact, paid clinical work was sometimes hard to come by, and colleagues therefore undercut each other by underbidding for contract work. Accordingly, clubs or societies seeking a contract doctor often pitted practitioners against each other, so that their earnings were low. In turn, many doctors chose to increase their income by taking on more patients than they could manage or neglected their contract patients in favor of fee-paying private patients. Thus, abuses on both sides were common. Notices detailing the frequent disputes were published in the medical journals.[27]

The very poor received some care – at least while they remained destitute – from underpaid, overworked, and seemingly contemptuous poor-law doctors, who were themselves often regarded with disdain by their better placed medical brethren. Poverty brought illness, for which help was often sought only as a last resort; illness, in turn, led to greater poverty.

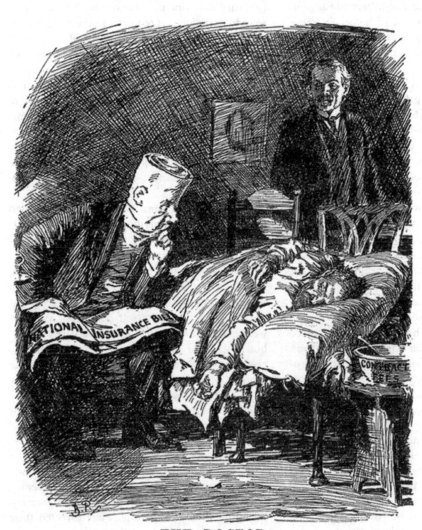

Figure 10.1 Cartoon based on the famous picture by Sir Luke Fildes, the Victorian painter whose *The Doctor* remains on display in London's Tate Gallery and in 1949 was reproduced in posters and on brochures by the American Medical Association in its campaign against President Harry Truman's proposal for nationalized medical care. In the cartoon, the patient (a general practitioner) is saying that Lloyd George's National Insurance bill will be the death of him. (Cartoon by Bernard Partridge, from *Punch*, June 14, 1911.)

THE DOCTOR.
(*With Apologies to Sir Luke Fildes, R.A.*)
PATIENT (*General Practitioner*). "THIS TREATMENT WILL BE THE DEATH OF ME.'
DOCTOR BILL. "I DARE SAY YOU KNOW BEST. STILL THERE'S ALWAYS A CHANCE."

In 1909 a Royal Commission on the Poor Laws, recognizing the inadequacy of the existing system, recommended in its Majority Report that healthcare for the poor should be reorganized on a contract (insurance) basis, although some members favored the provision of a full-time, salaried medical service, as outlined in the Minority Report authored primarily by Beatrice Webb, with the help of her husband Sidney. There were other, fundamental differences between the two groups. The majority believed that the cause of poverty related to moral factors and that the Poor Laws should be retained but reformed and renamed. The minority argued that poverty was a social issue requiring a multifaceted approach for its prevention and relief, with separate administrative departments to deal with specific issues such as health, employment, and education. Their proposals provide one of the earliest accounts of a modern welfare state.

The British Medical Association, within a few months, set out certain principles concerning the healthcare issues, but its main concern was to ensure the adequate remuneration of doctors rather than the welfare of the public. It was in this context that, early in 1911, David Lloyd George, as chancellor of the exchequer, introduced a National Insurance Bill that was divided into a part concerned with healthcare of wage-earners and a second part providing protection against unemployment (for which the young Winston Churchill, while president of the board of trade, deserves credit). The health provisions, which are the focus of the present commentary, were based in part on the experience in Germany and favored an expanded but reformed version of the contract system. The bill initially received support from both major parties in parliament, and rapid enactment seemed likely, but the proposals met with much opposition in the country.

The workers were angered by the proposed compulsory weekly contributions, which were four pence from the employee, three pence from the employer, and tuppence from the state – "nine pence for four pence" as the slogan went. The doctors also were divided – many thought their private practices would be ruined and protested bitterly at an extension of contract practice that would cause them to be overworked and underpaid. Although general practitioners were finding it difficult to manage financially in the existing system, apprehension about change and misconceptions about the nature of the proposed changes led to hostility and rejection of the proposal. An added concern was that the system would be abused by mendacious foreigners coming to Britain for free treatment, echoes of which would be heard repeatedly over the rest of the century as the welfare state and a national health service evolved.

In the words of Lloyd George, "Never was legislation more needed. Never was it less wanted." The bill originally provided for care using the contract model through "approved societies," with which the chancellor was soon consulting. Within a few weeks, the British Medical Association drew up a list of demands (its "cardinal principles") to be met if its members were to participate. It required an income limit for those entitled to benefits, the right of the patient to choose his doctor, the involvement of insurance companies (rather than friendly or mutual societies) in administering benefits, adequate medical representation on the administrative panels of insurance companies, an agreed level of payments to doctors, and an agreed method of payment. Some twenty-seven thousand doctors eventually signed a pledge not to take part in the scheme except in accordance with the policy of the association.

During negotiations, the association obtained most of the concessions that it sought. The bill was passed in December 1911, but its medical provisions did not come into full effect until January 1, 1913, leaving another year for further negotiation, especially on fees. Everyone earning less than three pounds per week was to be covered, but not their family or the self-employed. Workers were entitled to free treatment by a panel doctor, but hospital or specialist services were not covered. They could also receive paid sick leave for six months, with men receiving ten shillings weekly for the first three months and five shillings per week thereafter, the corresponding numbers for women being seven shillings and six pence and three shillings, respectively.

The doctors, of course, had the right to distance themselves from the scheme if they chose, but clearly they were needed for it to operate. Many remained hostile, their grievances becoming more heated with time. They directed their fury not only at the government but also at the association and its council, which they roundly and readily denounced. In early December 1911, the council met to discuss an offer from the prime minister's office for Mr. Smith Whitaker, its medical secretary, to serve as deputy chairman of the National Health Insurance Commission as established by the act. It agreed (by thirty-eight votes to three) that Whitaker was free to accept the offer, for it served the association's interests to have a friend in a leadership position within the new organization. Doctors opposed to the government's proposals were furious, speaking publicly of a "shameless betrayal" of the profession. An acrimonious correspondence followed in the columns of *The Times* and the medical journals, though Horsley and others pointed out that Whitaker's acceptance of the appointment in no way affected the position of the association in its negotiations with the government.[28,29]

Worse was to follow. On December 19, three days after the National Insurance Bill was finally enacted, some two thousand angry doctors met at the Queen's Hall, in Langham Place, London, believing that the original six cardinal points of the association had not been guaranteed satisfactorily by the act. The special correspondent of *The Times* described the assembly as resembling "a political meeting at election time, when party feeling is running high."[30] The meeting began after a one-hour organ recital that ended with "Rule Britannia," the audience standing to sing the chorus of "Britons never shall be slaves." As the meeting got under way, cries of "Smash the Act" and "Strike" filled the air, inflaming the crowd. Horsley, sitting quietly at the back of the hall, eventually stood to defend the official policy of the association but was hissed and booed, called a traitor, and told to "go to your Lloyd George."[30,31] He was invited onto the platform, and then "was howled down." The few words that he spoke were met with derision and interrupted by hecklers, and the obvious hostility of the crowd forced him to stop within a few minutes.[30] In the end, he wrote to *The Times* to get his views across, concluding:

> The irresponsible statements made at the Queen's Hall meeting do not represent the position of the British Medical Association towards the Insurance Act. The mover of the first resolution (Dr. F. J. Smith) admitted to the meeting that he had read nothing on the subject until the last three weeks, not even the minutes of the three representative meetings held during

the last nine months. Such ignorance of public affairs is only too common, and to ignorance alone and not to intentional discourtesy do we ascribe the unfortunate intolerance of the Queen's Hall meeting.[32]

Horsley felt privately that the demonstration against him had been planned, in part because of his liberal political views. He was hurt that he did not receive support from some of the other senior doctors present at that fateful event and angered that the leaders of the profession had not attempted to ensure freedom of speech. William Osler wrote to him from Oxford that he "was disgusted that they should have treated you so badly." Horsley responded bitterly that as "no public protest of any kind has appeared from you or any other 'leader' of the profession the public can only assume that you endorsed the conduct which had been organised beforehand."[33]

Negotiations continued into 1912. Lloyd George commended the association for trying to find an equitable solution (even though it simply repeated the same demands time and time again), but was disappointed in the Royal Colleges of Surgeons and Physicians for their "curt, undignified, discourteous refusal to meet a Government department to discuss matters affecting the profession which they officially represented."[34] By July, he was able to write that all but two of the original cardinal points of the association had been conceded.[35] Letters for and against the bill were published in the medical and lay press, sometimes with extravagant claims that were difficult even to understand. The master of a Cambridge college, for example, claimed quite sincerely that Lloyd George's bill would stop the progress of preventive medicine,[36] a puzzling point that Horsley easily refuted.[37] Some were disturbed by the expense involved. Others disapproved on more philosophical grounds, describing the bill as "a long step in the downward path towards socialism."[38] The individual initiative of wage-earners would diminish, it was argued, accompanied by an increase in "that spirit of dependency which is ever found in degenerate races. This spoon-fed race will look more and more to a paternal government to feed and clothe it, and not require it to work more than a few hours daily. They will be further encouraged to multiply their breed at the expense of the healthy and intellectual members of the community."[38] Thus spoke the president-elect of the British Medical

Association. Perhaps not surprisingly, Sir James Barr was also an ardent supporter of eugenics. "The race" he said in his presidential lecture "must be renewed from the mentally and physically fit, the moral and physical degenerates should not be allowed to take any part in adding to the race. Above all, we must breed for intelligence."[38]

The chancellor finally agreed to an increased annual capitation fee of nine shillings per patient, of which at least seven shillings (rather than the original four shillings and sixpence) was for the doctor, and the balance for medications (previously one shilling and sixpence). With this, he believed he could now enroll sufficient doctors for the scheme to move forward. Still, some doctors objected. The dispute in the medical profession became increasingly bitter, with abuse, intimidation, pickets, threats of social ostracism, and professional isolation all being used to influence the outcome. There were dark murmurings in the press about a relatively well-off group trying to challenge parliament and frustrate the will of the people. In fact, many doctors, especially the younger ones and those in the poorer districts, now favored the scheme, which represented a significant increase in their income. The chancellor encouraged them to take on assistants and partners as needed, offering to send in doctors to complete understaffed panels or even to appoint salaried doctors in certain areas.[25] So many doctors volunteered for these salaried appointments that opposition to the panel scheme finally broke. Early in 1913, the British Medical Association realized that it had to release its members from their pledge: the battle was over.

So what of the outcome? The liberal *Westminster Gazette*, in a commentary that probably reflected pretty fairly the public and political opinion at the end of 1912, when the issue was not yet fully resolved, said: " We all admire people who do not know when they are beaten, but the difficulty about the British Medical Association is that it doesn't know when it has won."[7] Somewhat unfortunately, many people gained the impression that the association was simply against the whole concept of national insurance. Certainly there was much bitterness among its members when the revolt collapsed.[25]

Nevertheless, since that time the British government has accepted the association as the organization representing the entire medical profession. As for Horsley, his support of national

health insurance and of the council's policy cost him dear. Much of the bitterness of the profession turned on him. His relations with the association deteriorated, for many council members had changed their views, opposed the government's scheme, and attacked him for his support of it.[39] Once a hero among doctors for his long service in safeguarding their welfare, he came to be resented as a socialist, a traitor to the profession, and a lapdog of Lloyd George. His clinical practice suffered as patient referrals declined as the result of a professional boycott. A bewildered profession was casting him out even as he took up new challenges in support of women's suffrage and continued with increased vigor his activities for the temperance movement. After 1912, Horsley had little to do with the association except for continuing to work on the issue of school medical services, discussed earlier.

Parliamentary Candidate

Horsley's interest in politics and his drive to reform many aspects of life in Edwardian Britain made it inevitable that he would stand for election to parliament. Few doctors had attempted to enter parliament before 1910, if only because there was no financial or professional incentive to do so and it was generally necessary to have private means of support.[40] Some would-be politicians might have been put off by their experience with the British Medical Association, but in Horsley's case the experience seems to have whetted his appetite for public service and social reform. He became increasingly concerned with the welfare of the unemployed, with obtaining relief for taxpayers, and with arbitration for settling civil disputes.[41]

Despite the gibes of those who opposed his support of national health insurance, Horsley was certainly not a socialist. He believed in free enterprise and in the right of the individual to personal property and wealth, even as he favored progressive reforms to help those in need. He stood as a Liberal candidate for the University of London in 1910 but was opposed for his support of the suffragists and of the temperance movement. The antivivisectionists deliberately set out to prejudice his candidacy by distributing a hostile circular to electors; they were led, among others, by Miss Lind af Hageby, who had figured in the Brown Dog affair just a few years earlier (see Chapter 11).[42] In any event, he was defeated by the incumbent, his former tutor, Sir Philip Magnus. He had not helped himself by his refusal to compromise, the abrasive manner in which he sometimes advanced his views, and the lack of subtlety with which he challenged personally those who opposed them. Nevertheless, his candidacy was important in bringing home to many liberals that "a man may care supremely for social improvement and at the same time for scientific progress" and that social progress is limited without a scientific basis for change.[43]

In 1911 he was adopted as the prospective Liberal candidate for North Islington (London), but he resigned in favor of standing as the Liberal candidate for the Harborough Division of Leicestershire early in 1913. By the end of the year he had been dropped as candidate, primarily because his views on female suffrage were not appreciated as widely in the country as they were among the sophisticated intellectuals of the metropolis, and it was thought – wrongly as it happened – that he supported the "lawless methods of the militants."[44,45]

The Liberal member of parliament for Poplar (in London) resigned in 1914. Alfred William Yeo, who had worked in local government for many years and was at one time mayor of Poplar, was selected to replace him as the Liberal candidate. His preference over Horsley upset the chairman of the local Liberal Association, who resigned in protest. Indeed, there was "very considerable dissatisfaction" in Liberal circles at the choice.[46] In any event, Yeo succeeded in holding the seat for the Liberals but by a greatly reduced majority. During 1914 and the first months of 1915, Horsley was approached as a potential candidate by several other constituencies, the last being Gateshead, which he declined on May 17, 1915: "[I am] certainly anxious to get into Parliament … but am just, in half an hour, embarking with a division of the Dardanelles Force as Surgeon-in-Chief of a Hospital."[47] He had also been asked to stand for parliament as liberal candidate for Huddersfield, the party offering to wait until his return from the war, but it was not to be.

Horsley was a public but controversial figure whose support of liberal causes, which included proportional representation and home rule for Ireland,[48,49] brought him enemies as well as friends, letters of opposition and of support, of explanation and regret. He was, it seems, too honest to be a party politician, for he would not sacrifice principle for expediency and would have found it difficult to toe the party line. In any event, his political aspirations were interrupted by the outbreak of World War I, a war that he did not survive.

Notes

1. Anon: Deputations to the Privy Council relative to the proposed new charter of the Royal College of Surgeons of England. *Br Med J* 1887; **2**: 1110–1117; Anon: The Royal College of Surgeons. *Br Med J* 1888; **2**: 1053–1054, 1118–1119, 1170–1171, 1234–1235 [four parts]; Correspondence: Royal College of Surgeons. *Br Med J* 1889; **1**: 437–438; Anon: The Royal College of Surgeons and its members. *Br Med J* 1889; **1**: 603 and 606; Anon: Parliamentary Bills Committee. Government of the College of Surgeons. *Br Med J* 1890; **1**: 740–743; Anon: Royal College of Surgeons of England. Annual meeting of fellows and members. Direct representation of members on the council. *Br Med J* 1907; **2**: 1624. [Similar articles can also be found in the *Lancet* over this same time period.] Horsley twice introduced resolutions for the direct representation of members on the college council [Anon: Royal College of Surgeons of England. Annual meeting of fellows and members. *Lancet* 1912; **180**; 1532–1533; Anon: Annual meeting of the Royal College of Surgeons. Representation of members. *Br Med J* 1914; **2**: 951.]

2. Horsley V: The conference on medical politics at Newcastle-on-Tyne. *Lancet* 1899; **2**: 1474–1477.

3. Little EM: *History of the British Medical Association 1832–1932*. British Medical Association: London, 1982.

4. Horsley V: Conference on medical organisation at Manchester. The Medical Acts. *Lancet* 1900; **1**: 1302–1303; Conference on medical organisation. The Medical Acts. *Br Med J* 1900; **1**: 1123–1124.

5. Anon: British Medical Association. Extraordinary General Meeting. *Br Med J* 1900; **2**: 189–191.

6. Horsley V: Reconstitution of the Association. Sixty-eighth annual meeting of the British Medical Association, held at Ipswich, July 31st, August 1st, 2nd, and 3rd. *Br Med J* 1900; **2**: 320–321.

7. Manknell A: The British Medical Association and its work for the general practitioner. *Br Med J* 1928; **2** (Suppl. 1258): 125–128.

8. Cox A: Obituary of Sir Victor Horsley, C.B., F.R.S., M.B., F.R.C.S. Work for the British Medical Association. *Br Med J* 1916; **2**: 164–165.

9. Horsley V: The journal. Sixty-eighth annual meeting of the British Medical Association, held at Ipswich, July 31st, August 1st, 2nd, and 3rd. *Br Med J* 1900; **2**: 316–317.

10. Williams D: The journal. Sixty-eighth annual meeting of the British Medical Association, held at Ipswich, July 31st, August 1st, 2nd, and 3rd. *Br Med J* 1900; **2**: 317–318.

11. Heggie V: Lies, damn lies, and Manchester's recruiting statistics: Degeneration as an "urban legend" in Victorian and Edwardian Britain. *J Hist Med Allied Sci* 2008; **63**: 178–216.

12. Newman G: *The Building of a Nation's Health.* pp. 194–195. Macmillan: London, 1939.

13. Robinson W: Historiographical reflections on the 1902 Education Act. *Oxf Rev Educ* 2002; **28**: 159–172.

14. Earl of Mansfield, Cochrane T, Glen-Coats T, Craik H, Stewart MHS, Alston JC, Fergusson JB, McCrae G, Ogston A: *The Royal Commission on Physical Training (Scotland). Volume 1. Report and Appendix.* His Majesty's Stationery Office: Edinburgh, 1903.

15. Anon: The Royal Commission on Physical Training (Scotland). *Br Med J* 1903; **1**: 817.

16. Inter-Departmental Committee on Physical Deterioration: *Report of the Inter-Departmental Committee on Physical Deterioration. Vol. 1: Report and Appendix.* His Majesty's Stationery Office: London, 1904.

17. Anon: Medical inspection of school children. *The Times (Lond)*, March 17, 1911, p. 6.

18. Anon: Parliament: House of Commons. Tuesday March 21. Medical inspection in schools. *The Times (Lond)*, March 22, 1911, p. 12.

19. Anon: Medical treatment of school children. Mr. Runciman and the London County Council. *The Times (Lond)*, June 28, 1911, p. 4.

20. Anon: Medical inspection and treatment of school children under the London County Council. Deputation from the British Medical Association to the President of the Board of Education. *Br Med J* 1912; **1** (Suppl. 422): 545–547.

21. Anon: Medical inspection of school children. *The Times (Lond)*, November 14, 1912, p. 3.

22. Gilbert BB: *The Evolution of National Insurance in Great Britain: The Origin of the Welfare State.* pp. 149–152. Joseph: London, 1966.

23. Macdonald JA: Matters referred to divisions. Medico-political committee. Medical inspection of school children. Report: Provision for treatment of children found, upon medical inspection, to be defective. *Br Med J* 1908; **2** (Suppl. 222): 41–42.

24. Anon: Medical treatment of school children. The distribution of grants. *The Times (Lond)*, April 11, 1912, p. 11.

25. Turner ES: *Call the Doctor: A Social History of Medical Men.* Joseph: London, 1958.

26. Medico-Political Committee of the British Medical Association: An investigation into the economic conditions of contract medical practice in the United Kingdom. *Br Med J* 1905; **2** (Suppl. 66): 1–29.

27. Anon: Contract medical practice. Notice as to districts in which disputes exist. *Br Med J* 1905; **2**: 207–208.

28. Goodall EW, Horsley V, Keay JH, Rice-Oxley AJ, Shaw LE: The great "betrayal." A reply to Dr. Smith. [Letter to the editor.] *The Times (Lond)*, December 7, 1911, p. 10.

29. Goodall EW, Horsley V, Keay JH, Rice-Oxley AJ, Shaw LE: The great betrayal. Policy of the doctors. [Letter to the editor.] *The Times (Lond)*, December 11, 1911, p. 10.

30. Anon: The doctors' protest. Enthusiastic meeting in London. Sir Victor Horsley refused a hearing. *The Times (Lond)*, December 20, 1911, p. 9.

31. Horsley V: The profession and politicians. [Letter to the editor.] *Br Med J* 1912; **1**: 462.

32. Horsley V, Keay JH, Rice-Oxley AJ, Shaw LE: The Council's position. The Association and the profession. [Letter to the editor.] *The Times (Lond)*, December 20, 1911, p. 10.

33. Osler W: Note to Horsley, dated December 20 [1911]; Horsley V: Draft of reply to Osler. Section A54, Horsley Papers, Special Collections, UCL Library Services (London, UK). See also Dunnill MS: Victor Horsley (1857–1915) and national insurance. *J Med Biogr* 2013; **21**: 249–254.

34. Anon: National Insurance: The Chancellor of the Exchequer on the medical aspects. *Br Med J* 1912; **1** (Suppl. 408): 177–180.

35. Lloyd George D: The National Insurance Act. An open letter from Mr. Lloyd George. *Lancet* 1912; **180**; 124–125.

36. Marsh H: Medicine: individual and social. The value of prevention. [Letter to the editor]. *The Times (Lond)*, June 4, 1912, p. 4.

37. Horsley V: Medicine and the Insurance Act. [Letter to the editor.] *The Times (Lond)*, June 8, 1912, p. 6.

38. Barr J: President's Address, delivered at the eighteenth annual meeting of the British Medical Association. *Br Med J* 1912; **2**: 157–163.

39. Turner EB: Reply to Sir Victor Horsley. Obligation of the pledge. [Letter to the editor.] *The Times (Lond)*, December 28, 1912, p. 6.

40. Cooter R: The rise and decline of the medical member: Doctors and parliament in Edwardian and interwar Britain. *Bull Hist Med* 2004; **78**: 59–107.

41. Papers on political matters. Section C, Horsley Papers, Special Collections, UCL Library Services (London, UK).

42. Papers on the 1910 general election. Section C4, Horsley Papers, Special Collections, UCL Library Services (London, UK).

43. Barlow, Sir Thomas: Letter to Victor Horsley dated January 7, 1911. Section C4, *Horsley Papers, Special Collections*, UCL Library Services (London, UK).

44. Anon: Sir Victor Horsley. Attitude towards suffragettes. *Daily Telegraph (Lond)*, November 15, 1913, p. 12; Harborough division. Radical candidature. *Daily Telegraph (Lond)*, November 24, 1913, p. 11.

45. Anon: Sir Victor Horsley's denial. *Daily Mail (Lond)*, November 21, 1913, p. 5.

46. Anon: London by-elections. Opening of short campaigns in the east. Polling days fixed. *The Times (Lond)*, February 13, 1914, p. 8.

47. Paget S: *Sir Victor Horsley: A Study of His Life and Work*. p. 208. Constable: London, 1919.

48. Papers on tariff reforms, free trade, and home rule. Section C5, Horsley Papers, Special Collections, UCL Library Services (London, UK).

49. Proportional Representation Society: *Report for the Year 1914–15*. P.R. Pamphlet No. 27: London, 1915.

Antivivisectionist Claims and Clamor

Horsley's work over the years had involved much experimentation in animals, and this inevitably brought him the opprobrium of a certain segment of the general public. He took on with seeming relish those crusading against such experimentation, becoming the *bête noire* of the antivivisectionists as he responded to their jibes and insults, always concerned to have the last word.

During the nineteenth century, an organized antivivisection movement had developed in Britain. An influential and typically prosperous segment of the general public – among them Queen Victoria, the wealthy philanthropist Angela Burdett-Coutts, members of the aristocracy, and ministers of the church and crown – became increasingly concerned about alleged cruelty to animals in the supposed interest of humanity. In response to their clamor, in 1875 the government set up a Royal Commission of Enquiry into Vivisection, which accepted the necessity of animal experimentation but led to regulatory legislation in the following year. Experiments were only to be conducted in approved laboratories and under specified conditions by approved researchers. Nevertheless, the use of experiments on live animals increased with growth in the biological sciences, and this led to the establishment of several societies or associations concerned with the welfare of animals. Among them was the Victoria Street Society, which later became the National Anti-Vivisection Society, with Stephen Coleridge, a barrister and a distant relative of the poet, as its honorary secretary, and Lord Shaftesbury as its president.

Other humanitarian groups were also forming, for example, to protect children from abuse or exploitation, and an increasing number of people began to press for the abolition of blood sports such as foxhunting. It was a time of change, of new values. With regard to animal rights and the push against vivisection, women – many of whom were also suffragists – seemed to play a particularly important part. The Irish writer Frances Power

Cobbe (1822–1904) had a leading role in the antivivisection movement, as also did Anna Kingsford (1846–1888), an English woman who studied medicine in Paris but was sickened by the animal experiments of the physiologists and scientists she encountered there, men such as Claude Bernard, Brown-Séquard, and Louis Pasteur. Others prominent in the antivivisection movement included Louise ("Lizzy") Lind af Hageby, discussed later; Charlotte Despard, suffragist, novelist, and sister of Sir John French, who for a time during World War I commanded the British expeditionary force on the Western Front and then the home forces; Margaret Damer Dawson, who went on to found the British Women's Police Service during the war; Gertrude Colmore, the writer; and Isabella Ford, the social reformer and activist.[1]

The antivivisectionists became increasingly aggressive in late Victorian and Edwardian times. They held angry rallies to publicize their cause, published hostile articles about animal researchers, and listed hospitals where these researchers were on staff, hoping thereby to restrict the appointments available to licensed experimenters and to diminish public support for hospitals employing them.[2] They even sent circulars to the subscribers of such hospitals, attempting to divert funds to other institutions.[3] But their indignation inevitably focused on London's University College, the focal point in Britain of the experimental approach to physiology and medicine during the early twentieth century, and on Victor Horsley, one of its most visible exponents.

The Nine Circles

Horsley and Cobbe had clashed in the correspondence columns of *The Times* in 1885 with regard to the utility of vivisection.[4,5] In early 1892, *The Nine Circles of the Hell of the Innocent*, compiled by a Mrs. G. M. Rhodes under Cobbe's direction, was published.[6] Cobbe planned the book, wrote the preface, and intended it to show the horrors of vivisection. The book contained verbatim extracts from published scientific papers and reports, including several by Horsley. Cobbe believed that "the reader who will spend but half-an-hour over this volume will . . . be better qualified to pass judgment on the character of the practice of vivisection" and she ended her preface with the hope that "God move the hearts of those who read this sickening book to pity and rescue."[7]

A few months later, in October 1892, the annual congress of members of the Church of England was held in Folkestone, on the south coast of England. The issue of vivisection had been placed on the agenda despite objections that it was a medical question and a somewhat unseemly topic to discuss in Folkestone, the birthplace of the physician-scientist William Harvey who first described in detail the circulation of the blood. The discussion took the form of a debate on morality: "Do the interests of mankind require experiments on living animals, and, if so, up to what point are they justifiable?" The meeting hall was packed in anticipation of a spirited dialogue. Bishop Alfred Barry and Dr. F. S. Arnold, a man with a medical degree from Oxford and a member of the Royal College of Surgeons, spoke against vivisection; Horsley spoke for it, as did Dr. M. Armand Ruffer, a pathologist and the first director of the British Institute of Preventive Medicine, later renamed the Lister Institute. Horsley, intent on showing the anti-vivisectionists in their true colors, stole the show.

He did not tread lightly. Experimental observations in the laboratory or at the bedside were the only means of extending knowledge of the processes and phenomena of life. This was the reason,

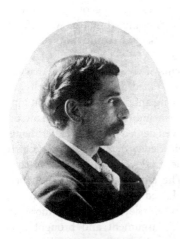

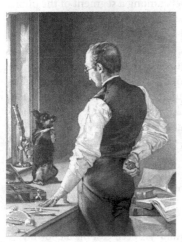

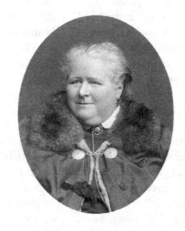

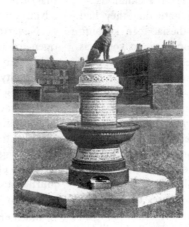

Figure 11.1 *Top left*, Victor Horsley, aged about thirty, defender of vivisection as a means of advancing medical science. *Top right*, Frances Power Cobbe, the Irish social activist and founder of the British Union for the Abolition of Vivisection. Horsley and Cobbe clashed over *The Nine Circles* affair. *Bottom left*, A dog in a laboratory begs a vivisector for mercy, part of an emotional appeal against vivisection. (Engraving by D. J. Tomkins, 1883, after a painting by J. McClure Hamilton.) *Bottom right*, the famous statue of the brown dog that led to student demonstrations and near-riots. (Images from the Wellcome Collection, London.)

he said, that at the International Medical Congress held in London in 1881, there was unanimous support for the resolution that "experiments on living animals have proved of the utmost service to medicine in the past and are indispensable to its future progress."[8,9] Indeed, he went on, the British Medical Association just two months earlier had adopted unanimously a resolution for transmission to the Church congress that "the continuance and extension of such investigations [experiments on living animals] is essential to the progress of knowledge, the relief of suffering, and the saving of life." As the Church was concerned with the moral aspects of vivisection, Horsley stressed the morality of scientific experimentation in its pursuit of truth. Medical men were particularly upset when experimentation caused pain to their animal subjects, but the morality of their work was not invalidated thereby. It was not considered immoral to kill animals for food, he pointed out, and accordingly it should not be considered wrong to kill animals to gain knowledge, especially when in the latter case they first are anesthetized.

Dismayed by unjust attempts to discredit animal experimentation, Horsley went on to accuse senior churchmen of being "culpably ignorant" because they based their objections on information provided by "sources of notoriously tainted character" instead of visiting university laboratories to gain first-hand knowledge of what transpired there. As an example of such sources, he referred to Miss Cobbe's book, describing it "as one of the rankest impostures that had for many years defaced English literature," with its seemingly deliberate and fraudulent misrepresentations of experiments by omitting to state that they had been performed under anesthesia.[8,9] In keeping with usual practice at the congress, no vote was taken at the conclusion of the debate, but certainly there was sympathy for Horsley's view among many in the audience.

The argument was continued in the correspondence columns of *The Times*, particularly by Horsley and Cobbe. She offered to apologize for "a small number of omissions" but this did not satisfy Horsley, who pointed out that she had purposely omitted the words "chloroform" and "morphia" in twenty of twenty-six cases cited in her book.[10] Cobbe responded that the book had been compiled for her, not by her, and that she could not be held responsible for any omissions or other

errors,[11] even though – as Horsley observed – in its preface she had affirmed its accuracy.[12] Their unfortunate exchange continued, with Horsley calling her a liar and claiming that for sixteen years she had been "falsely accusing medical men of murder, cruelty, falsehood, &c., ... while supporting such charges by fraud."[13]

Horsley's forthright language did not help his cause: concern about his allegations became obscured by dismay about the manner in which he made them. Thomas Huxley, Charles Sherrington, and Charles Ballance added their support, however, as did several influential medical knights, including James Paget, Andrew Clark, Samuel Wilks, and George Humphry. Bishop Barry conceded that the use of anesthetics had been omitted from *The Nine Circles* in a number of cases but remained opposed to vivisection.[14] Three days later, while accepting that vivisection did not "spring out of cruelty," the hapless bishop announced that he was sailing immediately for India and could not continue with the discussion.[15]

Other opponents of vivisection alleged that the use of anesthetics failed to prevent cruelty in experiments on living animals and, somewhat fantastically, some – including the surgeon Lawson Tait (p. 106)[16] – even denied that such experiments had advanced knowledge or cures for disease. It eventually became fruitless for the dispute to continue in print. The antivivisection agitation had indeed been conducted with culpable carelessness as pointed out by Horsley, but his manner had detracted from his argument and brought him particular notoriety among a segment of the public that believed it was unnecessary to use animals to advance medical science.

Nevertheless, Horsley had not hesitated to open his laboratory to journalists "to allow the public any opportunity to judge for themselves the cruelty of our methods." The correspondent of the *New York Times*, for example, arrived unexpectedly at his laboratory but was allowed to witness an ongoing operation on an anesthetized cat, and also to visit "the sick bay, convalescent ward and menagerie [animal house]" in the laboratory. Horsley elaborated on his frustration to the journalist:

Much opprobrium has been cast on me for my characterization of Miss Cobbe's action. But no one considers the provocation I have received.

For ten years Miss Cobbe, with her blind, unreasoning, narrow-minded malice, has carried on this unfair crusade against our body by means of constant willful falsification of evidence, not in occasional instances only, but in all cases![17]

Ten years later, Horsley again was in the spotlight as antivivisectionist agitation flared in the Brown Dog affair.

The Brown Dog Affair

In December 1902, Professor Ernest Starling (1866–1927) of University College London, while studying diabetes, tied off the pancreatic duct in an anesthetized brown terrier, which was then allowed to make a full recovery. Two months later, in early February, the dog underwent a second operation under anesthesia in which the pancreas was exposed and inspected, and the salivary duct was cannulated. The animal, still anesthetized (with alcohol, chloroform, and ether – ACE mixture – via an endotracheal tube), was then taken to a lecture theater where William Bayliss (1860–1924), an assistant professor of physiology, stimulated the nerve to the salivary gland before a class of students in an unsuccessful attempt to show that the pressure at which the saliva is secreted exceeds the blood pressure. Finally, the animal was removed and sacrificed by Henry Dale (1875–1968) – then a research student but a future Nobel Prize winner – who took its pancreas for further examination.

Among the students in the lecture hall on that February day were two Swedish activists, Lizzy Lind af Hageby and Leisa K. Schartau, who recounted that the experiments had been painful and conducted without anesthesia, that the students had laughed and joked during them, and that an unlicensed researcher had killed the unfortunate dog with a knife.[18] They claimed that the animal had tried to lift itself up during the experiment and that they had not smelled or heard any anesthetic being delivered. These claims were publicized by Stephen Coleridge of the National Anti-Vivisection Society, who read out a statement that described the alleged events at a meeting of the society in May, concluding eloquently: "If this is not torture, let Mr. Bayliss and his friends, Lord Lister and Sir Victor Horsley, tell us, in heaven's name, what torture is."[19,20,21] His statement was reported in a radical broadsheet, the *Daily News*. A detailed account also appeared in a book written by the two women, *The Shambles of Science*. When Bayliss heard of it and that Coleridge had accused him of torture, he demanded an apology and retraction, but these were not forthcoming. Starling and, especially, Horsley therefore encouraged him to take matters further, with Horsley allegedly commenting, "The Lord has delivered them into our hands."[22] Bayliss sued for libel and slander.

The case was heard in the law courts in November 1903 before Lord Alverstone, the lord chief justice. It aroused widespread interest and was reported extensively in the national press.[23,24] Mr. Rufus Isaacs, appearing for Bayliss, emphasized that his client held a license to perform

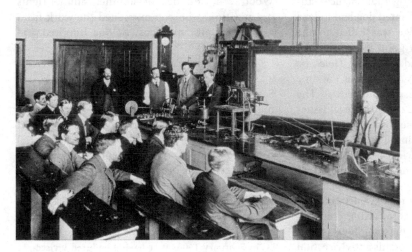

Figure 11.2 The experiment in the lecture theater at University College that led to the brown dog affair. Behind the table are Henry Dale (a future Nobel laureate), Ernest Starling, and William Bayliss (*extreme right*). The photograph shows a mock-up of the experiment and was used as evidence at the trial. (Image from the Wellcome Collection, London.)

experiments on living animals and that all the rules had been followed. In fact, as Bayliss pointed out, the experiment could not have been performed without the animal anesthetized. Coleridge was defended by John Lawson Walton, another well-known barrister, who cross-examined Bayliss intently about his experimental procedure, the need for experimenting on living animals, and the reason that a demonstration to students was deemed necessary. Unlike mechanics, which might be taught from a textbook or by word of mouth, Bayliss explained, physiology could only be taught on living organisms. Starling, called as a witness, indicated that the original experiment was to help understand a disease of the pancreas, to which the judge responded amid laughter that he had no idea where his own pancreas was even located. The proceedings were further enlivened by repartee when Horsley, who enjoyed the adversarial challenge of cross-examination, was called as a witness. Horsley stood his ground well in supporting the need for and benefits of experiments in animals, and loud applause broke out in the court when he responded to a point of Lawson Walton by questioning why there should be any limitation to the loss of animals for educational purposes, when there was none to their destruction for food. Horsley also explained that any twitching observed during the experiment related to the canine chorea that follows distemper, which the dog was known to have, and that such movements are not abolished by anesthesia, except preterminally. Horsley had himself devoted two of his Brown lectures to the topic in 1886 (see Chapter 3).

Other witnesses, including four medical students, confirmed that the ill-fated dog had indeed been anesthetized. Coleridge was called to the stand, but did not make a good impression. In the words of the correspondent of *The Times*, he "did as much damage to his own case as the time at his disposal for the purpose would allow."[2] The judge was concerned to focus on the legal issues rather than allowing the case to be influenced by sympathy for animal suffering. From his instructions to the jury, it seemed clear that a verdict for the plaintiff was the only one possible, based on the evidence.

The jury was out for about twenty minutes before finding for Bayliss and awarding him two thousand pounds in damages, plus costs. Contributions to Coleridge and his antivivisection society from animal-lovers all over the country more than covered the amount he owed within a few weeks. As for Bayliss, he donated the awarded money to support research in the physiology department at University College, and is remembered for his pioneering work there on hormones. Some suggested sardonically that his donation be named "The Stephen Coleridge Vivisection Fund."[25] Ernest Bell, the publisher and printer of *The Shambles of Science* hastily announced that the book was withdrawn from circulation, that all copies in stock would be given to Bayliss, and that he regretted his involvement with it,[26] but the book reappeared within a few months with the offending passages replaced by an account of the trial. Lind af Hageby, the grand-daughter of the chamberlain of Sweden, continued to agitate for reform, standing particularly for women's rights, animal welfare, and pacifism until her death in 1963. Rufus Isaacs went on to become successively a member of parliament, the lord chief justice of England, viceroy of India, and the marquess of Reading; he died in 1935.

The real winner of the lawsuit is unclear because the publicity it engendered brought the morality of vivisection out into the open once more, filling many column inches in the newspapers. It united at least temporarily a somewhat divided antivivisectionist movement[27] and led eventually to another royal commission to examine the issue. It also led to civil commotion and near-rioting when a monument was erected to the brown dog at the center of the affair. The idea for the monument had originated with Anna Louisa Woodward, founder of another animal-rights organization, who commissioned the work from a local sculptor at a cost of one hundred and twenty pounds.[27]

The monument was unveiled in Battersea, a working-class area in south London, in September 1906, by the mayor before a crowd of mainly women and children and in the presence of Louisa Woodward, Charlotte Despard, and – it is said – George Bernard Shaw. The memorial consisted of a drinking-fountain surmounted by an eighteen-inch bronze statue of a terrier dog sitting on its haunches. The inscription read:

In memory of the brown terrier dog done to death in the laboratories of University College in February 1903, after having endured vivisection extending over more than 2 months and having been handed over from one vivisector to another till death came to his release. Also in memory of the 232 dogs vivisected at the same place during the year 1902.

Men and women of England, how long shall these things be?

The wording of the inscription infuriated many, but for a while all was quiet. The authorities at University College considered their legal options, but these appeared to be limited. Then, in November 1907, ten medical students were arrested for attempting to damage the sculpture. The magistrate fined them each five pounds, pointing out that the memorial was legitimate, that there were two sides to the issue, and that any more students appearing before him for a similar offence would be jailed for two months with hard labor. His comments made things worse and, on the following day, more than five hundred students marched through central London bearing the magistrate in effigy, which they solemnly set alight to the accompaniment of hisses and boos and then – according to accounts in different newspapers – either hanged it on a lamp-post overlooking the Thames or threw it into the river. Traffic was brought to a standstill and passers-by took shelter, while the police attempted in vain to control the situation. The students then marched to Guy's Hospital and stormed its gate, before finally being persuaded to disperse.[28]

Over the next few days, there were other demonstrations, sometimes quite ugly, by angry students, chanting and carrying poles bearing figures of brown dogs. The antivivisectionists also held rallies for their cause. At one such rally held in London's famous Caxton Hall, Miss Lind af Hageby affirmed the truth of the statue's inscription, some-one else called the Brown Dog story a lie, and the meeting was then interrupted when a band of medical students broke into the hall, shouted down the speakers, and sang "Rule Britannia" until the meeting broke up in disorder. The students then marched in procession to Trafalgar Square, singing "Little Brown Dog" until dispersed by "a posse of constables."[29] More demonstrations and near-riots followed, as much against the fines imposed on the students who had damaged the memorial as against the memorial itself.

Medical students were joined in their protests by other students, and it became increasingly clear that the offending monument, or at the very least its inflammatory inscription, would have to come down. However, the antivivisection societies, certain trade unions, many of the working-class youths of Battersea, and some local politicians insisted that the memorial remain, even though the cost of its protection by six police constables was about seven hundred pounds annually. The cost was such that questions were raised in parliament, but Mr. Herbert Gladstone, the home secretary and youngest son of William Gladstone, could see no immediate solution, finding no reason to introduce legislation concerning the erection of controversial monuments or the cost of their protection.[30]

The controversy continued for many months, showing no sign of going away. Then in March 1910, after the election of a new local council, the statue was quietly removed by council workers during the early hours of the morning in the presence of a strong police detachment, despite objections and rallies of support for the little brown dog. After various legal challenges, the council had it destroyed in the hope of putting the matter finally to rest. In 1985, however, a new memorial to the brown dog was unveiled in Battersea Park. It was removed in 1992 – to be restored two years later following agitation by antivivisectionists. It remains a silent and little noticed memorial to an unsettled national controversy.

Horsley and Hadwen: A Curious Correspondence

The year 1908 saw many startling happenings. At the end of June a meteor that exploded high above the ground flattened some eighty million trees over eight hundred square miles in Siberia (the Tunguska event). The night sky glowed for several days with an unusual brightness visible even in England and Western Europe. Panicked people thought the world was ending. London that summer was hosting the Olympic Games, the highlight of which was the marathon, run on a very hot day from Windsor Castle to the new White City stadium. Several runners collapsed with the heat. Dorando Pietri of Italy was the first to enter the stadium, but he tottered in the wrong direction and then stumbled several times as he staggered on, still in the lead; when finally he fell forward close to the finishing line, an official helped him to the tape. Pietri, though disqualified because of this assistance, became an instant hero because of his courage and was presented with a special gilded silver cup by Queen Alexandra.

Despite these and many other newsworthy events, space was found in the columns of the *Daily Mail* to publish in September a rather strange series of letters between Horsley and, supposedly, Walter R. Hadwen, a medical man who opposed vaccination and was an honorary secretary of the British Union for the Abolition of Vivisection. It began when, in response to the query of another reader, the newspaper published a letter from Horsley on the part played by experiments on animals in relieving suffering. Hadwen felt obliged to respond, countering Horsley's comments. The series of letters that followed was very wide-ranging, with Hadwen seeming to dispute the germ theory of disease and the concept of antisepsis, unable to accept that tuberculosis was caused by an infective organism, and disparaging Pasteur's work on rabies. Horsley attempted, apparently unsuccessfully, to fill "all the hiatuses in Dr. Hadwen's medical education,"[31] but the columns of a newspaper were not the place to do so, and the editor soon brought matters to a halt. The abolitionists then published the correspondence in a twenty-page pamphlet, including the "suppressed" (unpublished) letters of Hadwen.[32]

In January 1909, a short unsigned note in the *Daily Mail* stated simply that the correspondence had actually been between Horsley and Coleridge, Hadwen being "merely an intervener."[33] If correct, the reason that Coleridge chose this means of communication is unclear. Perhaps he could not resist the opportunity to challenge Horsley but felt that people had heard enough from him already. It is also unclear why Hadwen agreed to serve as an intermediary and who it was that revealed his role in the correspondence.

The Royal Commission

In 1906 a Second Royal Commission on Vivisection was appointed. With this in mind, a meeting was held of delegates from various interested medical and scientific societies, and a committee was formed, with Starling as chairman, to organize the presentation of evidence concerning the history and value of experiments on living animals. For two days in November 1907, Horsley appeared before the commission as a witness representing the British Medical Association, during which time he emphasized the value of animal experimentation both in advancing medical knowledge and practice and as a means of teaching students the essentials of physiology, pathology, pharmacology, and surgery.[34] He believed that knowledge of pathology was best acquired by experimental work on the living rather than through morbid anatomy. For example, he held that the subject of inflammation should be taught by causing inflammation experimentally so that it could be studied in a living animal.[35] Horsley even submitted to the commission drafts of an application form that he suggested could be used by those requesting a license to perform experiments on living animals and another for annual reporting of the experiments so performed.[36]

Coleridge, in giving evidence to the commission before Horsley, took the opportunity to single out the experiments performed in Horsley's laboratory at University College for particular criticism. The young George Crile (see p. 91) had worked there in 1895, studying surgical shock induced in anesthetized dogs by a variety of injuries and surgical procedures that included crush injuries of the paws or testicles, surgical amputations, and nerve and brain injuries. The work, which Crile continued over the following two years in Cleveland and won for him an award,[37] was described by Coleridge as "repulsive" and "loathsome," causing "disgust and horror" to decent people. Some of Crile's dogs were said to be in a state of "incomplete anesthesia," Coleridge went on accusingly, taking this to mean that they could feel pain when the procedures were performed. As was his wont, he then proceeded to attack Horsley more directly.[38]

Horsley, in turn, explained that he had suggested to Crile the need to know more about the condition of the circulation during and after injuries or surgical procedures in humans, and that the experiments in dogs were performed with this in mind and to test various possible remedies for circulatory collapse. The crush injuries of the paws, for example, were performed to simulate the operation of tarsectomy as performed in humans. As for "incomplete anesthesia," this was synonymous with "light anesthesia" – it did not mean that the animal could feel pain but simply that certain reflex movements were preserved in the unconscious animal. Horsley took great trouble to clarify these various issues for the commissioners, even though he had gone over them with Coleridge on several occasions in the past, for example in correspondence published in *The Times* in 1902.[39]

Horsley also pointed out to the members of the commission that Coleridge had charged government "officials with placing a certain vivisector [namely, Horsley] ... beyond the reach of the safeguards erected by the Act ... by giving him permission to vivisect in private places, thereby placing him beyond the possibility of legal inspection." Aware of Coleridge's malicious misrepresentations and refusal to correct false statements, Horsley explained the circumstances. In late 1893, he had been given leave by government officials to inoculate blood from a patient with filariasis into two monkeys. Filariasis is a disease caused by certain roundworms that release their embryos into the blood stream, where they are taken up by a blood-sucking mosquito to be passed on to another host. Because the living embryos are present in the blood mainly at night, the inoculation had to be done at a time when laboratories are generally closed. Accordingly Sir Patrick Manson, the parasitologist who had requested the inoculation, brought the patient to Horsley's private house for this purpose. No embryos were present in the blood, however, and the experiment therefore ended before it could start, with no inoculations being performed. Horsley affirmed that he otherwise had never done any experiments on animals at his home or in an unregistered place, and had received no preferential treatment from the government.[40] He had certainly never received "unrestricted leave to do experiments when I liked, where I liked, and what I liked," as Coleridge had alleged.

The royal commission published its findings in 1912 and required no fundamental alterations in the approach to vivisection, making only some minor administrative and restrictive changes. Experimentation on living animals, it concluded, is morally justifiable and, with certain safeguards, should not be prohibited by legislation.

As for Starling's committee, it dissolved itself after all the evidence had been presented to the commission and after creating in 1908 a Research Defence Society to oppose the antivivisection movements and publicize the benefits of experiments on animals. From the outset, Horsley stressed the need for the new society to include as many members of the lay public as possible.[41] Membership was open to anyone on payment of a small annual subscription (five shillings). Many distinguished scientists, physicians, and surgeons joined the new society, as also did members of the aristocracy, parliament, church, and universities, as well as writers and artists. Its inaugural president was the earl of Cromer. Horsley's wife Eldred was to become a member of its management committee and – some years after his death – the honorary secretary (1920) and then honorary treasurer of the society (1921–1928). The society continued for one hundred years and then merged in 2008 with the Coalition for Medical Progress to form a new advocacy group. Its aims are to support ethical and humane research involving living animals so that the medical and biological sciences can continue to advance.

Notes

1. Kean H: The 'smooth cool men of science': The feminist and socialist response to vivisection. *Hist Workshop J* 1995; **40**: 16–38.

2. Anon: Editorial [Bayliss v. Coleridge]. *The Times (Lond)*, November 19, 1903, p. 9.

3. Anon: The West London Hospital and the National Anti-Vivisection Society. *Lancet* 1899; **154**: 427–428.

4. Horsley V: Surgery and vivisection. [Letter to the editor.] *The Times (Lond)*, January 16, 1885, p. 7.

5. Cobbe FP: Surgery and vivisection [Letter to the editor.] *The Times (Lond)*, January 22, 1885, p. 6.

6. Rhodes GM: *The Nine Circles of the Hell of the Innocent: Described from the Reports of the Presiding Spirits.* Sonnenschein: London, 1892.

7. Cobbe FP: Preface. pp. vii–xv. In: Rhodes GM : *The Nine Circles of the Hell of the Innocent: Described from the Reports of the Presiding Spirits.* Sonnenschein: London, 1892.

8. Anon: The church congress. *The Times (Lond)*, October 7, 1892, p. 6.

9. Anon: The Church Congress. The utility and morality of experiments on living animals. *Br Med J* 1892; **2**: 817–819.

10. Horsley V: Mr. Victor Horsley and Miss Cobbe. [Letter to the editor.] *The Times (Lond)*, October 12, 1892, p. 12.

11. Cobbe FP: Mr. Victor Horsley and Miss Cobbe [Letter to the editor.] *The Times (Lond)*, October 15, 1892, p. 12.

12. Horsley V: Mr. Victor Horsley and Miss Cobbe. [Letter to the editor.] *The Times (Lond)*, October 17, 1892, p. 7.

13. Horsley V: Professor Horsley and Miss Cobbe. [Letter to the editor.] *The Times (Lond)*, October 20, 1892, p. 14.

14. Barry A: Professor Horsley and Miss Cobbe [Letter to the editor.] *The Times (Lond)*, October 24, 1892, p. 11.

15. Barry A: Miss Cobbe's "Nine Circles" [Letter to the editor.] *The Times (Lond)*, October 27, 1892, p. 12.

16. Tait L: Experiments on living animals. [Letter to the editor.] *The Times (Lond)*, November 8, 1892, pp. 3–4.

17. Anon: The vivisector's battle. Prof. Horsley's laboratory for studying the live beast. *N Y Times*, October 30, 1892, p. 1.

18. Lind af Hageby L, Schartau LK: *The Shambles of Science: Extracts from the Diary of Two Students of Physiology*. Bell: London, 1903.

19. Anon: Bayliss v. Coleridge. *Lancet* 1903; 162: 1445–1446.

20. Anon: £2,000 Damages. Result of the vivisection libel case. Excitement in court. *Daily Mail (Lond)*, November 19, 1903, p. 3.

21. Anon: High Court of Justice. King's Bench Division. (Before the Lord Chief Justice and a special jury.) Bayliss v. Coleridge. *The Times (Lond)*, November 12, 1903, p. 13.

22. Henderson J: *A Life of Ernest Starling*. p. 63. Oxford University Press: New York, 2005.

23. Anon: High Court of Justice. King's Bench Division. Bayliss v. Coleridge. *The Times (Lond)*, November 12, 1903, p. 13; November 14, 1903, p. 6; November 18, 1903, p. 3; November 19, 1903, p. 3.

24. Anon: Vivisection of dogs. Eminent scientists in the law courts. Experiments described. *Daily Mail (Lond)*, November 14, 1903, p. 3; Vivisection of dogs. Evidence of the Swedish lady students. *ibid* November 18, 1903, p. 3; £2,000 Damages. Result of the vivisection libel case. Excitement in court. *ibid* November 19, 1903, p. 3; The outlook. An exemplary verdict. *Ibid* November 19, 1903, p. 4.

25. Emanuel W: The anti-vivisection case. [Letter to the editor.] *Daily Mail (Lond)*, November 28, 1903, p. 4.

26. Hempsons, Solicitors for Dr. W. M Bayliss: "Bayliss v. Coleridge." [Letter to the editor.] *The Times (Lond)*, November 30, 1903, p. 12.

27. Mason P: *The Brown Dog Affair: The Story of a Monument that Divided a Nation*. Two Sevens Publishing: London, 1997.

28. Anon: Tumult in London. Medical students stop traffic in the Strand. *Daily Mail (Lond)*, November 23, 1907, p. 7.

29. Anon: Uproarious students. Anti-vivisectionist's "Brown Dog" challenge. *Daily Mail (Lond)*, December 17, 1907, p. 3.

30. Anon: House of Commons. The Brown Dog. *The Times (Lond)*, February 7, 1908, p. 9.

31. Horsley V: Experiments on animals. Sir Victor Horsley's reply to criticism. [Letter to the editor.] *Daily Mail (Lond)*, September 15, 1908, p. 8.

32. Horsley V, Hadwen WR: *A Correspondence in "The Daily Mail" between Sir Victor Horsley and Dr. Walter R. Hadwen on Vivisection, September 1908: Suppressed Letters*. British Union for the Abolition of Vivisection: London, 1908.

33. Anon: Vivisection. *Daily Mail (Lond)*, January 16, 1909, p. 2.

34. Horsley V: Witness testimony, November 13, 1907. pp. 118–149. In: *Royal Commission on Vivisection. Appendix to Fourth Report of the Commissioners. Minutes of Evidence, October to December, 1907*. His Majesty's Stationery Office: London, 1908.

35. Crile G: *George Crile: An Autobiography*. p. 68. Lippincott: Philadelphia, 1947.

36. Horsley V: Appendix A: Forms I. and II. pp. 308–310. In: *Royal Commission on Vivisection. Appendix to Fourth Report of the Commissioners. Minutes of Evidence, October to December, 1907*. His Majesty's Stationery Office: London, 1908.

37. Crile G: *George Crile: An Autobiography*. pp. 74–75. Lippincott: Philadelphia, 1947.

38. Coleridge S: Witness testimony: June 19, June 26, July 3, 1907. pp. 143–207. In: *Royal Commission on Vivisection. Appendix to Third Report of the Commissioners. Minutes of Evidence, April to July, 1907*. His Majesty's Stationery Office: London, 1907.

39. Horsley V: Anti-vivisection methods. [Letter to the editor.] *The Times (Lond)*, March 12, 1902, p. 12 and March 20, 1902, p. 12.

40. Horsley V: Witness testimony, November 13, 1907. pp. 128–129. In: *Royal Commission on Vivisection. Appendix to Fourth Report of the Commissioners. Minutes of Evidence, October to December, 1907*. His Majesty's Stationery Office: London, 1908.

41. Horsley V: Letter to Schäfer E, dated February 1908, cited by Paget S : *Sir Victor Horsley: A Study of His Life and Work*. p. 188. Constable: London, 1919.

Chapter 12

Bitter Tears: Horsley and the Suffragist Movement

Although many women did not work outside the home in late Victorian and Edwardian Britain, more options than domestic service, factory work, or nursing were becoming available for those seeking a job. Shop assistants and clerical workers were in demand, and new opportunities had arisen in teaching and a few other professions. By 1901, for example, there were more than two hundred female doctors, almost a tenfold increase over the number twenty years earlier. Nevertheless, women continued to face disadvantages and prejudices. They therefore agitated for greater involvement in public affairs, the right to vote in parliamentary elections, and to receive the same pay as men for equal work. Both Eldred and Victor Horsley shared these wishes, although Eldred may well have influenced the extent and intensity of her husband's views.[1] Victor became involved in supporting the suffragists to an extent that involved him in controversy with professional colleagues and the government, and contributed to his failed attempt to be elected to parliament (Chapter 10). It was thought – wrongly as it happened – that he supported the lawless methods adopted by some of the more activist suffragists. In fact, he simply agreed with their beliefs and held that they should be treated with dignity and respect by the authorities.

A number of local societies and associations had been formed in the latter half of the nineteenth century to advance women's rights, but despite greater public awareness of the issues, little was gained. Some of these local organizations subsequently amalgamated, and in 1903 the steely Mrs. Emmeline Pankhurst and her daughter Christabel founded the Women's Social and Political Union. The Pankhursts soon decided that more militant strategies by "suffragettes" were required to achieve their aims.* The resulting civil

---

* A journalist of the *Daily Mail* newspaper coined the term "suffragettes" to refer to these activists, but it is avoided here because it is sometimes taken to be derogatory.

unrest summarized here focuses on the context of Horsley's involvement, and is not intended to be a history of the suffragist movement in Britain.

In addition to speaking at street corners and holding rallies, demonstrations, and protest marches, militant activists began heckling public speakers, chaining themselves to railings, and vandalizing property. Initially they focused on government buildings, but later they attacked private property, smashing shop windows and setting fire to letter boxes and then the houses of the wealthy, as well as public buildings such as schools and churches. They targeted unoccupied premises wherever possible, to avoid harming individuals. They managed to pour flour over the head of the prime minister, H. H. Asquith, from the visitors' gallery at the House of Commons, and smashed two of the windows at his official Downing Street residence. The chancellor of the exchequer, David Lloyd George, fared even worse, for in February 1913 activists planted a bomb in a country house being built for him and destroyed several rooms. A few months later, a suffragist named Emily Davison died after running in front of the king's horse at the Epsom Derby.

When caught, these activists were imprisoned. Under the Prison Act of 1898, the courts had the power to classify prisoners into three divisions based on type of offence and the offender's record, and this affected the conditions of their confinement. The suffragists were not regarded as first-division (political) prisoners and thus did not receive the better treatment reserved for such prisoners.[2] They protested by going on hunger strike. The government, concerned that death would make martyrs of them and cause a public scandal, tried feeding them forcibly. Forcible feeding had become common in mental institutions, where psychiatric patients were deemed to have lost their reasoning ability, but the same could not be said of the suffragists, who regarded it as punishment and a form of torture. In these circumstances, the procedure raised ethical issues about the role of doctors and their duty to nonconsenting, uncooperative, but sane prisoner-patients. There were also safety concerns. The struggling suffragist had to be held down by several wardresses while a rubber tube was inserted into the stomach through the nose or, after the mouth had been forcibly opened with a wooden or steel gag, through the throat. A liquid, such as a mix of milk and raw eggs, was then poured quickly into a funnel and down the tube. Retching and choking, bruised and sometimes bleeding, the helpless woman was left covered in vomit and sometimes went on to develop an aspiration pneumonia that could be life threatening.

Horsley strongly disapproved of the militant methods of the suffragists but, equally, was opposed to feeding them forcibly when they were on hunger strike – he believed this was a travesty of medical care and that the underlying motive was to punish them. In October 1909, Horsley and one hundred and fifteen other doctors, the majority of them women, wrote to the prime minister and members of his cabinet about the dangers and brutality of the procedure.[3] Horsley was one of the prime movers and his is the first signature on the memorandum, requesting that the practice of forcibly feeding suffragist prisoners should be stopped. Over the next few weeks, a lively discussion on the issues took place in the correspondence columns of the newspapers and the *British Medical Journal* (summarized elsewhere[4]).

Leigh versus Gladstone

Two months later, before the lord chief justice of England and a special jury, Mrs. Marie (or Mary) Leigh, a working-class woman from the midlands – and one of the first of the suffragists to be forcibly fed – sued Herbert Gladstone, the home secretary, as well as the governor and medical officer of the Winson Green Prison in Birmingham, for assault in feeding her against her will. She sought a restraining order to prevent repetition of such assaults. She had been sentenced to four months' imprisonment with hard labor for disturbing a meeting at which Mr. Asquith was speaking and then resisting arrest, and had previously been

convicted for throwing a stone through the prime minister's window. She objected to being treated as a criminal rather than political offender, however, and thus went on the hunger strike that led to her being fed forcibly through the mouth or nose, sometimes three times daily, for several weeks until her early release. Weak, starving, and ill, she was set free without even the means to get home, and was taken to a nursing home where she recovered.

Horsley appeared as a medical witness but, surprisingly given his previous experience as a medicolegal consultant, did the case more harm than good. He told the court that in hospitals, feeding through the nose was uncommon and to be avoided as far as possible because it caused depression and other complications, such as the passage of food into the airways. Unaccountably, he then added that "the usual method [of feeding in hospitals] was through the bowels," a comment that Lord Alverstone, the judge, interpreted as a suggestion to prison officials and one which no jury would have ever sanctioned.[5] Further, Horsley agreed that, in order to preserve life, he would not hesitate to feed forcibly a patient who was refusing to take food. The government's defence was that the assault was committed to save Leigh's life, and the court decided that there was indeed a legal duty for the authorities "to keep alive those in their charge." The fact that Leigh had refused food for only three days when the feeding commenced, and that her life was therefore not in jeopardy, was quietly ignored.

Accordingly, the question posed to the jury was whether the means adopted were appropriate for this purpose. It took them two minutes to decide that they were, and a precedent was set for the continuation of forcible feeding of the suffragists.[6] Meanwhile, Horsley wrote to *The Times*, explaining that he was against any form of forcible feeding of suffragists and that the lord chief justice had misconstrued the remarks he had made in court.[7,8] Nevertheless, they were picked up by others, including Bryan Donkin, consulting physician to the Westminster hospital and a commissioner of prisons,[9] and mockingly by Charles Mercier, a psychiatrist.[10] In his enthusiastic rejection of the forcible feeding of suffragists, Horsley had put his foot in his mouth by his ill-considered and contradictory statements in court. He did not come out looking good.

Forcible Feeding and Its Consequences

Forcible feeding continued, but adverse publicity led the government to consider other strategies. Winston Churchill, who in February 1910 became home secretary in Asquith's Liberal government, introduced Rule 243A, which allowed certain second- or third-division prisoners, who ordinarily were kept under harsher conditions, to receive first-division privileges without having the status of political prisoners. The hunger strikes stopped and did not resume until 1912, when political status again became an issue.[4]

In 1912, Reginald McKenna, an urbane and meticulous bureaucrat who had succeeded Churchill as home secretary, received a memorandum from Horsley and others, reiterating the points made previously. In his response, he claimed that he had also received a letter signed by various unnamed medical dignitaries indicating that forcible feeding was "neither dangerous nor painful." After pointing out the several inconsistencies in his statement in a letter published in the medical journals,[11] Horsley – together with Agnes Savill, a Harley Street dermatologist, and Charles Mansell Moullin, a general surgeon – decided to examine the issue for themselves. They considered the statements of one hundred and two suffrage prisoners, of whom ninety had undergone forcible feeding, examined a large number personally after their release from jail, and communicated with the doctors of those who required medical care upon release. They reported a variety of physical and psychological effects, not only from the forcible feeding but in many cases also from having been in solitary confinement and from "the mental anguish caused by hearing the cries, choking, and struggles of their friends" as they were fed against their will. Most had evidence of "neurasthenia," which, from the description provided, today would be labeled as post-traumatic stress disorder. Local injuries to the tissues of the nose and throat were common.[12]

This study seems to have been the first serious attempt to examine the effects of forcible feeding but, despite the findings, the medical establishment chose to regard the issue as a political rather than a medical one. A lengthy correspondence was published in the British Medical Journal, much of it hostile to the suffragists or objecting to the use of a medical journal to air political views, although a few correspondents wondered about the utility or ethics of forcible feeding.[13] Charles Mercier, the forensic psychiatrist who had opposed Horsley on a similar issue in 1909, actually authored a satirical piece parodying the Horsley study, suggesting that the forcible bathing of prisoners was dangerous.[14] Mercier, despite being in constant pain from osteitis deformans, had a sparkling wit and a caustic pen, which he could use to great effect. Nevertheless, many doctors gradually became more accepting of Horsley's views about forcible feeding, while rejecting the suffragists and their cause.

It was the disruptive actions of the suffragists that a large segment of the public found difficult to accept, although some were vigorously opposed to the very idea of women's suffrage. Among the latter was Sir Almroth Wright (1861–1947), a noted immunologist and a founder of modern vaccine therapy who, in a lengthy letter published in The Times in March 1912, argued that they did not merit the vote. "To give the vote to women is to give it to voters who as a class are quite incompetent to adjudicate upon political issues," he opined,[15] but without rhyme or reason. A Conciliation Bill, extending the franchise to women of certain means, was having its second reading in parliament at the time, and his letter may well have helped its narrow defeat.[16] In 1913 he authored The Unexpurgated Case Against Woman Suffrage, claiming preposterously that women have a physical, intellectual, and moral "disability" that renders them unfit for the vote.[17] He concluded that a "failure to recognise that man is the master, and why he is the master, lies at the root of the suffrage movement." No justification was provided for his beliefs, which he expressed as facts and which – if they had represented a common viewpoint – almost provided a justification for the militancy to which the suffragists were driven. Horsley described these beliefs as "most repulsive in the debased picture they present of women in her relation to man,"[18] in a letter that he, in turn, wrote to The Times in response to Wright's letter. Elizabeth Garrett Anderson (1836–1917) – the first qualified woman to practice medicine in Britain and after whom a London hospital was named – wrote to Horsley thanking him for having done so, declaiming that Wright ought to be "hounded out of the profession" and, somewhat curiously, questioning whether he was "a Turk" as his name (Almroth) had "an Eastern note."[19]

The Lilian Lenton Case

On February 20, 1913, Lilian Lenton was charged with setting fire to a building in Kew Gardens, and remanded to Holloway Prison, a fortress-like structure in north London, where she went on an immediate hunger strike. After three days, she was fed forcibly by a tube that was passed through her nose despite her violent struggles. Two to three hours later, she collapsed and – weak and starving – was released from the prison in case she died on the premises. She had developed an aspiration pneumonia. The prison authorities and doctors now denied that she had aspirated, claiming that she had experienced episodic chest pain and shortness of breath for some months before she was jailed.

This prompted a letter to *The Times* in which Savill, Mansell Moullin, and Horsley charged that the home secretary, McKenna, had deliberately misled the public and parliament by issuing a statement on the matter in which no mention was made of Miss Lenton being forcibly fed or that this resulted in her subsequent decline until she was "in imminent danger of death." Instead, they pointed out, her collapse was attributed by McKenna to her self-inflicted hunger strike.[20] McKenna, in turn, claimed that it was Horsley's account that was misleading and that he was in no position to contradict statements made by the prison doctors who had been directly involved in her care. The correspondence became increasingly bizarre, Horsley quoting the home secretary's words as published in *Hansard*, and McKenna and his assistants denying that these were his words or suggesting that they were taken out of context.[21] Horsley continued: "If you wish to suggest that your quoted words do not convey what they appear to do, I must require you to forward me as soon as possible what you consider them to mean."[22]

The home secretary angrily wrote to the Royal College of Surgeons, claiming that statements made by Horsley and Mansell Moullin – both of whom were fellows of the college – reflected seriously and unjustly on the professional conduct and skill of the two involved prison medical officers, and enclosing copies of all the correspondence.[23] McKenna refused, however, to communicate his complaint, or even the gist of it, to Horsley himself, as he stated when questioned by Lord Robert Cecil in parliament.[24] Horsley was also unable initially to obtain any information from the college.

He eventually complained publicly about this secrecy "as a citizen of a country which prides itself on the fact that every one who is accused is entitled to know at once exactly what charges are made against him with a view to being enabled to reply to them should he wish to do so."[25] He believed passionately that "unanswered slanders should not be bandied about secretly ... and concealed from the accused persons."[26] It was only after repeated inquiries that the correspondence of the home office eventually was published as a parliamentary white paper, and then quite probably in the hope that it would reflect badly on Horsley.[23]

Horsley's protests eventually led the president of the Royal College of Surgeons – Rickman Godlee, his former colleague and the man who had first operated on a brain tumor in 1884 – to respond. He let it be known that the college council was unable to resolve the ethical issues raised by the home secretary because the evidence was conflicting, and therefore that the college would take no further action. In such circumstances, Godlee explained, the college was under no obligation to reveal the specifics of the complaint but, as a courtesy, had finally given Horsley access to the relevant documents and told him the substance of its response to the home secretary.[27] It is possible, however, that the college council's decision may have related to fear of Horsley, who was even then trying to reform it so that it was more representative of the membership. At the same time, the reluctance of the council and its president even to speak with him about the matter until he forced the issue may also have related to their animosity towards him because of his support of the National Insurance Bill, discussed in Chapter 10.

Whither Forcible Feeding?

In 1913, to counter the adverse publicity that forcible feeding had generated, the government passed the Prisoners (Temporary Discharge for Ill-Health) Act. Suffragists on hunger strike were no longer to be fed against their will but, once weakened and ill from starvation, were to be released from prison. As soon as they had recovered, they would be re-arrested and returned to prison, the process being repeated as often as necessary until their sentences were served. This seemingly adroit legal maneuver to deal with hunger strikers became widely known as the Cat and Mouse Act, but it led to further problems when temporarily released suffragists eluded re-arrest and gained public sympathy by appearing to have been tortured or persecuted by the authorities.

In 1914, Frank Moxon, an eye doctor who was disturbed at the silence of leaders of the medical profession, provided a horrifying account of the medical aspects of forcible feeding that drew on the experience of several suffragists. He argued that the prison doctors were violating their professional ethics by forcing unwanted treatments on their charges because of government pressure.[28] Other accounts followed. But even as feelings escalated concerning the suffragists' cause and government's response in the context of an ever-increasing spiral of civil disobedience, retaliatory imprisonment, defiant hunger-strikes, and release and re-arrest under the Cat and Mouse Act, other events were occurring that were to lead to a world war.

With the outbreak of hostilities, Emmeline Pankhurst ordered a stop to further acts of defiance and the government ordered the unconditional release of all imprisoned suffragists. She and her daughter Christabel now returned to England from France, where they had fled to avoid the reach of the authorities. They returned home even as civil unrest ceased, young men queued up to enlist, and many thousands of British soldiers were ferried across the channel to serve under the command of Field Marshall Sir John French, the brother of a leading suffragist and pacifist, in the war to end all wars. Like so many other suffragists, in the months that followed they lent their aid to the war effort, becoming active in recruitment campaigns and rallies. Women now gathered to hand out white feathers to shame young men who had not signed up for military service, and to demand war-work and the chance to fill the jobs of those who had enlisted.

It was not until 1918 – as the war drew to its close in a devastated continent, as revolution added to the chaos and influenza to the death toll – that women over the age of thirty finally obtained the right to vote in Britain, and then only if they met certain property and other requirements. In the same year, women gained the right to stand for election to parliament. Ten years later, the voting right was extended to all women over the age of twenty-one, regardless of property requirements. Men and women finally had the vote on equal terms. The forcible feeding of mentally competent prisoners on voluntary hunger strike remains a contentious issue, but it is generally regarded as medically unethical and a contravention of international human rights laws.

Notes

1. Walshe FMR: Personal communication, July 15, 1966.

2. Purvis J: The prison experiences of the suffragettes in Edwardian Britain. *Women's Hist Rev* 1995; **4**: 103–133.

3. Horsley V, 115 others: The dangers of forcible feeding. Opinions of medical experts. Memorial signed by one hundred and sixteen doctors. *Votes for Women (Lond)*, October 8, 1909, p. 19.

4. Geddes JF: Culpable complicity: The medical profession and the forcible feeding of suffragettes, 1909-1914. *Women's Hist Rev* 2008; **17**: 79–94.

5. Anon: High Court of Justice. King's Bench Division. Before the Lord Chief Justice of England and a special jury. Leigh v. Gladstone and others. Feeding by force: Suffragist's action. *The Times (Lond)*, December 10, 1909, p. 3.

6. Raeburn A: *The Militant Suffragettes.* p. 132. Joseph: London, 1973.

7. Horsley V: Forcible feeding. Leigh v. Gladstone and others. [Letter to the editor.] *The Times (Lond)*, December 11, 1909, p. 4.

8. Horsley V: Forcible feeding. [Letters to the editor.] *The Times (Lond)*, December 18, 1909, p. 12; December 21, 1909, p. 10; December 23, 1909, p. 8.

9. Donkin HB: Forcible feeding. [Letters to the editor.] *The Times (Lond)*, December 18, 1909, p 12; December 22, 1909, p. 8.

10. Mercier C: Forcible feeding. [Letters to the editor.] *The Times (Lond)*, December 15, 1909, p. 12; December 17, 1909, p. 10; December 23, 1909, p. 8; December 24, 1909, p. 8.

11. Savill A, Mansell Moullin C, Horsley V: Forcible feeding. [Letter to the editor.] *Br Med J* 1912; **2**: 100–101, 151.

12. Savill AF, Mansell Moullin CW, Horsley V: Preliminary report on the forcible feeding of suffrage prisoners. *Lancet* 1912; **180**: 549–551; *Br Med J* 1912; **2**: 505–508.

13. Various authors: Forcible feeding of suffrage prisoners. [Letters to the editor.] *Br Med J* 1912; **2**: 659–661.

14. Mercier C: Preliminary report on the forcible bathing of prisoners. *Lancet* 1912; **180**: 801–802.

15. Wright AE: Suffrage fallacies. Sir Almroth Wright on militant hysteria. [Letter to the editor.] *The Times (Lond)*, March 28, 1912, pp. 7–8.

16. Cope Z: Wright's views on feminism. pp. 140–143. In: *Almroth Wright: Founder of Modern Vaccine-Therapy*. Nelson: London, 1966.

17. Wright AE: *The Unexpurgated Case Against Woman Suffrage*. Hoeber: New York, 1913.

18. Horsley V: Sir Almroth Wright's letter. Reply by Sir Victor Horsley. [Letter to the editor.] *The Times (Lond)*, April 1, 1912, p. 6.

19. Garrett Anderson E: Letter to Sir Victor Horsley dated April 1, 1912. Section C6, Horsley Papers, Special Collections, UCL Library Services (London, UK).

20. Savill A, Mansell Moullin C, Horsley V: The case of Miss Lenton. [Letter to the editor.] *The Times (Lond)*, March 18, 1913, p. 6.

21. Case of Miss Lilian Lenton. Correspondence of the Home Office with the Royal College of Surgeons and Sir Victor Horsley with regard to the case of Lilian Lenton. II. – Correspondence of the Home Office with Sir Victor Horsley. *Lancet* 1913; **181**: 192–193.

22. Horsley V: Letter to the Secretary of State, dated May 14, 1913. Reprinted in *Lancet* 1913; **181**: 192.

23. *Correspondence of the Home Office with the Royal College of Surgeons and Sir Victor Horsley with Regard to the Case of Lilian Lenton.* His Majesty's Stationery Office: London, 1913. Reprinted in *Lancet* 1913; **181**: 189–193.

24. Anon: Medical notes in parliament. Sir Victor Horsley. *Br Med J* 1913; **1**: 1293.

25. Horsley V: A constitutional point. [Letter to the editor.] *Br Med J* 1913; **1**: 1299.

26. Horsley V: A constitutional point. [Letter to the editor.] *Br Med J* 1913; **2**: 48–49.

27. Godlee RJ: A constitutional point. [Letter to the editor.] *Br Med J* 1913; **1**: 1351; Sir Victor Horsley and Mr. McKenna. [Letter to the editor] *Lancet* 1913; **181**: 1762.

28. Moxon F: *What Forcible Feeding Means.* The Women's Press: London, 1914.

Chapter 13

Last Orders: The Temperance Movement

In 1911, when the *Daily Mail* announced that Horsley had won the international Lallelongue Prize for surgery, it added a personal anecdote. At his club, a friend had asked him whether he could say what whisky was. "Certainly," remarked Sir Victor, "it is the most popular poison in the world."[1] Horsley is remembered for his strong views on alcohol and for his monumental row about its effects with Karl Pearson, a man who was as fond of controversy and as outspoken as Horsley. Pearson, professor of applied mathematics (and later the first Galton professor of eugenics) at University College, had established there a biometrics laboratory and the Francis Galton Laboratory for National Eugenics and was interested in the relative importance of heredity and environmental factors in evolution.

Contemporary Beliefs on the Alcohol Problem

Pubs, taverns, and alehouses had an important social role in Victorian Britain, especially for the working and lower middle classes who gathered there for warmth, companionship, and good cheer. Alcohol was also important in the lives of other classes. Naval personnel received a daily rum ration, and the well-to-do took alcohol liberally with meals and at social events in their homes and exclusive clubs. Students were known for their drinking prowess, and among them the ability to consume large quantities of alcohol was often seen as a sign of manliness. Everywhere, it seemed, alcohol was an important social catalyst, serving to initiate or cement friendships.

The health benefits and problems associated with alcohol consumption were unclear even in the early twentieth century. The published evidence was contradictory and could be used to support or challenge almost any medical or social belief. Many held that alcoholism was an important cause of madness, as well as of crime, poverty,

unemployment, and illness, and that it could cause heritable degenerative physical and mental conditions.[2] As the consumption of alcohol, and particularly of spirits such as cheap gin, had increased over the years, drunkenness had increased with it. Because drunkenness was common among the insane, alcohol came to be regarded by a twist of logic as a common cause of insanity, especially as both drunkenness and insanity were characterized by irrational behavior, violence, and "immorality."[3] Even so, others believed that alcohol was a food, a medicine and restorative, and even a cure for insanity.[3]

The situation was even stranger with regard to the possible effects of alcohol on the next generation. Some doctors did not hesitate to prescribe alcohol to treat the morning sickness of pregnancy and certain other gestational complaints,[4] but insobriety in women was blamed as a cause of infant mortality. Advocates of temperance believed that alcohol was also a cause of physical "degeneration" in the offspring of heavy drinkers, leading to a higher prevalence of epilepsy and "idiocy" through unknown mechanisms, although it was equally plausible that these were hereditary disorders unrelated to alcohol intake. Taking it one step further, some held that alcohol caused the physical deterioration (or so-called racial degeneration) that made many recruits unfit for military service during the Boer War (see Chapter 10). Finally, there were concerns that the next generation would have a particular fondness for alcohol, either on a hereditary basis or because of the example set by alcoholic parents.

Horsley's Views on Alcohol

Horsley had been opposed to alcohol and tobacco use since his student days, but was very partial to sweets, which he consumed in great quantities. Although he did not drink alcohol himself, there was a time when he would take a bottle of wine on picnics for those of his companions who did not share his opinion.[5] Nevertheless, his views evolved until he came to consider that anyone who had taken a drink was necessarily drunk, and he became increasingly involved in lecturing about the ill effects of alcohol, in crusading for total abstinence, and in campaigning for government action to limit exposure to alcohol. In 1900 he was invited to give the second annual Lees and Raper Memorial Lecture, a lecture series devoted to the medical, legal, or economic aspects of the temperance movement. He discussed the slowing of various mental processes that occurs with even small quantities of alcohol, as well as the unsteadiness and slurred speech that relate to its effect on the cerebellum.[6]

Articulate, enthusiastic, and socially prominent, he was soon recruited to office in temperance organizations, bringing to them his scientific prestige. In 1892 he became a vice president of the National Temperance League, and then successively the president of the British Medical Temperance Association (1896), the International Association of Abstaining Physicians (1909),[7] and the National Temperance Federation of temperance associations and societies (1913). He was one of several doctors belonging to the Society for the Study of Inebriety[8] who endeavored to raise public awareness about the adverse effects of alcohol,[9,10] and particularly its effects on the developing fetus and on the children of parents who drank alcohol liberally. Their activities helped to reveal the extent of alcohol consumption, especially by working-class women who spent hours in pubs and alehouses, often accompanied by their babies and small children who would be pacified with sips of beer or weak gin.[11] They stressed that even the medicinal use of alcohol, as in treating fever, was ineffective and had been abandoned by the experts.[10]

These medical advocates of temperance included such leaders of the profession as Sir Thomas Barlow, later president of the Royal College of Physicians; Sir Thomas Clifford Allbutt, regius professor of physic at the University of Cambridge, inventor of the modern clinical thermometer, and later president of the British Medical Association; and Sir Lauder Brunton, who developed an effective treatment for angina pectoris. Together with Horsley, they urged that the teaching of general science in schools be revised to include the principles of hygiene and temperance, and that these topics therefore should be taught in all training colleges to student teachers.[12,13] Indeed, they formed part of a medical committee, established in 1903 under the chairmanship of Sir William Broadbent, a well-known physician, which obtained the supporting signatures of some fifteen thousand doctors in favor of these aims, gained the approval of the British Medical Association, and sent deputations to meet with the president of the board of education.[13] Although not incorporated into the national curriculum, many local schools did indeed go this far,[11] and the 1908 Children's Act finally restricted children from premises licensed to sell alcohol (see Chapter 10).

His views on alcohol brought out in Horsley attitudes that conflicted with his strong feminist views and sometimes led him to oppose the concept of equal opportunities for women. In February 1905, for example, he hosted a meeting of influential medical leaders opposed to the employment of young women in public bars.[14] His opposition related in part to concerns about exposing women of childbearing age to the temptations of alcohol when they might become pregnant or already have children at home, but also to concerns that a small quantity of alcohol might expose them to "vice" and to the "most loathsome diseases."[14]

In 1907 Horsley's book, *Alcohol and the Human Body*, was published.[15] Written with Mary Sturge, a physician, the book was quite successful and went into several editions, selling more than twenty thousand copies before Horsley's death. The first edition was written by the two of them mainly on Sunday afternoons in Horsley's drawing room, where a background of music and family chatter and the inevitably frequent interruptions made concentration difficult; revisions for subsequent editions were undertaken largely by Horsley alone. The book's theme was that alcohol is a drug and poison that affects the brain and other organs, even in small doses, and Horsley and Sturge detailed the various ill effects that result. Their views, however, were not universally accepted. Indeed, in 1907 a note was published in the *Lancet* that stated succinctly:

> As an article of diet we hold that the universal belief of civilised mankind that the moderate use of alcoholic beverages is, for adults, usually beneficial, is amply justified.

We deplore the evils arising from the abuse of alcoholic beverages. But it is obvious that there is nothing, however beneficial, which does not by excess become injurious.[16]

This became known as the *Lancet* Manifesto. Its sixteen authors formed an august group that – unlike Horsley – did not deplore the use of alcohol, but only its abuse. Among them was William Gowers, Horsley's great neurological colleague. When an outpouring of letters followed in the medical journals and lay press, adding support to or opposing these views, Gowers attempted to reassure the public that the declaration really meant very little,[17] but to no avail. The controversy continued, based mainly on personal opinions and anecdotal experience. It received much attention at the August meeting of the British Association, where certain medical men made the most outrageous statements in favor of alcohol, such as that alcohol did not cause cirrhosis because Scotsmen were exempt and cats very liable to it.[18] Horsley spoke at the meeting, pointing out that the hospitals had been giving up alcohol steadily over the last thirty years and called on the entire profession to "perform the national and patriotic duty of abolishing it root and branch."[18]

Out of concern that alcohol might be contributing to the physical (racial) deterioration of Britons, he also sent letters to various secondary schools, including well-known public schools such as Eton, Oundle, Lancing, and Marlborough, to enquire whether the boys customarily drank alcohol or water with their principal meals, and – if the former – what percentage of boys took alcohol.[19] The responses were varied and not especially helpful. At Eton, for example, all were allowed beer whereas at Oundle alcohol was not available, at Lancing twenty percent of the boys took beer, and at Marlborough a very light beer was available with lunch but taken by only about ten percent of the boys.

In 1909, at a dinner for brewers, Horsley's views on the evil nature of alcohol were publicly challenged with a demand that he provide proof of his assertions. His response[20,21] which simply referred readers to his book with Mary Sturge, failed to satisfy his critics, for the book did not provide proofs but simply stated beliefs and assertions that had not convinced other physicians or scientists, as indicated by the *Lancet* Manifesto.[22,23]

Horsley and Sturge wrote in their book about the effects of alcohol on the next generation:

The brunt of the evil heritage caused by alcoholism falls upon the nervous system of the next generation. ... With regard to mental development, many children of alcoholic parentage show signs of stupidity, mental deficiency, moral instability, and lack of normal control, whilst others exhibit idiocy, epilepsy, and hysteria, together with various unbalanced cravings. The characteristic mental trait of the child of the inebriate mother is a warped or stunted intelligence accompanied by impulsive, uncontrolled actions. Parental intoxication tends to produce 'impulsive degenerates' and moral imbeciles.[24]

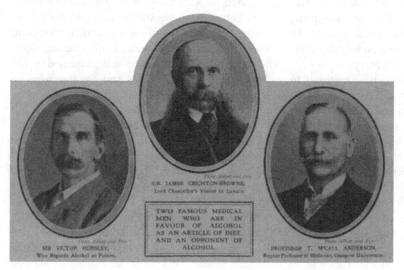

Figure 13.1 The section titled *Science Jottings* (p. 556) in the *Illustrated London News* of April 13, 1907 included an article on the alcohol question, which cited the *Lancet* Manifesto (see text). Its accompanying illustrations included this figure of Horsley (*left panel*), "who regards alcohol as a poison" and two famous medical men "in favor of alcohol as an article of diet" – Sir James Crichton-Brown (*center panel*), the lord chancellor's visitor in lunacy, and McCall Anderson (*right panel*), professor of medicine in Glasgow.

These were strong words, but they were based on prejudice and supposition rather than evidence or any factual analysis.

The Row with Karl Pearson: Alcohol and Pregnancy

Horsley's views were challenged by Karl Pearson (1857–1936), a colleague at University College. Pearson was a brilliant polymath who, after earning a first-class degree in mathematics at Cambridge, studied science, philosophy, metaphysics, medieval history and literature, and socialism in Germany, before returning to London to become a barrister. He never practiced the law. In 1884 he was appointed professor of applied mathematics and mechanics at University College and is widely remembered for developing some of the major analytical techniques of modern statistics (including the standard deviation, p-value, chi-squared test, and correlation coefficient), giving statistics its scientific respectability. His influential book, *The Grammar of Science*, anticipated themes that were to become part of the theories later developed by Einstein and others. Pearson was appointed the first Galton Professor of Eugenics at University College in 1911 and remained in that position until he retired in 1933. Some of his views were provocative and racist, as when he advocated "war with inferior races" to cleanse the human race of "feeble stock" or opposed Jewish immigration to Britain for fear of weakening the native population. Like Horsley, he had a dominating personality and often attributed intellectual differences to the stupidity of others, thereby disrupting friendships by bitter controversies. Indeed, he took pleasure in fights as well as friendships. He was therefore a formidable adversary.

Pearson used rigorous statistical methods to examine whether parental alcoholism did indeed affect the physical characters and abilities of their offspring. The first of his communications (1910), prepared by Ethel Elderton, his assistant, analyzed data derived from a report of the Edinburgh Charity Organization Society; the information was collected by social workers and related to children attending a specific school that supposedly was "widely representative" in character, although it was located in a poor part of the city. The report also included an analysis of data obtained from a survey of families with children attending a special school for the "mentally defective" in Manchester.[25]

For the analysis, parents were divided into those who were completely abstinent or usually sober, and those who were suspected or known to be heavier drinkers ("alcoholics"). A slightly higher death rate occurred among the offspring of alcoholic parents, especially when the mother was the drinker, but there was little difference in family size because the alcoholic parents had more children. Importantly, parental alcoholism did not seem to have much effect on children's intellect, physique, or disease. In other words, there was no evidence to support the belief that parental alcoholism affected the health of their offspring.[23] Elderton and Pearson concluded, for example, that low intelligence in the children of alcoholic parents probably related to parental intelligence rather than alcohol intake.

The first criticisms came from the influential economist Alfred Marshall,[26] and were dismissed by Pearson.[27] It was the criticisms of Marshall's protégé, John Maynard Keynes (1883–1946), that stung. Keynes claimed that both sets of data were invalid, the Manchester set because of the presence of "feeblemindedness" in the families, and the Edinburgh set because it was derived from a poor district and thus not truly representative of the general population. He concluded therefore that the work was almost valueless and certainly misleading, primarily because the original data sets were not suited to the problem under study.[28,29] His criticism of the complex statistical methods of the study led to a tart rejoinder that reflected on Keynes' ignorance of modern statistics. Both sides – the statisticians and the economists – had some justification for their views but, overall, Pearson may have come out on top.[30] A series of letters by others was published in *The Times*, with various claims and counterclaims to which the undaunted Pearson responded briskly.

Horsley and Sturge also objected to Pearson's study. In their first response, a letter to the editor of the *British Medical Journal*, who seemingly had endorsed Pearson's study, their main concern was whether alcoholism had preceded or followed childbirth, for if the latter the findings could be discounted.[31] They were irked by Pearson's response, which seemed to involve playing with the numbers to justify his claims.

Pearson and Elderton replied in greater detail to their medical critics later in 1910. They showed that the various criticisms leveled at their own work applied equally to the earlier studies on which Horsley and others relied to support their claims for the adverse effects of alcohol.[32] They accused Horsley of mistaking association for causation.

Horsley and Sturge responded in kind. They accused Pearson of being personally offensive, claimed that statements in his publications were self-contradictory, and charged him with using scientific or technical terms inaccurately. They quarreled, for example, with his use of the word "offspring" or the definition of "sober" and "alcoholic." Some of their comments, however, altered the emphasis and changed the nuance of Pearson's text and thereby misstated it. Further, Horsley appeared to confuse matters by raising minor or irrelevant points whereas – as Pearson pointed out – his study was an attempt to answer a specific question. In addition, certain methodological aspects seem to have been misunderstood by Horsley, as they were also by Marshall and Keynes. Nevertheless, Horsley and Sturge raised some important issues and returned repeatedly to the point that the data analyzed by Elderton and Pearson did not relate to alcohol consumption *before* conception but only to consumption some years later, so that their children could not be classified properly. In other words, the data were of uncertain validity. They also lamented the lack of adequate controls, the use of a non-representative population, and – somewhat courageously given Pearson's statistical expertise – the presence of statistical inaccuracies. They accused Pearson of "carelessness and inaccuracy" and of "creating statistics where real data did not exist." Horsley and Sturge concluded their ten-page, nineteen-column letter in the *British Medical Journal* on a personal note:

> It seems to us, therefore, that these writers constitute a national danger ... [T]he questions of parental alcoholism, of the wage-earning efficiency, physique and mentality of the alcoholic workman and his children, remain exactly where they were before Miss Elderton and Professor Pearson began publishing in May, 1910. Consequently those social reformers who have been led by their publications to believe that previous information and knowledge on this subject was wrong may rest satisfied that it is not.[33]

The Times now published an editorial summarizing the controversy and lamenting the language employed by Sturge and Horsley, which "practically amounts to an accusation of bad faith against their adversaries; an accusation which, unless it be thoroughly substantiated, is always liable to recoil upon those by whom it is advanced." The public, it continued magisterially, looked forward to a clarification of the issues by further study "away from the din of controversy."[34]

Pearson's blood was aroused. He responded with a cold invective as he went point by point through Horsley's criticisms, indicating apparent misrepresentations and misquotations. He concluded that "Sir Victor Horsley accuses me of fabrication and dishonesty; the only charge I make against him is that his partisanship for a special theory has wholly destroyed his scientific balance."[35,36]

Horsley's misgivings were spelled out again in detail, and seemed to gain weight by their repetition.[37,38] The editor of the *British Medical Journal*, who had previously been convinced by Pearson – "the assailants of Professor Pearson have been somewhat over-hasty" – now confessed that his judgement had been premature and his words ill-chosen.[39] Horsley's charges were beginning to stick despite his manner, goaded as he was by Pearson.

Slowly the controversy came to be forgotten, for it remained unclear how it could be resolved and by what means alcohol might affect the developing fetus, and because the defects ascribed to alcohol might indeed have been inherited independently of maternal intake. Even so, occasional reports continued to be published concerning differences due to alcohol use (rather than to heredity) in the offspring of mothers who had or had not consumed alcohol during pregnancy. It was not until the 1960s and 1970s that a distinct fetal-alcohol syndrome was delineated. Babies born of alcoholic mothers may have a characteristic facial appearance and other congenital abnormalities including reduced intelligence. Alcohol was recognized also as teratogenic in animal studies. It is now recommended that women avoid any alcohol consumption during pregnancy.

Alcohol and Driving

In 1912, Horsley became embroiled in a further discussion in the correspondence columns of *The Times*, this time regarding tests of drunkenness. His main point – that total abstinence from alcohol was the safest qualification for all drivers – would be widely accepted today but was challenged angrily at the time.[40] He had therefore to amplify:

> The fact that even a small so-called dietetic quantity of alcohol appreciably lengthens the time of our response by movement to a sudden stimulus, and blunts the sharpness of our perception, shows that total abstinence from alcohol or any other like drug should be made a necessary condition of service among all motor drivers.[41]

The law in many developed countries is evolving to a position very much in line with that elaborated by Horsley more than one hundred years ago.

The Rum Ration

With the outbreak of war in 1914, Horsley became preoccupied with many other issues, but he reverted to the alcohol question when the British government decided to reintroduce the rum ration for the troops of the British Expeditionary Force. In the past, front-line British forces had received a ration of alcohol before and during battle as a means of fortifying them, relieving stress, and encouraging greater efforts, but whether this improved or impaired their operational efficiency was unclear. The controversial practice was reintroduced in 1914. Front-line French troops also received an alcohol allowance (*vin ordinaire*) during the war, as did the Germans (beer or brandy), whereas in Russia the sale of vodka was prohibited to prevent drunkenness among the troops.[43]

The rum ration for British troops was two and one-half fluid ounces daily for those "on active operations in the field," such as serving in the trenches, and, exceptionally, for those drenched or chilled while on military maneuvers or training exercises.[43] The alcohol was popular with the troops for the feeling of warmth that it provided. It did not take long, however, for Horsley – now a captain in the Royal Army Medical Corps (Territorial Force) – to point out that the alcohol had no nutritional or medicinal benefits, that it impaired efficiency, and that the medical profession was not responsible for the policy or its implementation.[44] The rum, which was supplied by the quartermaster and not the medical service, was supposed to make cold, wet soldiers feel warm and dry, whereas – he stressed – it actually lowered their resistance to cold. The reintroduction of the rum ration also undermined the army reforms of the previous forty years, he pointed out, leading to disorderliness, intolerance of discipline, impaired judgement, errors and accidents, diminished physical endurance, and reduced accuracy in shooting.[44] Rather than rum, Horsley proposed that the troops receive warm nourishment such as with hot milk flavored with coffee or chocolate or hot thick soups. There was sympathy for his views in certain quarters, especially as the effects of alcohol on the war effort and industrial production at home were also raising concerns. In early 1915, Lloyd George, the chancellor of the exchequer, declared that "Britain is fighting three enemies – Germany, Austria and Drink," while Kitchener, secretary of state for war, had pasted in every soldier's paybook the exhortation that "you may find temptations in both wine and women. You must resist both." The king himself pledged to give up alcohol until the war was over.[45]

Others felt Horsley's suggestions impractical. "Where no fires at all are allowed; where everything is water-logged; where fighting takes place at intervals all night, and no one can approach, how is hot coffee to be obtained?"[46] Moreover, it was not for its nutritious benefits that the rum was provided, and Horsley was taken to task for "striving to rob" the men "of an undoubted luxury and pleasure" because of his teetotal principles.[47] The discussion continued in the columns of the *British Medical Journal*, becoming anecdotal or increasingly offensive depending on the correspondent, and was not really advanced by the caustic wit of Charles Mercier, the British psychiatrist who seemed to take every opportunity to spar with Horsley and his causes (see p. 139).[48]

This was another battle that Horsley was clearly destined to lose but was determined to fight. His views had merit and are well worth remembering. Some still claim that alcohol assists in cohesive bonding during military training and has a positive effect on morale,[42] but consumption is likely to be excessive and problematic with the stress that precedes, accompanies, and follows battle. The rum ration itself was eventually abolished.[49] There is now little doubt that alcohol indeed impairs efficiency and function, and officers typically restrict its use during active engagements. Abuse of alcohol and other substances is common among former military personnel with posttraumatic stress disorder, but whether the alcohol consumption is the cause or the consequence of mental illness is debatable. Probably both views are correct.

Horsley maintained his stance against alcohol to the very end. While himself on military service in Egypt, he received a copy of the new edition of *Alcohol and the Human Body*, his book with Mary Sturge. In eager anticipation, he pulled the wrapping off and proudly opened the book at a spot marked by one of those small cardboard bookmarks advertising some product or another. Turning over the little card, he glanced casually at the woodcut advertising a Scottish insurance society, and there, under a grapevine, was a young couple drinking a glass of wine, with Cupid beneath them.[5]

Notes

1. Anon: Sir Victor Horsley. Great international prize for surgery. *Daily Mail (Lond)*, February 10, 1911, p. 7.

2. Bynum WF: Alcoholism and degeneration in 19th century European medicine and psychiatry. *Br J Addiction* 1984; **79**: 59–70.

3. McCandless P: 'Curses of Civilization': Insanity and drunkenness in Victorian Britain. *Br J Addiction* 1984; **79**: 49–58.

4. Pauly PJ: How did the effects of alcohol on reproduction become scientifically uninteresting? *J Hist Biol* 1996; **29**: 1–28.

5. Walshe FMR: Personal communication, July 15, 1966.

6. Horsley V: *The Effect of Alcohol upon the Human Brain: A Lecture. The Second Lees and Raper Memorial Lecture.* p. 10. Lees and Raper Memorial Trustees: London, 1900. Abstracted by Anon: The effect of small doses of alcohol on the brain *Br Med J* 1900; **1**: 1126–1128; *Lancet* 1900; **155**: 1271–1273; The effect of small doses of alcohol on the brain. *Quart J Inebr* 1900; **22**: 306–311.

7. International Association of Abstaining Physicians: Invitation to serve as president, dated July 20, 1909. Section C2/1, Horsley Papers, Special Collections, UCL Library Services (London, UK).

8. Anon: Society for the Study of Inebriety: Jubilee celebration. *Br Med J* 1934; **1**: 681–682.

9. Horsley V: Alcohol and commercial efficiency. *Lancet* 1905; **165**: 739–740.

10. Horsley V: *What Women Can Do to Promote Temperance.* An address delivered at the Annual Meeting of the Women's Union (C.E.T.S.). Church of England Temperance Society: London, 1906.

11. Gutzke DW: 'The Cry of the Children': The Edwardian medical campaign against maternal drinking. *Br J Addiction* 1984; **79**; 71–84.

12. Anon: Political notes. *The Times (Lond)*, November 12, 1906, p. 8.

13. Anon: The teaching of hygiene and temperance in elementary schools. Deputation to the President of the Board of Education. *Br Med J* 1906; **2**: 1412–1414.

14. Anon: Anti-barmaid movement. *Daily Mail (Lond)*, February 15, 1905, p. 3; February 1, 1908, p. 3.

15. Horsley V, Sturge MD: *Alcohol and the Human Body. An Introduction to the Study of the Subject.* Macmillan: London, 1907.

16. Anderson TM, Barrs AG, Bennett WH, Crichton-Browne J, Dixon WE, Duckworth D, Fraser TR, Glynn TR, Gowers WR, Halliburton WD, Hutchinson J, Hutchinson R, Owen E, Pye-Smith PH, Roberts FT, Venning E: The use of alcoholic beverages. *Lancet* 1907; **189**: 894.

17. Anon: Letter from London. *NY Med J* 1907; **85**: 840–842.

18. Anon: Doctors and drink. Divergent views at the British Association. Speech by Sir Victor Horsley. *Daily Mail (Lond)*, August 6, 1907, p. 3.

19. Horsley V: Letter sent to various secondary schools dated March 23, 1907. Section C2/1, Horsley Papers, Special Collections, UCL Library Services (London, UK).

20. Horsley V: Brewers' challenge to teetotalers. [Letter to the editor.] *The Times (Lond)*, February 22, 1909, p. 10.

21. Horsley V: Brewers' challenge to teetotalers. [Letter to the editor.] *The Times (Lond)*, February 25, 1909, p. 10.

22. A Moderate Drinker: Alcohol and total abstinence. [Letter to the editor.] *The Times (Lond)*, February 25, 1909, p.10.

23. Barclay E: Brewers' challenge to teetotalers. [Letter to the editor.] *The Times (Lond)*, February 26, 1909, p. 7.

24. Horsley V, Sturge MD: *Alcohol and the Human Body. An Introduction to the Study of the Subject.* pp. 319–320. Macmillan: London, 1907.

25. Elderton EM, Pearson K: *A First Study of the Influence of Parental Alcoholism on the Physique and Ability of the Offspring.* Dulau: London, 1910.

26. Marshall A: Alcoholism and efficiency. [Letters to the editor.] *The Times (Lond)*, July 7, 1910, p. 12; August 2, 1910, p. 4; and August 19, 1910, p. 4.

27. Pearson K: Alcoholism and efficiency. [Letters to the editor.] *The Times (Lond)*, July 12, 1910, p. 11 and August 10, 1910, p. 10.

28. Keynes JM: Review of *A First Study of the Influence of Parental Alcoholism on the Physique and Ability of the Offspring*, by Ethel M. Elderton with the Assistance of Karl Pearson. *J R Stat Soc* 1910; **73**: 769–773.

29. Keynes JM: Influence of parental alcoholism. [Letters to the editor.] *J R Stat Soc* 1910; **74**: 114-121and 1911; **74**: 339–345.

30. Stigler SM: *Statistics on the Table: The History of Statistical Concepts and Methods*. pp. 13–50. Harvard University Press: Cambridge, MA, 1999.

31. Sturge MD, Horsley V: Alcoholism and degeneration. [Letters to the editor.] *Br Med J* 1910; **2**: 1656, 1817–1818, 1946–1947, 2048–2049.

32. Pearson K, Elderton EM: *A Second Study of the Influence of Parental Alcoholism on the Physique and Ability of the Offspring: Being A Reply to Certain Medical Critics of the First Memoir and an Examination of the Rebutting Evidence Cited by Them*. Dulau: London, 1910.

33. Sturge MD, Horsley V: On some of the biological and statistical errors in the work on parental alcoholism by Miss Elderton and Professor Karl Pearson, F.R.S. *Br Med J* 1911; **1**: 72–82.

34. Anon: Parental alcoholism. *The Times (Lond)*, January 13, 1911, p. 9.

35. Pearson K: Alcohol and degeneracy. *Br Med J* 1911; **1**: 278–281.

36. Pearson K: Alcohol and degeneracy. [Letter to the editor.] *The Times (Lond)*, January 16, 1911, p. 7.

37. Sturge MD, Horsley V: Alcoholism and degeneracy. *Br Med J* 1911; **1**: 112, 333–336, 404.

38. Horsley V: Alcohol and degeneracy. [Letter to the editor.] *The Times (Lond)*, January 16, 1911, p. 7.

39. Anon: Editorial comment. Alcoholism and degeneracy. *Br Med J* 1911; **1**: 336.

40. Horsley V: Tests of drunkenness. [Letter to the editor.] *The Times (Lond)*, November 8, 1912, p. 16.

41. Horsley V: Tests of drunkeness. [Letter to the editor.] *The Times (Lond)*, November 1, 1912, p. 15.

42. Jones E, Fear NT: Alcohol use and misuse within the military: A review. *Int Rev Psychiatry* 2011; **23**: 166–172.

43. Anon: *Regulations for the Allowances of the Army*. pp. 15–16. His Majesty's Stationery Office: London, 1914.

44. Horsley V: On the alleged responsibility of the medical profession for the reintroduction of the rum ration into the British Army. *Br Med J* 1915; **1**: 203–206.

45. Haslam S: A literary intervention: Writing alcohol in British literature 1915–1930. *First World War Studies* 2013; **4**: 219–239.

46. Woodman EM: The rum ration. [Letter to the editor.] *Br Med J* 1915; **1**: 448.

47. Ogilvie G: The rum ration. [Letter to the editor.] *Br Med J* 1915; **1**: 529.

48. Mercier CA: The rum ration. [Letter to the editor.] *Br Med J* 1915; **1** :489–490.

49. In the Royal Army, the allowance was discontinued gradually in different units after World War I although alcohol was issued intermittently in various later campaigns or situations, including in certain circumstances during World War II. The situation was different in the Royal Navy, where personnel received a daily allowance of rum to compensate for the arduous nature of their life; this was abolished after a parliamentary debate in 1970.

Syphilis and the Public Health

During and after the late 1890s, Horsley turned increasingly from diseases of the individual to the ills of society, as discussed in earlier chapters. Prominent among his concerns were attempts to limit the extent and spread of venereal diseases (defined then as syphilis, gonorrhea, and soft chancre or chancroid) and to improve the certification system for disease.

Syphilis and Other Venereal Diseases

Syphilis – the great pox – probably made its appearance in Europe during the fifteenth century; ever since, it has remained an expensive consequence of sexual contact with an infected partner. Called a venereal disease after Venus, the Roman goddess of love, syphilis has had many other names, many based on traditional national enmities or rivalries – thus the French pox to the British, the Spanish disease to the French, the Polish disease for the Russians, the Chinese pox to the Japanese, and so on. It is now known drily as a sexually transmitted disease.[1]

The early symptoms of infection include genital sores or ulcers, skin rashes, pains, malaise, headache, fever, enlarged lymph glands, impaired vision, and abnormalities of liver, kidney, and neurological function. After several years, other horrors may develop – some combination of heart failure, aortic aneurysm and other vascular diseases, strokes, seizures, progressive dementia, severe stabbing pains, weakness or paralysis, gait disturbances, and disease of the bone, liver, and kidneys. Disabled, disfigured, and demented, the victims of late syphilis come to a miserable end. Equally horrifying, children of an infected mother may be stillborn or delivered prematurely; they may be deformed and can become blind, deaf, mentally impaired, and diminished by a variety of other abnormalities.

Gonorrhea ("the clap"), by contrast, is often asymptomatic but may cause pain on urination and a purulent discharge (urethritis) or other urogenital symptoms; infertility may result in women and occasionally in men. Infants born to untreated mothers can develop gonorrheal conjunctivitis, which sometimes progresses to blindness. Chancroid – which is not considered further in this chapter – leads to painful genital ulceration and may cause swelling and abscesses in the lymph glands of the groin.

The development of arsenical drugs (Salvarsan and then Neosalvarsan) in the early years of the twentieth century, and their subsequent combination with small quantities of bismuth or mercury, finally provided an effective treatment for syphilis that was widely utilized until the advent of penicillin. Gonorrhoea, regarded as less serious, was often treated by lotions, herbal remedies, or the introduction of caustic solutions into the urethra before antibiotics became available. With both diseases, the cessation of symptoms in treated patients was thought incorrectly to indicate a cure.

During Edwardian times, these infections aroused mixed feelings in the general public and even among doctors. Venereal diseases (as then designated) were regarded, even by well-meaning doctors, as the price exacted by an angry divinity for sexual liberty and sinful behavior. (A similar viewpoint was common in the last quarter of the twentieth century concerning infection with the human immunodeficiency virus.) Thus, a sense of guilt and disgrace came to be associated with them, such that many doctors used euphemisms rather than stating the true cause of disease or death to their patients or to officialdom. There was consequently an unfortunate lack of statistics concerning the incidence and prevalence of sexually transmitted diseases, particularly among the civilian population, making it difficult to gauge the breadth of the problem by those anxious for reform.

Horsley had seen cases of syphilis at the very start of his medical career, and in 1882, while surgical registrar at University College Hospital, he described, at a meeting of the Pathological Society of London, the autopsy findings in a patient with destruction of the facial bones and widespread involvement of other parts of the body including the brain.[2] His report was not quite as arresting as it might have been, however, for it was preceded by a somewhat exotic account of abscesses in the liver of a kangaroo and a python.[3]

Agitation for Reform

In 1896 a physician was consulted by a woman with a highly contagious form of syphilis. Other than warning her that she was a danger to anyone with whom she might come into contact, no other steps could be taken to protect the five little children who were under her care. The physician did, however, discuss the case with a visitor at a Lock hospital, which specialized in treating patients with venereal diseases. She apparently raised the possibility of persuading the government to set up an enquiry into these diseases, and was given an introduction to Horsley with this in mind.[4] Thus began the agitation that would lead eventually to a royal commission of enquiry, although Horsley's role in it remains in the shadows. A clue is provided, however, by the comments of the chairman of council of the British Medical Association in 1916 while moving a resolution to place on record the deep regret of council at the death of Horsley. He stated:

> Twenty years ago the fight to get the Royal Commission on Venereal Diseases began, and it was seen that a man was required of forceful nature who would give time, trouble, and energy, who would collect, collate, and put forward the mass of medical information that was needed to convince the public. Sir Victor Horsley was described to him (the Chairman) by a great mutual friend – George J. Romanes, the biologist – years ago as a man who had in him of the spirit of the old Crusader. Sir Victor threw himself into the campaign, spoke at meetings, spoke and helped to wear down the opposition. Whatever good came from the Commission's work, the whole nation would owe to Sir Victor Horsley an enormous debt of gratitude for what he did.[5]

When, a few years later (1904), an interdepartmental committee was set up by the government to study the causes of the physical deterioration that supposedly had affected certain segments of the population (see p. 119), Horsley appeared before it.[6] He stressed the need for an inquiry into the prevalence and best means of checking the spread of venereal disease. Many syphilitics were not ill enough to require hospitalization, he pointed out, and they therefore continued with their usual activities, becoming a source of infection to others.[7] He also emphasized the need for death certificates to be a private document and doctors to be protected from charges of libel if the certification were to be accurate. The committee went on to recommend – at the urging of Horsley and others – that another body should be established to examine the prevalence and effects of syphilis. The political climate was such, however, that little further was accomplished for several years.[4]

In 1913, Sir Malcolm Morris, a well-known dermatologist, published an eloquent plea for the establishment of a royal commission to inquire into the venereal diseases,[8] a viewpoint that received much support in the Lancet.[9] On July 22, a letter from Morris to the same effect appeared in The Morning Post, co-signed by many distinguished members of the medical profession, including Horsley.[10]

The Royal Commission

A royal commission of inquiry was appointed almost immediately, chaired by Lord Sydenham of Combe and with Morris one of fourteen other members, including members of parliament, civil servants, doctors, clergymen, the widow of a former bishop, and an expert on mentally handicapped children.[11] Its aims were to examine the prevalence, consequences, prevention, and treatment of venereal diseases in the United Kingdom, and it began its meetings later in 1913. The timing was propitious, for in the preceding few years the causal organism of syphilis had been identified, a diagnostic test (the Wasserman reaction) had been developed, and new treatments had become available. Reliable estimates of its prevalence were not available for the civilian population; in the armed forces, syphilis seemed to be on the decline, perhaps due to better education, a reduced incidence of alcoholism, and the provision of better recreational facilities for the men, but it remained a major problem.[12]

Toward the end of March, 1914, Horsley appeared as a witness before the commissioners.[13] His comments show him to be a liberal thinker who was ahead of his times on many important matters, but his advocacy might have been more effective if he had not tried also to promote the other causes on which he held strong views but which were beyond the commission's purview, such as temperance.

He highlighted for the commissioners the importance of providing sex education for children.[13,14] Such teaching, he believed, should not be left simply to parents; teachers also were ill-equipped for it, and doctors should not do it to avoid sex becoming "part of a medical mystery." Teaching by laymen or teachers with special training in the topic should begin gradually, starting with nature study for five-year-olds and moving on to reproduction in plants and then in animals so that, by the age of puberty, teaching – directed now at the individual child rather than the class as a whole – should focus on human sexuality and reproduction, and then on the sexually transmitted diseases. He stressed the inadequacies of the contemporary teaching of science (physics and chemistry), which did not attempt to train the mind, did not involve study of the biological sciences, and failed to educate children in the application of scientific knowledge. It was also important, he believed, to educate or otherwise instruct the public in lay terms about venereal diseases in the hope of reducing the spread and encouraging the treatment of infections, rather than participating in a conspiracy to "conceal the existence of these evils." He believed that "you destroy prurient curiosity by really informing them [people] of the facts."[13]

He also pointed out the difficulties faced by doctors in matters related to public health, not only because of their professional ethics but also because of the libel laws. For example, a doctor who warned some-one at risk from their partner of being infected with a venereal disease could, in turn, face an action for libel that might lead to ruin. Horsley declined to suggest how the libel laws might be amended, for he was not a lawyer, but he believed that, depending on the circumstances, it should be possible to release such confidential information to "people who had a right to demand it," specifically the nearest relative of the patient. He was also concerned that the duration of antisyphilitic treatment (two years) was inadequate and believed correctly that the resolution of symptoms did not necessarily signify freedom from disease. He was in favor of the confidential notification of all venereal diseases, but on questioning, conceded the difficulty in maintaining confidentiality if notification were to be acted upon by local medical authorities. He also proposed other fundamental reforms, such as the establishment of a ministry of public health to take over all medical duties then undertaken by several other departments (such as local government boards and national health insurance commissions, as he wrote in a letter to *The Times*[15]), and within which there would be a department of national statistics. It would not be until after Horsley's death, however, that a separate ministry of health was established in Britain, and later still before an independent office for national statistics was established.

His views of temperance colored some of his statements. He claimed that alcohol lowered the resistance to infections, including those causing venereal diseases, without offering evidence to support his statements, and contended that "the drink trade" was associated with prostitution and the spread of sexually transmitted diseases. In order to prevent the spread of these diseases, he remarked, other social reforms were needed – increasing the individual's wage-earning capacity would reduce prostitution, and the risks of infection would be diminished by reducing overcrowding in housing and by improving hygiene and cleanliness (for example, by the provision of public baths and of hot water for dwelling houses).[13]

Horsley made similar points at a meeting of the British Medical Association, emphasizing the need to improve the nation's vital statistics and for developing a real "nomenclature of diseases" in order to delete old, non-specific terms that had led to inaccurate certification; he urged also that there should be direct confidential certification of the cause of death, which should be separate from the death certificate.[16]

The Outcome

The commissioners received evidence from many other sources, confirmed the high prevalence of venereal infections in Britain, and in their 1916 report, made specific recommendations concerning the diagnosis and treatment of these diseases. These were carried speedily into law by the Public

Health (Venereal Diseases) Regulations of 1916 and the Venereal Diseases Act of 1917. Local government authorities were required to establish special free clinics for the confidential treatment of persons with venereal disease, unqualified persons were prohibited from treating these diseases, and advertisements for their prevention or treatment were banned, except those of the local authorities. Laboratory facilities for the diagnosis of sexually transmitted diseases were to be provided to all doctors without charge, and all medical students were to receive practical instruction in venereology.

The commissioners rejected any notification of disease that involved the naming of individual patients because of the need to maintain confidentiality, requiring instead that the numbers of patients with each disease should be reported. Such aggregate data were to be provided by all institutions receiving government grant support for the diagnosis and treatment of venereal diseases. They also recommended that registration of the cause of death should be confidential, that stillbirths with a gestational age of less than twenty-eight weeks should be notified, and that statistics should be kept of patients provided with Salvarsan or related compounds at public expense.[17]

Thus an effective system for managing venereal diseases was established in the United Kingdom. The subsequent development of antibiotics, the establishment of the national health service, the appearance of antibiotic-resistant organisms, and the advent of the human immunodeficiency virus (HIV) and the acquired immunodeficiency syndrome (AIDS) all led to further changes, but the basic principles of care had been established. Later changes in the regulations ensured that all sexually transmitted diseases were covered, and not just those previously designated as venereal diseases. The general registration of stillbirths came into effect in 1927.

Many of the issues that troubled Horsley, however, continue to concern doctors, ethicists, and the general public, such as the balance between the rights of an individual and the needs of society in general. It is in the public interest to ensure both patient confidentiality and the safety of others from dangers posed by an individual patient. When – if ever – is it acceptable to disclose personal information without the consent of the patient? Is it when there is a risk to the health

or life of an identifiable third party? Is it, as Horsley believed, when a patient with a sexually transmitted disease refuses to warn their spouse or partner about the risks of infection? And what is the legal liability if a doctor fails to breach confidentiality and an identified sexual partner becomes infected? Many countries or states now have regulations or legal precedents that bear on these or related issues, which remain controversial and troubling.[18]

Notes

1. Frith J: Syphilis: Its early history and treatment until penicillin, and the debate on its origins. *J Mil Vet Health* 2012; **20**: 49–58.

2. Horsley V: Case of severe syphilitic disease of the facial bones and viscera. – Death from pyaemia. *Trans Pathol Soc Lond* 1883; **34**: 208–209; Bone and brain disease in syphilis. [Abstract] *Br Med J* 1882; **2**: 1254.

3. Sutton JB: Disseminated abscesses in the liver of a kangaroo and of a python. [Abstract] *Br Med J* 1882; **2**: 1254.

4. Turner EB: The history of the fight against venereal disease. On the Final Report of the Royal Commission on Venereal Diseases. *Sci Prog* 1916; **11**: 83–88.

5. Anon: The late Sir Victor Horsley. Comments of the chairman. *Br Med J* 1916 (Suppl. 641); **2**: 41–42.

6. Horsley V: Witness testimony, March 16, 1904. pp. 384–387. In: *Report of the Inter-Departmental Committee on Physical Deterioration. Volume 1. – Report and Appendix*. His Majesty's Stationery Office: London, 1904.

7. Anon: The prevalence and prevention of syphilis. *Br Med J* 1905; **1**: 97–98.

8. Morris M: A plea for the appointment of a Royal Commission on Venereal Disease. *Lancet* 1913; **181**: 1817–1819.

9. Anon: Syphilis and the responsibility of the state. *Lancet* 1913; **181**: 1810–1811.

10. Anon: Public health. *Bost Med Surg J* 1913; **169**: 287–288. [This editorial republished a major part of the letter from the *Morning Post* concerning venereal diseases, of which Horsley was a co-author. The original has been difficult to trace.]

11. Oriel JD: *The Scars of Venus: A History of Venereology*. pp. 196–203. Springer; London, 1994.

12. Willcox RR: Fifty years since the conception of an organized venereal disease service in Great Britain: The Royal Commission of 1916. *Br J Vener Dis* 1967; **43**: 1–9.

13. Horsley V: Witness testimony, March 27, 1914. pp. 372–389. In: *Royal Commission on Venereal Disease. Appendix to First Report of the Commissioners. Minutes of Evidence: 7th November 1913 to 6th April 1914. Question 1 to Question 12,549.* His Majesty's Stationery Office: London, 1914.

14. Anon: Doctors and the Libel Law. Sir V. Horsley on the campaign against venereal disease. *The Times (Lond)*, April 20, 1914, p. 3.

15. Horsley V: Mothers of the race. A ministry of public health. [Letter to the editor.] *The Times (Lond)*, April 13, 1914, p. 5.

16. Anon: A new nomenclature of diseases. Doctors and reform in vital statistics. Sir Victor Horsley's views. *The Times (Lond)*, July 30, 1914, p. 13.

17. Commissioners, Royal Commission on Venereal Diseases: Section V. Summary of recommendations and general conclusions. In: *Royal Commission on Venereal Diseases. Final Report of the Commissioners.* pp. 62–66. His Majesty's Stationery Office: London, 1916.

18. Beresford HR: Legal process, litigation, and judicial decisions. pp. 35–61. In: Bernat JL, Beresford HR (eds): *Ethical and Legal Issues in Neurology. Handbook of Clinical Neurology, Vol 118.* Elsevier: Amsterdam, 2013.

A Surgeon Goes to War

15

In 1914, Europe blundered into war. Horsley regarded it as "an insane folly" and hoped that it would lead the peoples of Central Europe to rise up and remove their rulers from power, that democracy and universal suffrage would follow. He did not foresee that an uprising against the government would occur in Russia, one of the allies but a country that he detested because of its autocratic barbarism.

Within a few days of the declaration of war, Horsley – a captain in the territorial (reserve) force of the British Army since 1910 – was agitating enthusiastically for a transfer to active service, while his two sons enlisted with his approval in the Artists' Rifles and subsequently received commissions in the Gordon Highlanders. The war was supposed to be over by Christmas, but instead it followed a weary course for more than four years. Young men with heady ideas of honor and duty enlisted as if it were all a game, only to be let down by the failures of politicians and generals, to die on distant battle fields or to return home disfigured and dispirited. Victor Horsley was among the millions who lost their lives during the devastation of war. He died in a far-off and forgotten land, campaigning to the end for the welfare of the troops and against the culpable negligence and incompetence of those in command. It required a government commission of enquiry to show that the chaotic conditions to which Horsley had objected were indeed responsible for much preventable misery and unnecessary loss of life.

Research on Gunshot Wounds

Long before his wartime military service, Horsley's researches, undertaken years earlier, came to contribute to the British war effort and earned him the thanks of the secretary of state for war. As a young man, Horsley had liked to play with guns and enjoyed hunting and shooting. He had even contemplated a military career before deciding to become a surgeon. Guns fascinated him. Queen Victoria is said to have given him a shotgun as a child.[1] Early in his career, he began to examine the effects of gunshot wounds and made observations on the properties of bullets that became highly relevant when war broke out.

The Physics of Gunshot Wounds to the Head

As might have been anticipated given his interest in the brain, Horsley focused his studies on the effects of gunshot wounds to the head, hoping to understand why they often were fatal and to place their clinical management on a sound scientific footing. He spoke of his research to members of the Royal Institution in April 1894, fully twenty years before the start of the world war. For experimental purposes, he fired bullets into canisters filled with wet or dry lint or into blocks of modeling clay mixed with different amounts of water, and made casts of the resulting cavities by pouring liquid plaster-of-paris into them. Confirming and extending earlier observations, Horsley concluded that the destructive effect of a bullet on the brain was not due to the "wind of the shot" (the wave of compressed air that the bullet drives before it) or to the heat generated by the bullet, but rather was related to its momentum and cross-sectional area and to the water content of the tissues. The wetter the clay (so that it more resembled brain tissue), the greater was the destruction that occurred. He noted that the disruptive forces were at an angle to the path of the bullet.[2]

Additional experiments showed that a bullet fired at the head first depresses the bone at the contact site, causing a slight rise of intracranial pressure. As it enters the head, the bullet displaces its content, causing a more marked rise of pressure in the head. The generated forces burst the rigid skull or, failing that, drive brain tissue against the internal surface of the skull. Displaced brain and cerebrospinal fluid compress the brainstem, leading to a respiratory arrest and, initially, to a slight decline followed by a rise in blood pressure. Horsley believed that a respiratory – rather than cardiac – arrest was the primary cause of death.[2] He thus suggested that immediate treatment should be to assist ventilation rather than to administer cardiac stimulants, then the prevailing approach.

In 1897 he published a more detailed account with S. P. Kramer, later professor of pathology at the University of Cincinnati. They shot anesthetized dogs in the head with bullets of various calibers and confirmed that the primary cause of death was respiratory arrest, which could be countered by artificial ventilation; a secondary cause was increased intracranial pressure from hemorrhage.[3] Their emphasis on the need to maintain the airway and ventilation has since received wide support, and the death rate has declined because of early tracheostomy and other measures.[4]

Horsley subsequently found that maximal destruction occurred where the bullet at its highest velocity is surrounded by the largest mass of wet tissue.[5] The exit wound from the head is larger and more irregular than the entry wound, reflecting bullet tumbling (that is, yawing or turning from its trajectory) and the driving out of tissues and fluids by the bullet. Further analysis of the plaster casts suggested that water molecules are thrown off almost at right angles to the axis of flight.[5] This radial (outward) displacement of tissues is due to secondary pressure changes.[6,7,8] As the bullet passes through the brain, it creates a crush or permanent cavity; this expands temporarily as the relatively inelastic brain tissue moves away from the bullet's path. The skull limits the extent of the transiently expanded cavity, and pressure changes can then either burst the skull or damage tissues away from the bullet track, especially in the brainstem.[6,7,8]

Certain bullets are particularly likely to fragment on impact, causing even more damage because each fragment then acts as an individual projectile. With the onset of war in 1914, the Germans alleged that British soldiers were using such dumdum bullets. The British government denied this, its war office charging instead that it was the Germans – in Togoland (a German colony in West Africa) and in France – who were using an expanding soft-core bullet of the type expressly prohibited by the Hague Convention.[9] Horsley had examined the properties of the bullets used by the British forces in his experiments referred to earlier, concluding that their design and manufacture ensured that they were not easily flattened or deformed in shape and that they did not break into fragments to inflict a wound which, while "effecting its necessary object of disabling, caused unnecessary suffering."[10] His reports were attached to the government's response as two appendices,[11] and brought him the thanks of Lord Kitchener, then secretary of state for war and – more than that – a national hero, the symbol of military success.

Clinical Aspects of Gunshot Wounds to the Head

In a lecture given in February 1915, Horsley discussed various clinical aspects of the management of gunshot wounds to the head, stressing that these injuries are not always fatal despite the commonly held view to the contrary. He urged that intracranial pressure should be controlled, certain intracranial hematomas evacuated, fragments of bone removed from the brain, and wounds disinfected.[5] The correctness of this view and the need to debride gunshot wounds has since been recognized, particularly with the experience gained in subsequent wars.[12]

Horsley's practical approach involved excision of the affected area of the scalp to expose the injured area of skull, and removal of sufficient bone to expose normal dura mater around the entire circumference of the wound. Foreign bodies, blood, and pus were removed from the brain without breaking down protective adhesions. Over the years since then, based on his work and that of Harvey Cushing[13] and others, the general approach has been to remove completely any intracranial bone or metal fragments, if necessary by repeated surgeries, although less aggressive debridement has been favored by some.[14]

Military Service

Early in the war, Horsley recognized and criticized the many inadequacies in the medical services provided for the wounded. He pointed out that the enormous casualty rates made it impossible for the existing staff to keep patients clean and comfortable and to change their dressings as often as necessary to prevent septic complications. More medical and nursing staff and supplies were required, and he regarded it as shameful that motor ambulances and other resources had to be provided privately to prevent unnecessary suffering.[15] His concerns were justified, for private support became essential to the war effort – the British Red Cross, for example, helped to recruit medical and paramedical personnel and provided hospitals, rest stations, supplies and supply depots, and motor ambulances for use overseas, supported by a fund-raising campaign for which *The Times* newspaper donated advertising space almost daily through much of the war.[16]

Horsley also became involved in a public row with Rickman Godlee, who advocated the use of undiluted carbolic acid (phenol) to swab out recent wounds in the belief that this had been advocated by Lister. Horsley pointed out that tissue damage would likely result unless a weak (five percent) solution was utilized.[15,17] Their disagreement was heated, stoked by ill-feeling reflecting their differences over Lloyd George's National Insurance Bill, the lack of representation of members (as opposed to fellows) on the governing council of the Royal College of Surgeons (see Chapter 10), and Godlee's failure to support Horsley when the government complained to the college about him in the controversy over forcible feeding of suffragists (see Chapter 12).

Horsley, a man of action, was not content simply to criticize the medical arrangements for the troops during the war but went on to volunteer his own services. He did not feel his age, remained vigorous and energetic, wanted to share in the war effort, and believed his surgical expertise would be invaluable in dealing with casualties and improving the quality of medical care. It concerned him particularly that many head wounds were deemed by medical officers to be untreatable and thus were simply neglected. In discussing his military contributions here, a more general account of the war or of particular campaigns is not provided except to furnish necessary background information.

As a volunteer in the territorial force, Horsley was on the staff of the Third London General Hospital, housed in a Gothic-style Victorian building, formerly an orphanage, in Wandsworth, south London. The hospital was one in name alone until the outbreak of war, at which point its staff was mobilized. It had no equipment, and Horsley was soon involved in selecting the surgical instruments and supplies that would be needed. There was little else to do, however, and in mid-August he therefore asked for a transfer from the reserves to active service.[18,19] Realizing that sudden pressure on the base hospitals was likely as war casualties mounted, he suggested to the director-general of the Army Medical Service that experienced surgeons should be appointed to the expeditionary force as supernumeraries, to be sent to hospitals as needed.[18,19]

> The condition in which the wounded arrive here, the statements they make of the want of surgical attention during transport, especially in trains, the fact that many cases are prejudiced (some have even died) by being put on board ship when they should have been treated at a base hospital, are all clearly due to a shortage of experienced surgeons on the other side of the Channel.[18,19]

His advice, unsolicited and unwanted, was ignored – it would take many more months before the authorities took note of criticisms and constructive suggestions to improve the available medical services, by which time Horsley was himself a casualty.

France

While awaiting placement, he volunteered to work in the small (one-hundred bed), private British Red Cross hospital established late in 1914 at Wimereux, close to Boulogne in northern France by Sir Henry Norman, a Liberal politician, and his suffragist wife, Priscilla. The hospital was located in the rather squalid Hôtel Bellevue, close to a river, the railway – which helped in transporting the wounded – and a seaport, which facilitated the evacuation of the seriously injured to Britain. Horsley regarded it as almost an annex of No. 14 General Hospital, also at Wimereux. Beds, sterilizers, and equipment filled the small wards on the first two floors of the old hotel; the staff occupied the top floor. Lady Norman acted as the superintendent, and, in addition to Horsley, there were three other doctors, with one of whom – Captain Robinson – he became especially close. At first the hospital was only half filled, but that changed as its presence became better known. Patients did not stay long, either dying or passing on to other facilities.

Horsley became busy with both head cases and general surgical problems, performing amputations, dressing wounds, and countering sepsis. There was little time for recreation after the first days, but he made time to write home about daily events, the problems at the hospital, the inadequacies he now perceived in the Normans, the temperance movement, a sightseeing trip to Boulogne, and even about the Brotherhood Movement of the Free Churches, with its idealistic Christian appeal to non-churchgoers.

Early in 1915, Horsley was placed in charge of the surgical division of No. 21 General Hospital, which was destined for service in France. This meant he had to give up his voluntary work at Wimereux. It had been instructive, for his experience had confirmed his worst fears. Amateurism and charity were not sufficient to run a military hospital in wartime.

Egypt and Gallipoli

In the spring of 1915, the No. 21 General Hospital was ordered to Egypt, and Horsley, now appointed a major in the Royal Army Medical Corps (Territorials), left England with it on May 20. They sailed on *HMHS Delta*, a liner built in 1905 for the P&O Line, but now converted to a makeshift naval hospital ship, its cabins and cargo decks converted to wards.[20] The ship was painted white but with large illuminated red crosses to signal its identity.

Robinson wrote to him from Wimeraux: "If it is true you are going to Egypt I shall be sorry. It will make it impossible to see you soon again. Don't work so hard there as you did here. The heat would take it out of you. . . . "[21] His warning seems prophetic.

Horsley arrived in Alexandria, the base of the Mediterranean Expeditionary Force, at the end of May 1915. Several military hospitals – British, Australian, New Zealand, French, Indian, Greek, and local Egyptian ones – were located there, as were various convalescent facilities. The 21st General settled, after a great deal of hard work, into the dilapidated cavalry barracks at the royal Ras-el-Tin Palace on the Mediterranean coast. The first few days were spent in cleaning out the buildings with insecticides and other pesticides,

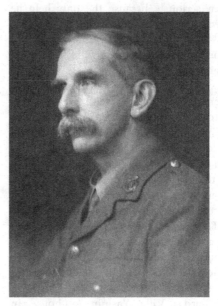

Figure 15.1 Victor Horsley in military uniform. Photograph by G. C. Beresford. (Image courtesy of the Queen Square Archives and Sir Victor Horsley's family.)

scrubbing down the walls and windows, and bringing in supplies, work in which the famous brain surgeon did his fair share. The equipment for the hospital was quite inadequate, and requests for essential supplies and X-ray equipment had to pass along the proper channels, with inevitable delays and requests for justification even as the wounded started to arrive. At a time when the hospital was barely operational, the staff were told to expect four hundred casualties although there were nurses for fewer than half that number. Horsley noted bitterly that inadequacies were dismissed as simply due to the war and that the needs of the men seemed to matter little to the authorities back home.

The aging neurosurgeon was struck by the heat and the flies, and by the noise, smells, and dirt of the city, and he may well have been disappointed by his lowly duties as a junior officer. He was entranced, however, by the colors, especially at sunset, and became popular with the men as he joined uncomplainingly in the work to bring the hospital into some sort of order. His own worth initially passed unrecognized. On one occasion, a surgeon at an Egyptian hospital requested the help of a brain surgeon to manage several patients with head injuries. Horsley saw them and gave his advice, but the Egyptian – not recognizing him – complained that his request had not been taken seriously because the only help he received was from an elderly junior officer.

The ill-fated Gallipoli campaign, intended to shorten the war by capturing the Ottoman capital of Constantinople and opening a sea route to Russia, had fared badly since its commencement in February 1915. Renewed military actions in June led to a medical crisis in Egypt because of the appalling increase in number of the sick and injured. Consequently, in mid-July, Horsley was appointed a consultant surgeon (with the rank of colonel) to the Mediterranean Expeditionary Force, and was based in Alexandria with a second consultant, Alfred Tubby, an orthopedic surgeon. They were required to operate whenever necessary and otherwise to oversee and advise on surgical matters in the various hospitals and other medical facilities in the region. The two surgeons became good friends, and each had rooms in Mme. Caillard's Villa Yasmin, a house in Glymenopoulo, near Ramleh in the eastern suburbs of the city. Horsley worked hard all day and continued without rest well into the night, adding to the records of head wounds that he was assembling.[20] Francis Walshe, one of his former house surgeons in London, was neurological specialist to the military forces in Egypt and helped greatly in dealing with obscure disorders of the nervous system.

Within a few weeks, Horsley had inspected the Egyptian hospital at Damanhur, east of Alexandria, and reported that its staffing, supplies, and treatment facilities were inadequate.[22] General William Babtie, director of medical services for the Dardanelles campaign, ignored him. David Semple, director-general of the public health department in Egypt, responded that Egyptian hospitals were not intended for Europeans and that nothing was amiss when he inspected the hospital. He queried acidly whether "Sir Victor Horsley is simply a consulting surgeon to these hospitals or whether he has some authority to act as an inspector?"[23] Semple, a protégé of Almroth Wright, was renowned for his work on rabies prevention in India and had established a Pasteur Institute in the foothills of the Himalayas.

Each of the several regional consultant surgeons, including Horsley, expressed a wish to go to the Dardanelles, and so were required to spend three weeks at a time there.[24] Horsley spent most of October in Gallipoli, visiting medical units,

field ambulances, and the makeshift dressing and casualty clearing stations on the front line and in the trenches. He met with the officers and men staffing these stations at Anzac Cove, Suvla Bay, and Cape Helles, listened closely to their accounts, and advised them on surgical issues. He impressed everyone by his physical fitness in clambering about the ravines and gullies of the peninsula, and by his courage and thoughtfulness. He noted the unfinished shelters, lack of warm clothing and blankets, and need for better provisions,[25,26] and he wrote to Sir Alfred Keogh, director of the Army Medical Service, to describe the poor conditions, which he likened to those in the Crimean War.[27] Indeed, he continued to send unsolicited reports about various inadequacies to his superiors throughout his military service as he visited other medical facilities. For example, he complained later in the year that the so-called "hospital ships" transporting the injured back to Egypt were completely unsatisfactory – lacking adequate equipment or medical facilities – and were often dangerously overloaded.[28] The people at home, however, seemed not to want to know of the problems and deficiencies that existed, focusing their attention more on the Western Front than on Gallipoli.

Horsley's personal courage cannot be doubted. He was mentioned in dispatches in December 1915 for his "gallant and distinguished services in the field," the certificate of appreciation being signed by the secretary of state for war, Winston Churchill, after the war was over, in 1919.[29]

Horsley had missed his family, but Eldred joined him in Egypt in August and, two months later, while he was away in Gallipoli, their twenty-one-year-old daughter Pamela also arrived. She had been a wonderful correspondent, sending chatty letters full of fun and trivia as well as family news, adorned with little sketches, and addressed to him as Alexander or by nickname ("Sanders").[30] The two women helped out at a neighboring hospital but, in November, Pamela came down with severe dysentery and had to be admitted to the Fifth Indian Hospital, where Major Robert McCarrison of the Indian Medical Service looked after her. McCarrison (1878–1960) had previously studied goiter and cretinism in Asia and thus had a common interest with Horsley (see Chapter 3); he went on to become a major-general and an international expert on nutritional deficiencies, and received many prizes and honors including a knighthood.

After recovering, Pamela went with Eldred to convalesce for ten weeks at Helwan, a suburb of Cairo opposite the ruins of Memphis, the capital of ancient Egypt, and then at Luxor, with its ancient temples. Walshe encountered her on one occasion at a local museum, sitting on a hard bench and sketching some of the specimens on display. She looked wan and drawn, but this apparently was Eldred's idea of a recuperative holiday.[31] Horsley wrote them frequent, gossipy notes and, with Walshe, was able to join them for a few days of rest and sightseeing at Luxor. The hotels and restaurants were on the east bank of the Nile, while on the opposite bank were the Valley of the Kings and various relics and ruins of interest to foreign tourists. To visit them it was necessary to cross the river and then proceed by trap or donkey. Horsley and Walshe were thus presented with a choice as they made plans for a daytrip, leading Horsley to start a protracted but unsuccessful search for Lady Horsley. Eventually he had to decide alone whether she would prefer to travel in the trap or ride by donkey. He opted for the trap but with a certain trepidation, remarking that whatever he chose would displease Eldred, who would then declare her strong preference for the other. And so it was, for when they finally found her and told her of the plans for the trip, she asked whether they thought her incapable of riding a donkey.[31]

Things quieted down at the hospitals in Alexandria with the withdrawal of British and French forces from the Gallipoli Peninsula in January 1916, and there was then little for Horsley to do other than follow the progress of his patients, enjoy the mild climate and flowering desert, and visit archeological ruins. The news about the ongoing Mesopotamia campaign, in which British and Indian forces faced the Ottoman army, was increasingly grim, however, at least as recounted by medical officers returning to Egypt on leave: disease was rife, facilities for treating the wounded were appalling, and supplies were lacking. Concerned about the welfare of the men and fearful about wasting his time in Alexandria, at the beginning of March Horsley approached General William Babtie, who directed medical services for the British Indian Army, volunteering for active service in Mesopotamia. Within a few days, he was on his way to India, mistakenly believing he would have a free hand.

He had made many friends in Egypt, learned something of the language and culture, and enjoyed the beauty of Alexandria, its museums, churches, catacombs, and antiquities. His military colleagues had enjoyed his company and gained much from his expertise and advice, which he gave without being in the least bit patronizing or condescending. He had been tireless in helping the injured, whose interests he always held at heart, but – true to form – he made enemies among those in command by his criticisms of the inadequate facilities to care for the wounded of Gallipoli. Despite the hostility of his superiors, early in 2016 he was made a Companion of the Order of the Bath (C.B.), military division, for his services with the Mediterranean Expeditionary Force.[32]

And so to Mesopotamia

Horsley reached Bombay on the P&O's SS *Arabia*, on March 25, 1916. He left after two weeks for Mesopotamia, reached Basra on April 16, and died three months later.

While in Bombay, he stayed with Lord Willingdon, its crown governor (later viceroy and governor-general of India) at Government House. His suite overlooked the bay, outlined at night by the lights of the city, sparkling with a romance and glamour that he could not share with Eldred. The city itself was colorful and lively, its people interesting, and he enjoyed his visit, even as he disliked the servants fussing over him.

The Indian government and army had directed the Mesopotamia campaign, and Horsley therefore met with the army commander-in-chief, Sir Beauchamp Duff, in Delhi and Simla, as well as with the director-general of the Indian Medical Service, Sir Pardey Lukis. Back in Bombay, he lectured stirringly to the medical students at Grant Medical College on poverty, disease, and racial poison ("alcohol being the commonest, the handmaiden of which [is] venereal disease"),[33] but his concern was for the apparent breakdown of medical arrangements in Mesopotamia.

In view of a mounting public outcry about the conduct of the campaign and the increasing number of casualties, the Indian government now appointed a commission to investigate the arrangements for the wounded and sick in Mesopotamia. The commission consisted of Sir William Vincent, a retired civil servant with judicial experience, Major-General A. H. Bingley, a staff officer of the Indian Army, and, later, E. A. Ridsdale, a London businessman and commissioner of the British Red Cross. Horsley, still in India and dismayed that a medical man was not included, regarded the investigation as bogus from the start. In fact, the commission spent several weeks in Mesopotamia and produced a damning report three months later (shortly before Horsley's death). Its findings, however, would not be published for another year.

Mesopotamia ("the land between the rivers") corresponds in the main to present-day Iraq. The Tigris and Euphrates rivers, which arise in the mountains to the north, traverse it and tradition places the Garden of Eden in the land between them as they run to the sea. The country is largely arid desert, except where it becomes marshy as the two rivers converge in their approach to the Persian Gulf. The confluence of the two rivers forms the Shatt al-Arab waterway, some of which now delineates part of the border between Iraq and Iran. In the early twentieth century, nomadic sheep and goat herders lived in much of Mesopotamia, but the land was farmed where it became more fertile along the rivers' edge and delta.

To the British, the only redeeming feature of this inhospitable, barren country – a part of the far-flung Ottoman Empire – was the possibility that it harbored oil, for there were vast reserves in adjacent Persia (Iran) and the Anglo-Persian Oil Company operated a major refinery at Abadan, close to the Persian Gulf.[34] With the Ottoman involvement in World War I and increasing local unrest, the British needed to protect their oil supplies and underline their imperial role. They sent troops to the area, secured the oil fields, and occupied Basra on the Shatt al-Arab. The troops then moved ambitiously toward Baghdad, but setbacks followed. At the end of April 1916, a large Anglo-Indian force, besieged at Kut-al-Amara, was forced to surrender to the Ottomans and marched into captivity. It was a humiliating and shattering defeat, brought on in part by uncertain priorities, ambiguity about the purpose of the campaign, failure to supply the means to achieve the desired ends, and the use of troops and a command structure without experience of the required operations.

In the first half of 1916, conditions in Mesopotamia were primitive and morale among the troops was low. Anticipated victories had turned into defeats. The wet season (November to March) was cold, muddy, and in itself dispiriting. In the dry season, the heat was almost unbearable, dust was several inches deep, and the banks of the rivers or waterways were made up of fissured clay as hard as concrete. All manner of insects were present including fleas, bedbugs, sand-flies, flying beetles, large dragonflies, and huge moths.[35] Flies were everywhere and got into every orifice. The mosquitos were insuperable. There was little fuel or drinking water, and at times almost no food for the troops. There were palm and fig trees along the banks of the waterways but no trees on the plain to shade the men. In the tents, the temperature sometimes reached 130°F, but – with little fluid to sustain them – the men could barely sweat. When they developed a high fever and headache, they were admitted to hospital, but no ice-making plants were available to counter the effects of the excessive heat and reduce the risk of death. Tents, beds, mattresses, medications, and even the simplest instruments were in short supply. Splints, for example, had to be made from empty packing cases. Diarrhea, dysentery, and cholera were constant problems due to the filth and improperly sterilized water; skin sores were common and took months to heal; beriberi and scurvy were widespread. Sand-fly fever and malaria added to the general misery. It was in these circumstances that Horsley arrived in mid-April, the beginning of the hot dry season.

Although the medical problems were enormous,[36] foremost among them was the difficulty in evacuating the sick and wounded to base hospitals. Ambulances were in short supply, stretchers had to be improvised, bearers were lacking, and transport along the waterway from the front to Basra utilized filthy river steamers and barges that were returning there after having ferried troops forward. The patients – exhausted, hollow-eyed, and gaunt – huddled miserably in crowded boats, with the most seriously injured laid out on the oft-flooded deck like sardines in a can, only occasionally shielded from the relentless sun by a single canvas awning, without clean drinking water, and with only a single latrine on each barge. Like everyone else, the medical personnel who attended to them were affected by the extreme temperature so that, by mid-morning, they were exhausted, their energy sapped, their initiative replaced by inertia. Reading and writing became an unwelcome chore, rational planning almost impossible. The exception was Horsley who, almost as soon as he arrived, began to write outraged reports that were cabled to the authorities in London and India.[37,38,39]

Unlike many senior medical officers, Horsley refused to confine himself to a base hospital but went right up to the trenches and the front. He stopped first in Basra, where the houses nudged down to a river congested with boats of all sizes going in all directions, and he wrote to Lukis in Simla and the authorities in London about the primitive transport arrangements and lack of even the most simple supplies.[40] Because of the climate, the troops were provided with a pith helmet and a cloth spine pad (that was attached to the shirt, and maintained in position by tapes tied round the trunk) in the belief that it was important to protect the nervous system from direct exposure to the sun. Horsley, however, often went about his duties with neither, believing that his teetotalism would protect him. Food was scarce and, due to the heat and lack of adequate storage facilities, perished rapidly. It was even more limited upriver, as Horsley discovered when he moved on after a few days, eventually stopping in Amara, some one hundred miles to the north, where there were seven general hospitals as well as smaller medical facilities. From Amara he went forward to the front when he pleased. Regardless of where he was, he helped to look after the injured and sick while he looked for problems, suggested solutions, and reported on the difficulties to those in charge.

He objected to the quantity of alcohol brought in, often in seeming preference to food or medical supplies, and he lost no opportunity to rail against this in his reports and letters home. But others differed with him on the alcohol question. Thus, Martin Swayne, a physician, wrote:

> It was almost a universal experience to find alcohol necessary in the evening. The mind was exhausted, food was unattractive, conversation was impossible, the passage of time immeasurably slow, and a restless irritation pervaded one until a dose of alcohol was taken. Its effect was humanising.[41]

In fact, Horsley was more understanding of the troops and their needs than is usually credited, and his objections were to the preferential transport of alcohol rather than more essential supplies. A New Zealand military surgeon later wrote of the time that Horsley spent as a guest in their small mess. "We felt very honoured to entertain a man of such eminence, but we were a little concerned as well, for we were aware of his strong views on tobacco and alcohol. However, he proved a most pleasant companion, and quite uncritical of the use of these solaces by us."[42]

The mail, when it came, was a means of reestablishing, for a few moments, a private life. Horsley wrote of the scandalous conditions, and of the local inhabitants, wildlife, forbidding countryside, and the supposed tomb of the biblical Ezra on the bank of the Tigris, illustrating his accounts with simple sketches. He wrote of the abuse of alcohol, of the political situation in Britain, of a future in politics. He wrote of the floating corpses contaminating the drinking water, the insects that made life a misery, the need to walk many miles to inspect medical outposts. He wrote from Basra, Amara, Shaik Sad, from the front close to the firing line. He finally heard from Eldred that she had arrived back in England and rejoiced.

The Death of Horsley

On July 14, just after he had returned to Amara from the front, Horsley began to feel unwell even as he continued to work. On the following day, having walked one and one-half miles back to camp over the open plain where the shade temperature exceeded 130°F, and the atmosphere was humid, he reached his tent only to hear about a sick officer about a half-mile further on. He went on to see the man, and returned with a headache.[43] Later that day, he was admitted to No. 2 (Rawal Pindi) British General Hospital with a fever and suspected paratyphoid, although the infection could not be confirmed bacteriologically. On July 16, his fever worsened, he lapsed into unconsciousness and he died that evening, officially of heatstroke, a diagnosis that seems quite appropriate in the circumstances.

The troops and medical staff felt his death deeply. His funeral the following evening was attended by eighty officers who walked the mile to the cemetery in columns of fours, the most junior in front. He was buried at the same time as seven other soldiers, one of whom had been his patient.[44] Because of the scarcity of wood, it was common for bodies to be buried sewn up in army blankets, but Horsley was given the privilege of a coffin. He was placed in a shallow grave after a brief ceremony. "Last Post" was played over his and the other new graves.[45] A cross of white marble was later placed on his grave.

Major George Grey Turner (later the first director of surgery at the British Postgraduate Medical School in London) was present with Horsley in Mesopotamia. He commented:

> It seemed fitting that after his work for the service Sir Victor should have found a soldier's grave; and as he was laid to rest the sun was setting in the direction of the distant battle line which he had visited, and the crack of a Maxim at practice accompanied the burial service. The coffin bore the simple inscription –
> *Colonel Sir Victor Horsley, A.M.S. Died 16/7/16.*[44]

The Amara War Cemetery, east of Amara between the river and the Chahaila Canal, contains four thousand six hundred and twenty-one graves from the Great War, three of them for winners of the Victoria Cross. In 1933 all the headstones, which were crumbling, were removed

and a screen wall was erected with the engraved names of those buried in the cemetery.[46] The cemetery itself was quietly forgotten in the West, however, at least until the Iraq invasion of 2003.[47] Reports have since described a vandalized and looted site, "an unsightly expanse of mud, weeds and uncut grass the size of four or five football pitches. The smashed remains of the traditional Cross of Sacrifice are piled in the middle. Plaques naming the dead have fallen off the commemorative wall."[48]

A Letter from the Grave

But what of Horsley's complaints about the medical services? Were they justified?

In August, the editor of the *British Medical Journal* received a letter from Horsley, written while he was at the front, ten days before his death. He had not wished it published, but the information it contained was not confidential and formed the basis of a lengthy editorial.[49] As in his many reports from Mesopotamia, Horsley attributed the breakdown of medical services to government economies and "to the non-provision of transport. There never has been in this country [Mesopotamia] adequate transport for food, and

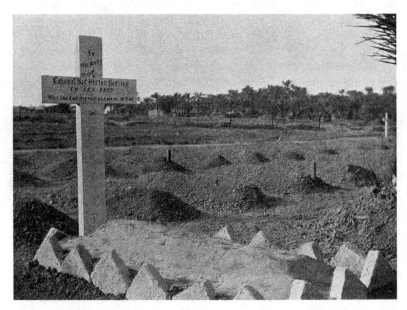

Figure 15.2 Horsley's grave at Amara. The inscription reads: "In memory of Colonel Sir Victor Horsley CB, FRS, FRCS, who died on service at Amara 16.7.16." (Photograph by Dr. Andrew Balfour; From Paget S: *Sir Victor Horsley: A Study of His Life and Work*. Constable: London, 1919.)

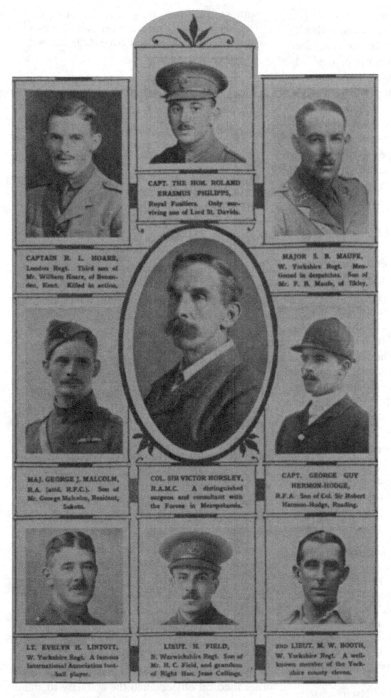

Figure 15.3 Portion of *For King and Country: Officers on the Roll of Honour*, published in the *Illustrated London News* of July 29, 1916, p. 139. Photographs of twenty-two fallen officers were shown on the page. Horsley's image was the centerpiece.

CAPT. THE HON. ROLAND ERASMUS PHILIPPS, Royal Fusiliers. Only surviving son of Lord St. Davids.

CAPTAIN R. L. HOARE, London Regt. Third son of Mr. William Hoare, of Benenden, Kent. Killed in action.

MAJOR S. R. MAUFE, W. Yorkshire Regt. Mentioned in despatches. Son of Mr. F. B. Maufe, of Ilkley.

MAJ. GEORGE J. MALCOLM, R.A. [attd. R.F.C.]. Son of Mr. George Malcolm, Resident, Sokoto.

COL. SIR VICTOR HORSLEY, R.A.M.C. A distinguished surgeon and consultant with the Forces in Mesopotamia.

CAPT. GEORGE GUY HERMON-HODGE, R.F.A. Son of Col. Sir Robert Hermon-Hodge, Reading.

LT. EVELYN H. LINTOTT, W. Yorkshire Regt. A famous International Association football player.

LIEUT. H. FIELD, R. Warwickshire Regt. Son of Mr. H. C. Field, and grandson of Right Hon. Jesse Collings.

2ND LIEUT. M. W. BOOTH, W. Yorkshire Regt. A well-known member of the Yorkshire county eleven.

there never (until March, when our solitary hospital steamer arrived) has been any medical transport whatever; nothing but the foulest store barges and steamers used on their return journey to the base to carry the sick and wounded." Independent sources confirmed his allegations, which neither the Indian government nor the war office in London could continue to deny.

In fact, in the week before he died and unknown to him, urgent questions were asked in parliament about the conduct of the mismanaged Mesopotamian campaign, including the "appalling collapse in the medical arrangements."[50] As a correspondent wrote in *The Times*, "Many, both in Great Britain and India, consider the facts connected with the breakdown of medical and other arrangements in Mesopotamia to constitute the greatest scandal that has occurred in our Empire for at least half a century."[51] The statement to parliament of the prime minister, Mr. Asquith, produced more questions than answers,[52] and in August a special commission of enquiry was set up by an act of parliament. Horsley's widow let it be known to Asquith that she would make his letters available to the commission.[53]

The former secretary of state for India chaired the new enquiry, assisted by five members of parliament, an admiral, and a general. Their report was published in 1917,[54] and included an appendix with the findings of the earlier Vincent–Bingley commission.[55] The extraordinary inadequacies of the military and medical services in Mesopotamia were recorded, but no blame was attached to the medical staff. The report pointed to a number of major deficiencies relating especially to the transport and evacuation of the wounded. The conditions in which the wounded arrived at Basra were not detailed "because of their sickening horror"[56] but were grotesque. A hint was provided by the harrowing testimony of a Major Carter, who had charge in Basra of a hospital ship awaiting the arrival of a small river steamer with two barges loaded with casualties. As the steamer

> came up to us I saw that she was absolutely packed, and the barges too, with men. The barges were slipped, and the *Medjidieh* [the river steamer] was brought alongside the *Varela* [the hospital ship]. When she was about 300 or 400 yards off it looked as if she was festooned with ropes. The stench when she was close was quite definite, and I found that what I mistook for ropes were dried stalactites of human faeces. The patients were so crowded and huddled together on the ship that they could not perform the offices of Nature clear of the edge of the ship, and the whole of the ship's side was covered with stalactites of human faeces. This is what I then saw. A certain number of men were standing and kneeling on the immediate perimeter of the ship. Then we found a mass of men huddled up anyhow – some with blankets and some

> without. They were lying in a pool of dysentery about 30 feet square. They were covered with dysentery and dejecta generally from head to foot.[56]

Carter had originally reported his observations to the authorities in Mesopotamia, but they had resented any implication of criticism, considered his comments "objectionable," and regarded him as a "meddlesome interfering faddist" whom they threatened with arrest and the loss of his hospital ship.[56] Not surprisingly, many medical officers – but not Horsley – accepted the futility of complaint in such circumstances.

The commission concluded that financial stringencies and defence cuts had limited general and medical preparations for the Mesopotamia campaign, with catastrophic consequences. Horsley's view, perhaps more intuitive than informed, had been similar. In its report, the commission caused something of a sensation by censuring various public figures including William Babtie and his successor as director of medical services in India, General James MacNeece; Lord Hardinge, the viceroy of India; and Sir Beauchamp Duff, the army commander-in chief. If Horsley had known, he would have felt vindicated.

Command of the campaign had moved from Delhi to London early in 1916 and led to an influx of resources, and especially of medical equipment and personnel. Hospital accommodation in Mesopotamia tripled between January and July, but was still insufficient.[58] New commanders and senior medical officers were appointed. Nevertheless, during Horsley's brief time there, conditions in Mesopotamia remained appalling and he was not satisfied with bland assurances that additional aid was on its way. He made a fuss. It is fair to conclude that without the vigilance of the press and the courage of individuals such as Horsley, the medical failings in the Dardanelles and Mesopotamia would have been far greater than they were.[59] Horsley, unlike most other medical officers, had the audacity to stand firm, taking his concerns to the highest levels of civilian authority and military command in the interests of the troops.

Just a few weeks after his death, Lloyd George, the secretary of state for war, responded to a parliamentary question about the Mesopotamia campaign. He informed the house that "an installation for sterilising water, recommended by the Director of Medical Services and the late Sir Victor Horsley, has already been provided on many ships and will be fitted to the remainder. . . . A large number of hospital river steamers and barges have also been ordered. As regards drugs, medicines, bandages and other medical appliances, all demands have been supplied. . . . I am satisfied that sufficient supplies are now available on the spot."

The follow-up question was peculiarly British – "Does that sufficiency of supplies include tea?"[60]

Notes

1. Kitchen N: Comments on Cybulski GR, Stone JL, Patel KJ. Sir Victor Horsley's contributions to the study and treatment of gunshot wounds of the head. *Neurosurgery* 2008; **63**: 812. The statement by Kitchen is based, in turn, on an account by Horsley's grandson, Victor Horsley Robinson, related to Michael Powell, FRCS (Powell, personal communication, 2017).

2. Horsley V: The destructive effects of small projectiles. *Not Proc R Inst Gr Br* 1894; **14**: 228–238; *Nature* 1894; **50**: 104–108.

3. Kramer SP, Horsley V: On the effects produced on the circulation and respiration by gunshot injuries of the cerebral hemispheres. *Philos Trans R Soc Lond B* 1897; **188**: 223–256.

4. Lewin W: Changing attitudes to the management of severe head injuries. *Br Med J* 1976; **2**: 1234–1239.

5. Horsley V: An address on gunshot wounds of the head. *Lancet* 1915; **185**: 359–362.

6. Hanna TN, Shuaib W, Han T, Mehta A, Khosa F: Firearms, bullets, and wound ballistics: An imaging primer. *Injury Int J Care Injured* 2015; **46**: 1186–1196.

7. Stefanopoulos PK, Hadjigeorgiou GF, Filippakis K, Gyftokostas D: Gunshot wounds: A review of ballistics related to penetrating trauma. *J Acute Dis* 2014; **3**: 178–185.

8. Stefanopoulos PK, Filippakis K, Soupiou OT, Pazarakiotis VC: Wound ballistics of firearm-related injuries – Part 1: Missile characteristics and mechanisms of soft tissue wounding. *Int J Oral Maxillofac Surg* 2014; **43**: 1445–1458.

9. Anon: The expanding bullet. British answer to German allegations. *The Times (Lond)*, November 18, 1914, p. 7.

10. Horsley V: Appendices to the memorandum communicated by the War Office respecting British and German service ammunition.

Appendix I: Memorandum on the .303 (174 grains) Mark VII British service rifle bullet in reference to explosive effects. Appendix II: Note on the flat-nose revolver bullet, Mark IV, in reference to the provisions of the Hague Convention. *Br Med J* 1914; **2**: 896.

11. Anon: British and German small arm ammunition. Memorandum communicated by the War Office respecting British and German service ammunition. *Br Med J* 1914; **2**: 895–896.

12. Aarabi B, Mossop C, Aarabi JA: Surgical management of civilian gunshot wounds to the head. *Handb Clin Neurol* 2015; **127**: 181–193.

13. Cushing H: A study of a series of wounds involving the brain and its enveloping structures. *Br J Surg* 1917; **5**: 558–684.

14. Pruitt B (ed.): Surgical management of penetrating brain injury. *J Trauma* 2001; **51** (Suppl.): S16–S25.

15. Horsley V: Care of the wounded. [Letter to the editor.] *Br Med J* 1914; **2**: 813.

16. British Red Cross: What we did during the war. Available at: https://vad.redcross.org.uk/What-we-did-during-the-war. Fundraising during the First World War [last accessed June 30, 2021].

17. Horsley V: Antisepsis and asepsis in war. [Letter to the editor.] *Br Med J* 1914; **2**: 861.

18. Horsley V: The wounded in the war. [Letter to the editor.] *Lancet* 1914; **184**: 1116.

19. Horsley V: The care of our wounded. [Letter to the editor.] *The Times (Lond)*, November 8, 1914, p. 9.

20. Tubby AH: *A Consulting Surgeon in the Near East*. Christophers: London, 1920.

21. Robinson EH: Letter to Victor Horsley dated May 15 or 16, 1915. Section E4/18, Horsley Papers, Special Collections, UCL Library Services (London, UK).

22. Horsley V: Report on the General Hospital, Damanhour, and related correspondence. Section B17, Horsley Papers, Special Collections, UCL Library Services (London, UK).

23. Dunnill MS: Victor Horsley (1857–1916) in World War I. *J Med Biogr* 2010; **18**: 186–193.

24. Babtie W: Letter to Major Sir Victor Horsley dated July 15, 1915. Section B1 (Miscellaneous documents), Horsley Papers, Special Collections, UCL Library Services (London, UK).

25. Horsley V: Draft letter to General Davis on conditions at the front, dated October 19, 1915. Section B23, Horsley Papers, Special Collections, UCL Library Services (London, UK).

26. Horsley V: Letter and report to Surgeon-General Babtie concerning tour of inspection

of the front, dated October 23, 1915. Section B24, Horsley Papers, Special Collections, UCL Library Services (London, UK).

27. Horsley V: Draft letter to Sir Alfred Keogh on conditions at the front, dated November 3, 1915. Section B26, Horsley Papers, Special Collections, UCL Library Services (London, UK).

28. Horsley V: Draft letters to General Babtie on hospital ships, dated December 22, 1915. Section B27, Horsley Papers, Special Collections, UCL Library Services (London, UK).

29. Churchill WS, Secretary of State for War: Certificate of the mention in dispatches of Colonel Sir VAH Horsley, FRS, MB, FRCS, on December 11, 1915. Certificate dated March 1, 1919. Section B1, Horsley Papers, Special Collections, UCL Library Services (London, UK).

30. Robinson PC: Letters to Victor Horsley, 1914–1916. Section E4/18, Horsley Papers, Special Collections, UCL Library Services (London, UK).

31. Walshe FMR: Personal communication, July 15, 1966.

32. Anon: Coronation Honours. *Br Med J* 1902; **2**: 75–76.

33. Anon: Sir Victor Horsley. Lecture to Bombay students. *The Times of India*, April 6, 1916, p. 8.

34. The Anglo-Persian Oil Company was renamed the Anglo-Iranian Oil Company in the 1930s and in 1954 became British Petroleum.

35. Begg RC: *Surgery on Trestles: A Saga of Suffering and Triumph.* Jarrold & Sons: Norwich, 1967.

36. MacPherson WG, Mitchell TJ: *History of the Great War Based on Official Documents. Medical Services: General History. Volume IV.* pp. 163–231. His Majesty's Stationery Office: London, 1924.

37. Copybook of original correspondence. Section B33, Horsley Papers, Special Collections, UCL Library Services (London, UK).

38. Horsley V: Correspondence, Mesopotamia, 1916. Section B34, Horsley Papers, Special Collections, UCL Library Services (London, UK).

39. Notebooks, Basra and Amara. Sections B35 and B36, Horsley Papers, Special Collections, UCL Library Services (London, UK).

40. Letters to Sir Pardy Lukis and to the Commander-in-Chief dated May 1916. Section B34, Horsley Papers, Special Collections, UCL Library Services (London, UK).

41. Swayne M: *In Mesopotamia.* p. 33. Hodder & Stoughton: London, 1917.

42. Moore AE: *Operation Lifetime: The Memoirs of a New Zealand Surgeon.* p. 99. Collins: Auckland, 1964.

43. Anon (a correspondent in Amara): Obituary. The late Sir Victor Horsley. *Br Med J* 1916; **2**: 343–344.

44. Grey Turner G: Obituary. The late Sir Victor Horsley. *Br Med J* 1916; **2**: 510.

45. Swayne M: *In Mesopotamia.* p. 109. Hodder & Stoughton: London, 1917.

46. Hughes JT: Sir Victor Horsley (1857–1916) and the birth of English neurosurgery. *J Med Biogr* 2007; **15**: 45–52.

47. Toodayan N: The death of Sir Victor Horsley (1857–1916) and his burial in Amarah. *J Hist Neurosci* 2017; **26**: 280–315.

48. Fletcher M: British war graves left to crumble in the dust. *The Times (Lond)*, April 25, 2016, p. 10–11.

49. Anon: A voice from the dead. *Br Med J* 1916; **2**: 261–262.

50. Anon: Responsibilities in Mesopotamia [editorial/leader]. *The Times (Lond)*, July 14, 1916, p. 9.

51. Hewett JP: Responsibilities in Mesopotamia. [Letter to the editor.] *The Times (Lond)*, July 18, 1916, p. 7.

52. Anon: Mr. Asquith and Mesopotamia [editorial/leader]. *The Times (Lond)*, July 19, 1916, p. 9.

53. Anon: Parliamentary intelligence. Medical arrangements in Mesopotamia: Sir Victor Horsley's letters. *Lancet* 1916; **2**: 212–213.

54. Mesopotamia Commission: *Report of the Commission Appointed by Act of Parliament to Enquire into the Operations of War in Mesopotamia, together with a Separate Report by Commander J Wedgwood, D.S.O., M.P., and Appendices.* His Majesty's Stationery Office: London, 1917.

55. Appendix I. "Vincent-Bingley" Report. Mesopotamia Commission: *Report of the Commission Appointed by Act of Parliament to Enquire into the Operations of War in Mesopotamia, together with a Separate Report by Commander J Wedgwood, D.S.O., M.P., and Appendices.* pp. 133–164. His Majesty's Stationery Office: London, 1917.

56. Mesopotamia Commission: *Report of the Commission Appointed by Act of Parliament to Enquire into the Operations of War in Mesopotamia, together with a Separate Report by Commander J Wedgwood, D.S.O., M.P., and Appendices.* pp. 76–77. His Majesty's Stationery Office: London, 1917.

57. Mesopotamia Commission: *Report of the Commission Appointed by Act of Parliament to Enquire into the Operations of War in Mesopotamia, together with a Separate Report by Commander J Wedgwood, D.S.O., M.P., and Appendices.* p. 81. His Majesty's Stationery Office: London, 1917.

58. Harrison M: *The Medical War: British Military Medicine in the First World War.* p. 222–227. Oxford University Press: Oxford, 2010.

59. Harrison M: *The Medical War: British Military Medicine in the First World War.* p. 203. Oxford University Press: Oxford, 2010.

60. Secretary of State for War (Mr. Lloyd George): Mesopotamia. Response to Sir John Jardine. Columns 1034–1035. In: *The Parliamentary Debates (Official Report) in the Sixth Session of the Thirtieth Parliament of the United Kingdom and Ireland.* Fifth series, Volume LXXXV, 1916.

Chapter 16

Aftermaths and Appraisals

Aftermaths

Horsley should have had charge of a center for head injuries in Western Europe or Alexandria, where his skills as a neurological surgeon could have been used to best advantage. Instead, the authorities foolishly allowed him to go to Mesopotamia, then a seeming outpost of the war, believing he would be a less visible nuisance, and there he died, pushing hard to improve the care of the needy. His death was something that he himself had considered. Even as he was leaving Egypt for Mesopotamia, he had said to Eldred: "I don't matter, I can't live forever, it's the young that matter."[1] Surprisingly, an administrative error resulted in a failure of the war office to notify his family that he had died, and Eldred only learned of it when she received a letter of sympathy from a friend.[2]

His will, made more than twenty years earlier with the expectation that he would die in England, had some curious provisions intended to advance medical science and education. He had directed that he was to undergo postmortem examination. He even prepared notes for the pathologist who was to perform the autopsy, emphasizing that he was born left-handed but became ambidextrous, that he had some thinning and a depression of the right side of his skull, which he attributed to being "thrown as an infant by a vindictive nurse," and that he might have a healed tubercular lesion in his right lung, based on symptoms that had occurred in the late 1870s.[3] His brain and skull were then to be preserved for future use by the Neurological Society of London, and the rest of his body given over to the pathology museum at University College, to be used at the discretion of its curator.[4] In the circumstances of his death, none of these directives, even if known, could have been met. His property, valued at a little under thirty-six thousand pounds, he left to Eldred.

The war and early post-war years were harsh on his family. Both of Horsley's sons, who had gone up to Oxford, had enlisted in the Artists' Rifles at the outbreak of war and were commissioned in the Gordon Highlanders. Horsley was proud of them. Siward was wounded and invalided out of the army late in 1915 with a recurrence of his previously well-controlled seizures, attributed by his doctor to his wound, the stress of life as an officer, and the hardships of life in the trenches.[5] He eventually returned to Oxford, graduated with a bachelor's degree in chemistry, and became a science teacher at Bedales, his old school.[6] On Christmas Day in 1920 his mother found him dead in the bathroom; he was naked, on his knees, with his chest on the side of the bath and his nose and mouth underwater. The coroner determined that he had had an epileptic seizure.[7] He left five thousand pounds to the school, with which science laboratories were built. As for Oswald, he was mentioned in dispatches from France in 1915, was wounded three times, and was awarded a Military Cross for conspicuous gallantry in action. He transferred to the Royal Flying Corps and was again awarded the Military Cross, this time for gallantry and devotion to duty while leading low-flying and bombing patrols, bringing down at least three and probably five enemy aircraft. He and his observer died in a flying accident attributed to mechanical failure in August 1918. Both Horsley boys are buried in the churchyard at Steep, where they had gone to school.

As for Pamela, in 1917 she married Edward Stanley Gotch Robinson (1887–1976), later a famous numismatist and authority on ancient Greek coins, who helped the art collector and millionaire Calouste Gulbenkian (1869–1955) with his acquisitions. He was knighted in 1972 and died four years later; Pamela died in 1980, aged eighty-four. They had two sons and four daughters.

Eldred lived on for twenty-five years after Horsley. Widowed and having lost both of her sons, she moved into a flat near Kensington Gardens and busied herself working for good causes such as child welfare. She died, aged eighty-six, on Christmas Eve in 1941.[8] The possibility of creating a memorial to Horsley was raised in 1920.[9] Eldred initially opposed the idea, upset that four years had elapsed since her husband's death and expecting only lukewarm support for the proposal. She urged that "the work he did be suffered to remain his real and only public memorial."[10] Explanations followed, the tardiness being attributed to the fact that many medical men had been away on war service.[11,12] Finally mollified, Eldred allowed the proposal to go forward. The memorial fund for Horsley was announced in 1921 by a committee chaired by Charles Ballance, the colleague who had assisted Horsley in his famous operation on a spinal tumor in 1887. The memorial itself was to take the form of a named triennial lectureship. Subscriptions came in from all over the world, from family, friends, former students, and colleagues, such that the list of subscribers reads like a "Who's Who" of medicine and science. A sum of well over one thousand pounds was collected. In today's terms, this translates to a sum of between forty thousand and just over four-hundred thousand pounds, depending on the measure used to calculate equivalency. Edward Sharpey-Schafer, "not only Horsley's oldest surviving scientific friend but also his first fellow worker" as he described himself[13] – in fact, his former teacher who had initiated their studies of cortical function – gave the first lecture in 1923, speaking on the relations of physiology and surgery, a topic that would have delighted Horsley.

Appraisals and Understanding

In his day, Horsley, a complicated man, evoked mixed feelings among his peers. Affection, respect, and awe were common among those close to him; anger and outrage followed the heated exchanges that sometimes marred disagreement. As a young surgeon, he was ambitious and driven, and his analytical curiosity paved the way for an academic career as a researcher. By contemporary standards he was successful, as evidenced by his numerous original publications, by his appointment as professor-superintendent of the Brown Institution while in his twenties, and by his election to fellowship in the Royal Society two years later. Although his research was solid and had important consequences, however, it followed directly from the work of others and did not in itself lead to novel insights that changed scientific thinking.

His work on the thyroid – to characterize the changes that follow its surgical removal – was an extension of that by Brown-Séquard, Moritz Schiff, Emil Kocher, and others, and helped to show that the thyroid has an endocrine function. His research on rabies helped to eradicate the disease in Britain but was based on and essentially confirmatory of the original studies of Louis Pasteur. He published surprisingly little on either of these topics, perhaps because he feared the work would have a difficult time in the review process preceding publication. His classic studies on cerebral localization extended those of David Ferrier and other physiologists and – while important – supported and extended those that had emerged already with the work of Ferrier and Jackson. Nevertheless, the work was sound, very detailed, and equipped him with the skills to advance the surgical treatment of diseases of the nervous system.

Although not the first to operate on the human brain, Horsley did so with an unusual confidence and technical facility born of his experience as an experimentalist. In addition to these assets, his willingness to apply the concepts of cortical localization as advanced in Britain particularly by Ferrier and then by his own laboratory work, and his utilization of a surgical approach based on the still-controversial Listerian principles of antisepsis, allowed him to operate on the brain safely and successfully. It helped that he was on the staff of University College Hospital, then the center of the scientific approach to medicine, and the National Hospital, the emerging hub of clinical neurology in Britain and its empire. Horsley thus seems to have invented – or at least had a major role in creating – neurosurgery, adding a new dimension to the surgical treatment of disease.

Horsley was more than a brilliant craftsman. He was an inspirational surgical pioneer who devised various instruments and operative approaches to enable the surgical aims to be achieved, and, in many instances, was the first to operate successfully on specific disorders of the

171

nervous system, as detailed in Chapters 5, 6, and 7. He did not hesitate to break new ground. His surgical skill, familiarity with the nervous system, and professional appointments enabled him to create the first major neurosurgical service in the world, and he was viewed with wonder by many lay people and medical colleagues for venturing into the magnificently supreme organ that is the brain.

Victor Horsley was nominated nine times for the Nobel Prize in medicine or physiology.[14] It is hardly surprising that the nomination was unsuccessful, for his work did not lead to the outstanding discoveries or novel biological insights that characterize the work of Nobel laureates. Rather, his work was based on the application of the emerging new concepts of functional cerebral specialization to the treatment of neurological disease, and this had a decisive influence on the path of clinical medicine.

Nearly twenty years after his death, the bishop of Chester, in paying a tribute to the medical profession, described an occasion when he saw Horsley, surrounded by his students, coming down the stairs at University College Hospital. "Talk of a general among his immediate staff, or a bishop among his clergy, they were not in it with the dignity of the surgeon and his ardent followers. I moved out of the way of them just as I would move out of the way of a royal procession."[15]

Harvey Cushing in Boston later made the new specialty his own, coming to be regarded by some as the "father of neurosurgery." In fact, the development of neurosurgery as a modern specialty was a collective enterprise, in which Horsley and Macewen (see Chapter 5) were the early pioneers. Not surprisingly, others were also beginning to explore the surgical treatment of neurological disorders, for the same interventional approach is likely to occur to more than one person in the right intellectual and scientific context. Cushing, who had yet to earn his medical degree, was a brilliant later exponent but did not always recognize his debt to his predecessors or contemporaries. Thus, he sometimes excluded from co-authorship of his papers those who had helped him with ideas and facilities, and failed to cite earlier studies on which his own work was based. His papers on the relationship between intracranial pressure, blood pressure, and heart rate, discussed in Chapter 7, angered

Mosso, Kocher, and Naunyn for this very reason. Cushing admired and authored a biography of Osler that won for him a Pulitzer prize, but even Osler was concerned when Cushing did not include his junior staff on certain papers reporting work in which they had been involved.[16]

Cushing's opinion of Horsley was ambivalent and ambiguous. Initially appalled by Horsley's seemingly reckless operative speed, he later appeared to appreciate the older man's genius and skill and he referred frequently to Horsley's work in some of his own early publications.[17] But in a private letter to Abraham Flexner, then secretary of the General Education Board of the Rockefeller Foundation, Cushing wrote on December 5, 1927, about "neurosurgical work in London which since Horsley's death is practically non-existent – and wasn't very much even then, though I would not want this opinion broadcasted."[18] Other contemporary American surgeons had more positive and admiring views about Horsley and his contributions to the field.[19]

Horsley's surgical brilliance later came to be overshadowed by his tireless endeavors as a social activist. Restless with ideas, he used his position as a medical celebrity to advance the various causes in which he believed. No cause was too small for him if he judged it worthwhile. No cause was too great for him if it would right some wrong. He was no bystander swept up by the swell for reform. Rather, he was a champion of the weak, the underprivileged, and the needy, troubled as he was by the inequities and social injustices of Victorian and Edwardian Britain. He was one of the few doctors who had the ear of the public, and he used this influence to advocate passionately for the causes in which he believed.

His was an intellectual life of vivid intensity, in which moral values were paramount. He performed many of his experimental studies in animals, and this brought him early into conflict with the antivivisectionists. He stood up to their attacks without flinching, declaring that experimentation in animals was the best way of advancing medical science, and brought on himself even more abuse and anger by exposing the distortions and half-truths used to promote antivivisectionist sentiment. It might be thought that he was acting out of professional self-interest, but his subsequent activities show that he was truly altruistic.

He worked hard to eradicate rabies from Britain once its cause was clear, and came thereby to appreciate the support of influential organizations and government agencies in this and other matters. His beliefs were based on the scientific evidence that he himself had helped to acquire. He did not hesitate to battle those who opposed him – not only the antivivisectionists but also the anti-muzzlers, which included animal welfare groups, farmers, the landed gentry, and many of his medical and veterinary colleagues. He seemed almost to relish the angry confrontations that followed, for compromise was not an option in this instance.

These confrontations, in which he challenged the prejudices of others by scientific reasoning, seemed to whet his appetite for medical politics. He enjoyed the cut and thrust of argument with his opponents and the support that he received from many of his contemporaries. Initially he focused on the interests of doctors and on protecting them from competition by the unqualified and from frivolous lawsuits, which often led to financial ruin. His increasing visibility caused his involvement with – and reform of – various British professional institutions. These included the Medical Defence Union, General Medical Council, and British Medical Association, which he helped to adapt so that they better served the physicians and surgeons whom they were supposed to represent. His various endeavors to help his professional colleagues led seamlessly to his becoming involved also with protecting the public from charlatans and unqualified or incompetent doctors, nurses, and midwives. The national prominence, intellectual challenge, and sense of accomplishment that resulted doubtless encouraged his further involvement with politics on a wider scale.

From his student days, he had been concerned about the ill effects of alcohol and he therefore embraced the temperance movement with fervor. He was troubled especially by the effects of alcohol on the health and development of children, and then became concerned more generally with their poor health. He thus became involved with attempts to establish the routine medical inspection and treatment of schoolchildren, policies with which few would argue today. He advocated also for the sex education of children as well as for measures to control the spread of sexually transmitted diseases, and did so many years before the need was recognized more generally. At the same time, his respect for individuals and for

a meritocracy caused him to support the suffragists and to oppose bigotry, discriminatory laws and regulations, and the forcible feeding of hunger-striking prisoners. Modern concepts of equal opportunities regardless of ethnicity or gender are now codified by law in many countries and would have met with his approval, while there is wide agreement that the forcible feeding of the mentally competent and of informed prisoners making an uncoerced choice to refuse nourishment is ethically unjustifiable. International codes of ethics, including that of the World Medical Association, thus support the views expressed by Horsley and others, views that brought them into conflict with the government of the day. He also championed national health insurance and various important public health measures that are now widely accepted but were contentious when first he advocated them.

He pursued these various interests with apostolic zeal, attacking those who opposed him with indignant and sometimes perplexing fury, at times careless of the feelings or needs of others. The antivivisectionists and the church met the full force of his opposition, as did Karl Pearson regarding the effects of parental alcoholism on children, John Troutbeck over the accountability of doctors, and the government regarding the rum ration. His concerns for the well-being of children and for the human rights of prisoners involved interactions – often angry – with local authorities and the national government, to the irritation of many politicians and officials. They at least recognized the sincerity of his views, which he held without thought of personal gain or benefit.

Horsley was an ardent supporter of the 1911 National Insurance Act that provided health insurance for wage earners as well as unemployment insurance for certain categories of worker. Many opposed it, however, because it conflicted with existing schemes and interests and because they regarded poverty as a sign of moral degeneracy in those unable to stand on their own two feet. In general, doctors initially opposed the measure, which they believed would impact them financially, and they did not forgive Horsley for supporting it. They came to regard him as a socialist and a traitor to the profession, and themselves only came around to the scheme when they realized that – with a revised fee schedule – it was in their interest to do so. Distrustful of Horsley, disillusioned by his politics, or believing incorrectly that he was withdrawing from clinical work to follow a career in public affairs, they took to referring patients elsewhere and his clinical practice therefore shriveled.

Clearly, then, Horsley put the welfare of his patients and of society in general above his own interests or the interest of the profession. He advocated for and supported laws that would help not just individuals but the most vulnerable segments of the population by improving the framework of society and various social determinants of health. He had the insight to perceive the limitations of the community in which he lived, to recognize adverse conditions that required correction, and to understand that only public advocacy would lead to change. Horsley believed that physicians have a professional obligation to take on the role of advocates for improvement in social conditions that otherwise lead to disease. He recognized that many factors contribute to ill-health or social injustice, and he opposed them vigorously. He also fought for reasoned accountability of doctors to patients, society, and each other. Public advocacy is recognized only now as an important aspect of the responsibilities of the medical profession, and is even part of the *raison d'être* of various professional organizations.[20]

Although Horsley's causes were all worthy, he sometimes behaved unwisely to attain his ends, as when he packed a protest meeting against the muzzling regulations with medical students, who heckled the speakers and then carried his motion in support of the regulations to limit the spread of rabies (see Chapter 3). On other occasions, his heated exchanges with opponents sometimes tempered the influence he might have had in advancing his causes. What – it might be wondered – sometimes led him to comment so injudiciously that government ministers, newspaper and journal editors, and even his own colleagues chided him for the tone of his remarks? In part, perhaps, it was because he felt unable to contain himself, believing that truth was paramount, regardless of the consequences. In part, also, it was probably a retaliatory response to the manner in which he felt he had been treated, based on the principle of an eye for an eye. In this regard, he appeared to be particularly vulnerable to criticism from his peers.

Despite his apparent self-confidence, he seemed to have a high-but-fragile self-esteem, which caused disagreements to become personal, as with Frances Cobbe, Stephen Coleridge, Karl Pearson, John Troutbeck, Rickman Godlee, and even Charles Sherrington, and sometimes led him to become impatient, imprudent, and unkind. To Horsley, his own opinions were then the only ones that really mattered and he seemed to lack empathy or even respect for those with opposing views.

His intense and uncompromising attitude almost certainly reduced the effectiveness of his advocacy and made the achievement of his ends more difficult. He failed to understand that in public affairs, courtesy and charm often win the day over truth, that style is sometimes more powerful than substance. Peaceful disagreement was difficult for him to accept, failing – as it did – to bring a resolution that was to his impatient liking. Spectacular verbal brawls sometimes followed. He was inflexible in insisting that his personal standards be met by others, always claiming to stand on the moral high ground. Those who disagreed came to regard him as sharp-tongued and opinionated, as someone who said too much, too often, too offensively.

The beliefs that he advanced with youthful vigor foreshadowed many bold ideas that came later to others, when the times were more propitious. Indeed, almost all of his suggestions were adopted eventually, although Horsley did not live to see them realized. His death on active military duty was a surprise, but that he should have volunteered for military service and for posting to Mesopotamia, when in his late fifties, was entirely in keeping with his character. He died fighting to improve the conditions and medical facilities for the forces fighting there. His death, shocking as it was, had an air of predictable inevitability about it, reminiscent of a Greek tragedy – a brilliant doctor who knowingly placed himself in danger to help others and believed that his teetotalism would protect him from the sun, only to succumb to heatstroke. Perhaps it was for the best, for it is difficult to imagine an elderly and infirm Horsley, relevant no longer, dependent on others, and dying in his own bed.

While away on military service, Horsley had made plans for the future he sought for himself when peace was restored. He intended to stand for parliament and – if elected – would have supported extension of the voting right to women on terms equal to those for men, would have wanted equal opportunities for all regardless of sex or ethnicity, and would have favored proportional representation and home rule for Ireland.[21,22] He would have advocated for the home delivery of sterilized milk from cows free of bovine tuberculosis. He would have focused on the welfare of the unemployed, on obtaining relief for taxpayers, and on using arbitration for settling civil disputes.[23]

Throughout his life, Horsley had set the fashion rather than following it. His self-confidence probably related at least in part to his upbringing in an influential, upper middle-class family. At school and university, he learned not only facts and figures but also to question seemingly unsupported beliefs, to develop an experimental approach, and to formulate his own opinions and convictions. He believed in the personal effectiveness of the individual and lived his life accordingly. As the British neurologist, Macdonald Critchley, described him during the centenary of the National Hospital in 1960, Horsley was "something of a superman."[24] He was certainly a man who shaped his own life and lived his own dreams, someone who above all showed great intellectual and physical courage, and whose life had enormous consequences, channeled as it was to help those less able to take charge of their own destiny. He had the strength to act on his moral beliefs regardless of whether they conflicted with those of the authorities. Ironically, Horsley the individualist fought to extend the reach of the state so that it could better protect the vulnerable and help them achieve a better way of life. He was therefore accused of weakening individual freedoms by creating a dependency on the state, by attempting to create what became widely known as the welfare state.

Horsley remains one of the most outstanding personalities of his times, at once a pioneering neurosurgeon, effective researcher, inspiring teacher, and principled social reformer, thereby exemplifying the modern ideal of the medical doctor and university professor. Much of his work "has long been incorporated into the general body of knowledge and has its lasting place,"[25] so that its origin is sometimes forgotten, while his efforts to create a better society have been dismissed or overshadowed by his medical triumphs. They surely deserve wider recognition and appreciation.

Notes

1. Paget S: *Sir Victor Horsley: A Study of His Life and Work*. p. 340. Constable: London, 1919.

2. Lyons JB: *The Citizen Surgeon: A Life of Sir Victor Horsley*. p. 283. Dawnay: London, 1966.

3. Horsley V: Notes to the pathologist of certain points at my autopsy. Section A63, Horsley Papers, Special Collections, UCL Library Services (London, UK).

4. Anon: Sir V. Horsley's will. *Daily Mail (Lond)*, October 12, 1916, p. 3; Anon: Sir Victor Horsley's will. *Daily Telegraph (Lond)*, October 12, 1916, p. 9.

5. Goadby KW: Letter to the War Office, 1915. Section K3, Horsley Papers, Special Collections, UCL Library Services (London, UK).

6. Anon: A brave life of service: The late S.M. Horsley. *The Times (Lond)*, January 6, 1921, p. 12.

7. Anon: Sir Victor Horsley's son: Found dead in a bathroom. *Daily Telegraph (Lond)*, December 29, 1920, p. 12.

8. Anon: Deaths: Horsley, Eldred. *The Times (Lond)*, December 29, 1941, p. 1.

9. Domville EJ: Proposal for a memorial to Sir Victor Horsley. [Letter to the Editor.] *Br Med J* 1920; **1**: 271.

10. Horsley E: Proposal for a memorial to Sir Victor Horsley. [Letter to the Editor.] *Br Med J* 1920; **1**: 418.

11. Anon, for the General Committee to Promote a Memorial to the Late Sir Victor Horsley: Memorial to Sir Victor Horsley. *Br Med J* 1921; **1**: 19.

12. Bowley AA, Paget S, Domville EJ, Sharpey-Schafer E, Lane WA: Victor Horsley memorial. [Letter to the editor.] *Daily Telegraph (Lond)*, January 6, 1921, p. 12.

13. Sharpey Schafer E: Victor Horsley Memorial Lecture on the relations of surgery and physiology. *Br Med J* 1923; **2**: 739–745.

14. Nomination Database, Nobel Prize in Physiology or Medicine. Available at: www.nobelprize.org/nomination/medicine/index.html [last accessed June 24, 2021].

15. Anon: A bishop's tribute. [Editorial.] *Br Med J* 1933; **1**: 475.

16. Feindel W: Osler and the "medico-chirurgical neurologists": Horsley, Cushing, and Penfield. *J Neurosurg* 2003; **99**: 188–199.

17. Cushing H: Surgery of the head. pp. 17–276. In: Keen WW (ed.): *Surgery: Its Principles and Practice*, Volume **3**. Saunders: Philadelphia, PA, 1908.

18. Cushing H: Letter to Abraham Flexner dated December 5, 1927. Cited by Fraenkel GJ: *Hugh*

Cairns: First Nuffield Professor of Surgery University of Oxford. p. 63. Oxford University Press: Oxford, 1991.

19. Lehner KR, Schulder M: American views of Sir Victor Horsley in the era of Cushing. *J Neursurg* 2019; **130**: 639–648.

20. Thomasson C: Physicians' social responsibility. *Virtual Mentor* 2014; **16**: 753–757.

21. Papers on tariff reforms, free trade, and home rule. Section C5, Horsley Papers, Special Collections, UCL Library Services (London, UK).

22. Proportional Representation Society: *Report for the Year 1914–15.* P.R. Pamphlet No. 27: London, 1915.

23. Papers on political matters. Section C, Horsley Papers, Special Collections, UCL Library Services (London, UK).

24. Critchley M: The beginnings of the National Hospital, Queen Square (1859–1860). *Br Med J* 1960; **1**: 1829–1837.

25. Trotter W: Victor Horsley Memorial Lecture on the insulation of the nervous system. *Br Med J* 1926; **2**: 103–107.

Appendix 1: Horsley's Procedure for Cranial Surgery

Horsley's neurosurgical approach to the brain is summarized here, based on his own published accounts.[1,2] In general, for cranial operations he placed the patient on the operating table with the head raised to diminish the pressure in the venous sinuses. For operations on the cerebellum, the portion of the brain at the back of the skull, the patient lay on one side with the uppermost arm drawn downwards. A headrest provided greater stability.

He scrubbed for surgery using soap and water, and then rinsed with an antimicrobial solution. He initially practiced antiseptic surgery, utilizing antimicrobial chemicals on instruments and the skin for disinfection; he also sprayed the operating field with a dilute carbolic solution or with a solution of mercuric chloride.[3] The rigorous aseptic techniques now preferred, which aim at eliminating or minimizing the presence of infectious organisms at the operative site, were introduced by others only later, and Horsley then accepted these newer approaches.

Operative Exposure

Horsley utilized from the first a curved scalp incision, turning back a skin flap with its blood supply preserved. This was an improvement on the older technique of making a cruciate skin incision centered on the site at which the skull was to be opened, because after wound closure over a skull defect, the replaced skin flap – "laid down again like the lid of a box"[1] – offered more resistance to "the upward pushing brain" due to brain swelling. With skin closure of a cruciate incision, "the point of meeting of four cross cuts" is the weakest part but faces the likely site of maximal bulging, where tension is greatest.[4]

With regard to opening the skull, he opposed a method then used abroad in which a mallet and chisel were used to create a large flap of bone with adherent soft tissues, believing that this was likely to harm the patient.[5] Instead, he removed the subjacent skull piecemeal using a saw and bone

forceps, with the least possible pressure applied to the brain and dura.[2] For operations on the cerebellum, he performed a suboccipital craniectomy, that is, he removed the bone at the base of the skull.

In an era that preceded even crude neuroimaging techniques, localization of the site of the cerebral lesion – whether a tumor or some other abnormality – was by clinical means and was neither precise nor reliable. Consequently, in many instances he had to enlarge the exposure progressively at operation, sometimes taking up one quarter of the skull, without any guarantee of success.

Staged Procedures

Horsley generally performed brain operations in two stages in order to reduce blood loss, surgical shock, and operative stress. In the first, he opened the skull to expose the underlying dura enveloping the brain, and initially made no attempt to save the bone for later replacement. He made the exposure large, finding that this gave him wider access and reduced complications arising from increased intracranial pressure. In the second stage, five to seven days later, he proceeded to operate on the brain itself.[3]

Hemostasis

The oozing of blood from the well-vascularized diploe of the skull-bones posed a particular problem during intracranial operations. Contemporary techniques to control bleeding from small vessels by hot saline douches and packs[4] were not particularly successful in the case of bone, and the sources of bleeding, which were not compressible, could be neither tied off nor cauterized. As discussed in Chapter 6, Horsley – in his experiments on animals – had adapted a little-used technique of smudging modeling wax on the cut and bleeding surface of the cranial bones to arrest any oozing of blood. In conjunction with P. W. Squire, the Oxford Street pharmacist, he subsequently developed a product composed of beeswax (seven parts) and almond oil (one part), plus salicylic acid, for use in humans.[6] Horsley's bone wax, modified in one way or another, has been used successfully by surgeons for the many years since then.

Despite his spectacular operative speed, Horsley took meticulous care to limit any bleeding regardless of its source. Blood vessels were tied with fine horse-hair or silkworm gut.[3] To control bleeding from the surface of the brain, he sprayed it with warm saline (at 110 to 115°F) and then applied gentle pressure with a sponge.[2] He also used muscle tissue to control bleeding from the brain (a forerunner of the modern Gelfoam, a commercially available, sterile, absorb-able surgical sponge).[7,8]

Finally, Horsley, in order to diminish the risk of bleeding, would also adjust the level of chloroform anesthesia to lower the blood pressure. He discour-aged the use of ether for anesthesia during neuro-surgical procedures both because of the hypertensive effects and increased risk of hemorrhage that he had noted during experiments in animals and because of the agitation that occurred during the recovery stage.

Incising the Brain and Dura

Horsley incised the dura mater around four-fifths of the circumference of the area exposed and about one-eighth of an inch from the edge of the bone, so that he could stitch the edges together afterwards. He opened it first with a scalpel, and then by blunt-pointed curved scissors, thereby protecting the underlying tissues.

Good visibility was essential during any opera-tion, and Horsley wore a strong headlight when he worked, using a spatula to move portions of the brain to one side in order to reach or view (often with a mirror) less accessible parts. Such retraction was important, but he cautioned that excessive force or the application of pressure too rapidly could cause local injury and bruising. He objected to the step favored by some "of removing portions and lobes of the encephalon if these impede the approach to the lesion."[2] Such excision for the convenience of the surgeon was, he stressed, to be avoided whenever possible.

When he needed to remove a portion of the brain or a tumor, Horsley incised the cerebral cortex perpendicular to its surface and cut into the subja-cent white matter in such a manner as to minimize damage to the adjacent nerve fibers. He was careful to preserve the blood vessels, pointing out that – as they run in the pia mater that envelops the brain –

they can be lifted off the surface of the brain and its sulci before the underlying cerebral tissue is removed.[1]

Closure and Drainage

If the dura mater was to be left intact, Horsley initially preserved portions of the bone he had removed in warm aseptic sponges and, at the end of the operation, divided them into small fragments that were then replaced between the dura and skin in a mosaic arrangement, as advised by Macewen. Later, he abandoned this fragmentation procedure and replaced larger portions of bone, as was the practice of contem-porary American surgeons.[9]

If the dura had been opened to allow the brain itself to be manipulated surgically, it was sutured and the scalp was closed with silk and horsehair stitches. Based on his initial experience, Horsley deemed drainage of clean wounds to be unnecessary apart from a temporary tube placed in the most dependent part of the incision for twenty-four hours.[1,2]

Notes

1. Horsley V: Brain-surgery. *Br Med J* 1886; **2**: 670–675.

2. Horsley V: Address in surgery on the technique of operations on the central nervous system. *Lancet* 1906; **168**: 484–490; *Br Med J* 1906; **2**: 411–423.

3. Sachs E: *Fifty Year of Neurosurgery: A Personal Story.* pp. 38–39. Vantage: New York, 1958.

4. Northfield DWC: Sir Victor Horsley 1857–1916. pp. 43–48. In: Bucy P (ed.): *Neurosurgical Giants: Feet of Clay and Iron.* Elsevier: New York, 1985; reprinted from *Surg Neurol* 1973; **1**: 131–134.

5. Horsley V: Discussion on the treatment of cerebral tumours. Remarks on the surgical treatment of cerebral tumours. *Br Med J* 1893; **2**: 1365–1367 (additional discussion, 1369).

6. Horsley V: Antiseptic wax. [Letter to the editor.] *Br Med J* 1892; **1**: 1165.

7. Bucy P: Editor's comments. pp. 49–50. In: Bucy P (ed.): *Neurosurgical Giants: Feet of Clay and Iron.* Elsevier: New York, 1985.

8. Horsley V: Note on haemostasis by application of living tissue. *Br Med J* 1914; **2**: 8.

9. Horsley V: Discussion on the treatment of cerebral tumours. Remarks on the surgical treatment of cerebral tumours. *Br Med J* 1893; **2**: 1365–1367 (additional discussion, 1369).

Appendix 2: Appointments, Honors, and Awards

1880

Member by examination of the Royal College of Surgeons of England

Appointed house surgeon to Professor John Marshall, University College Hospital, London (December 1880 to May 1881)

1881

Graduated with the degrees of bachelor of medicine and bachelor of surgery (MB, BS) from University College Hospital Medical School, London

1882

Appointed surgical registrar, University College Hospital, London (resigned 1884)

Appointed assistant professor of pathology at University College, London

1883

Fellow by examination of the Royal College of Surgeons of England

1884

Appointed professor-superintendent, Brown Animal Sanatory Institution, University of London (resigned 1890)

1885

Appointed assistant surgeon to University College Hospital, London

Elected foreign corresponding member, Société de Biologie, Paris

1886

Appointed to the staff of the National Hospital, Queen Square, London

Elected to fellowship of the Royal Society of London

1887

Appointed professor of pathology at University College, London (resigned 1896)

Appointed a special constable at a time of civil unrest

1890

Elected an honorary member of the American Surgical Association

1891

Appointed Fullerian professor of physiology and comparative anatomy, Royal Institution (until 1894)

Appointed vice dean of the medical faculty at University College London

Croonian Lecturer, Royal Society (with Francis Gotch)

1892

Elected president of the Medical Defence Union (until 1897)

1893

Appointed surgeon to outpatients, University College Hospital, London

Appointed dean of the medical faculty at University College London and chairman of the medical committee of the hospital (to 1895)

Awarded Cameron Prize for therapeutics from the University of Edinburgh

Elected corresponding member of the Royal Society of Physicians, Budapest

1894

Awarded Royal Medal of the Royal Society

Awarded honorary doctorate of medicine from the University of Halle

1895

Elected a corresponding member of the Société de Chirurgie de Paris

Elected fellow and awarded Fothergill Gold Medal by the Medical Society of London

1897

Elected to the General Medical Council as one of three direct representatives of the profession

Elected a fellow of the University of London and to the senate of the university

Appointed one of the managers of the Royal Institution of Great Britain (until 1898)

1898

Elected president, Neurological Society of London (vice president, 1896 and 1897; member of council, 1892, 1899)

1900

Appointed surgeon with charge of beds and professor of clinical surgery at University College Hospital, London (resigned 1906)

1902

Appointed knight bachelor by King Edward VII

Appointed honorary fellow, Imperial University of Yourief [formerly University of Dorpat; now of Tartu, Estonia]

Elected foreign honorary member of the American Academy of Arts and Sciences

1903

Elected first chairman of the Representative Body of the British Medical Association (to 1906)

Elected associate fellow, College of Physicians of Philadelphia

1906

Honorary degree of Doctor of Laws conferred by the University of Toronto.

Appointed to the consulting staff at University College Hospital, London

1907

Elected an honorary member of the Russian Surgical Society

Elected member, Royal Sanitary Institute (now Royal Society for Public Health), London

1908

Honorary PhD conferred by Physico-Medical Society of Vienna

1909

Appointed Linacre Lecturer, St. John's College, Cambridge University

1910

Elected a foreign associate of the French Academy of Medicine

Elected corresponding member of the Royal Prussian Academy of Sciences

Appointed president of the Section of Surgery of the British Medical Association

1911

Awarded Lannelongue Prize, French National Society of Surgery (now the French National Academy of Surgery)

Elected fellow, Royal Sanitary Institute, London

Elected honorary member of the Society of Psychiatrists, St. Petersburgh, Russia

Appointed lecturer in experimental neurology, University College London (resigned 1913)

1912

Elected a member of the Royal Society of Science of Uppsala in succession to Lord Lister

Elected an honorary fellow of the Italian Society of Neurology

Elected an honorary member of the Harveian Society of London

1914

Honorary degree of Doctor of Laws conferred by University of Aberdeen

1915

Appointed colonel, Army Medical Services, Mediterranean Expeditionary Force

Mentioned in dispatches for gallant and distinguished service in the field

1916

Awarded Companion of the Order of the Bath (C.B.), military division, for services with the Mediterranean Expeditionary Force

Appendix 3: Victor Horsley's Professional Publications

In preparing this bibliography, all citations have been verified personally except where indicated. Summaries, abstracts, or discussions of Horsley's papers, prepared by others, have not been included. Square brackets have been used to indicate material not in the original.

1880

Bastian HC, Horsley V: Arrest of development in the left upper limb, in association with an extremely small right ascending parietal convolution. *Brain* 1880; 3: 113–116.

1882

Mott FW, Horsley V: On the existence of bacteria, or their antecedents, in healthy tissues. *J Physiol* 1882; 3: 188–194, 296.

Horsley V: Zymotic: Zyme. pp. 1805–1806. In: Quain R (ed.): *A Dictionary of Medicine including General Pathology, General Therapeutics, Hygiene, and the Diseases Peculiar to Women and Children.* Longmans, Green: London, 1882.

Horsley V: Bacilli. pp. 1809–1810. In: Quain R (ed.): *A Dictionary of Medicine including General Pathology, General Therapeutics, Hygiene, and the Diseases Peculiar to Women and Children.* Longmans, Green: London, 1882.

Horsley V: On "septic bacteria" and their physiological relations. pp. 239–273. In: *Eleventh Annual Report of the Local Government Board 1881–82, Supplement containing the Report of the Medical Officer for 1881.* Eyre & Spottiswoode: London, 1882.

1883

Horsley V: Case of severe syphilitic disease of the facial bones and viscera. – Death from pyaemia. *Trans Pathol Soc Lond* 1883; 34: 208–209.

Horsley V: Adeno-sarcoma of testis with secondary growths in the viscera, occurring in a case of cardiac malformation. *Trans Pathol Soc Lond* 1883; 34: 161–167.

Horsley V: Note on the patellar knee-jerk. *Brain* 1883; 6: 369–371.

1884

Horsley V: Case of occipital encephalocele in which a correct diagnosis was obtained by means of the induced current. *Brain* 1884; 7: 228–243.

Horsley V: Consensual movements as aids in diagnosis of disease of the cortex cerebri. *Med Times & Gaz* 1884; 2: 214–215.

Horsley V: On the function of the thyroid gland. *Proc R Soc Lond* 1884; 38: 5–7.

Horsley V, Schäfer EA: Experimental researches in cerebral physiology. I. On the functions of the marginal convolution. (Preliminary communication.) *Proc R Soc Lond* 1884; 36: 437–442.

Horsley V: On substitution as a means of restoring nerve function considered with reference to cerebral localisation. *Lancet* 1884; 124: 7–10.

1885

Horsley V: Preliminary communication on the existence of sensory nerves and nerve endings in nerve trunks, true "nervi nervorum." (Abstract.) *Proc R Med Chir Soc Lond* 1885; 1: 196–198.

Horsley V: Acute septic peritonitis – operation – recovery. Remarks by Mr. Victor Horsley. *Med Times & Gaz* 1885; 2: 431–432.

Horsley V: The motor centres of the brain and the mechanism of the will. *Nature* 1885; 32: 377–381.

Horsley V: The motor centres of the brain, and the mechanism of the will. *Not Proc R Inst Gr Br* 1885; 11: 250–262.

Horsley V: The motor centers and the will. *Pop Sci Mon* 1885; 28: 100–112.

Horsley V: Myxoedema. [Letter to the editor.] *Br Med J* 1885; 1: 302.

Horsley V, Schäfer EA: Experimental researches in cerebral physiology. II. On the muscular contractions which are evoked by excitation of the motor tract. *Proc R Soc Lond* 1885; 39: 404–409.

Horsley V: Sur la fonction de la glande thyroide. *C R Soc Biol (Paris)* 1885; 37: 762–763.

Horsley V: The Brown Lectures on pathology. Lecture I. The thyroid gland: Its relation to the pathology of myxoedema and cretinism, to the question of the surgical treatment of goître, and to the general nutrition of the body. *Br Med J* 1885; 1: 111–115.

Horsley V: The Brown Lectures on pathology. Lecture II. – The thyroid gland: Its relation to the pathology of myxoedema and cretinism, to the question of the surgical treatment of goître, and to the general nutrition of the body (*continued*). *Br Med J* 1885; 1: 211–213.

Horsley V: The Brown Lectures on pathology. Lecture III. – Traumatic fever: Pyrexia following simple fractures. *Br Med J* 1885; 1: 419–423.

1886

Beevor CE, Horsley V: A minute analysis (experimental) of the various movements produced by stimulating in the monkey different regions of the cortical centre for the upper limb, as defined by Professor Ferrier. (Abstract.) *Proc R Soc Lond* 1886; 40: 475–476.

Horsley V: Brain-surgery. *Br Med J* 1886; 2: 670–674.

Horsley V: A case of a congenital canal in the raphe of the scrotum. *Trans Clin Soc Lond* 1886; 19: 325–326.

Horsley V: A case of suppuration of the mastoid cells complicated by thrombosis in the right lateral sinus with septic embolism of the heart and left lung, in which recovery followed trephining of the mastoid process, &c., with remarks on the prevention of septic embolism in such cases. *Trans Clin Soc Lond* 1886; 19: 290–295.

Horsley V: A further and final criticism of Prof. Schiff's experimental demonstration of the relation which he believes to exist between the posterior columns of the spinal cord and the excitable area of the cortex. (An answer to Prof. Schiff's "reply" in this issue.) *Brain* 1886; 9: 311–329.

Horsley V: Further researches into the function of the thyroid gland and into the pathological state produced by removal of the same. *Proc R Soc Lond* 1886; 40: 6–9.

Horsley V: M. Pasteur's prophylactic. [Letter to the editor.] *Br Med J* 1886; 2: 573, 654–655, 892.

Horsley V: Mr. Horsley's criticism on Prof. Schiff. [Letter to the editor.] *Lancet* 1886; 127: 227, 470–471.

Horsley V: On the relation between the posterior columns of the spinal cord and the excito-motor area of the cortex, with especial reference to Prof. Schiff's views on the subject. *Brain* 1886; 9: 42–62.

Horsley V: *Report to the Committee of the Brown Institution for the Year 1885*. University of London: London, 1886.

Horsley V, Schäfer EA: Experiments on the character of the muscular contractions which are evoked by excitation of the various parts of the motor tract. *J Physiol* 1886; 7: 96–110.

Semon F, Horsley V: Report to the Scientific Grants Committee of the British Medical Association. On an apparently peripheral and differential action of ether upon the laryngeal muscles. *Br Med J* 1886; 2: 405–407, 445–447.

Semon F, Horsley V: Paralysis of laryngeal muscles and cortical centre for phonation. [Letter to the editor.] *Lancet* 1886; 127: 1045–1046.

Horsley V: Translation of Robert Koch's monograph, "On the investigation of pathogenic organisms." In: Cheyne WW (ed.):

Recent Essays by Various Authors on Bacteria in Relation to Disease, pp. 1–64. New Sydenham Society: London, 1886.

Horsley V: Albuminoid Degeneration, pp. 29–31, Bacillus, pp. 123–124, Bacterium, p. 135, Fatty Degeneration, pp. 518–520, Hypodermic Injection, pp. 767–769. In: Heath C (ed.): *Dictionary of Practical Surgery, vol 1.* J. B. Lippincott Company: Philadelphia, PA, 1886.

Horsley V: Micrococcus, p. 20, Nerve-Avulsion, pp. 57–58, Nerve-Stretching, pp. 58–61, Neurotic Fever, pp. 71–72, Poisoned Wounds, pp. 224–229, Rigor, pp. 363–364, Sapraemia, pp. 367–369, Schizomycetes, pp. 386–387, Sepsin, pp. 416–417, Septic Diseases, pp. 417–423, Septicaemia, pp. 423–426, Shock, pp. 432–437, Surgical Fever, pp. 522–523, Traumatic Fever, pp. 660–662, Urea, pp. 711–713, Urethral Fever, pp. 722–724, Urinary Deposits, pp. 732–734, Urine, pp. 736–742, Vibrio, pp. 788–789. In: Heath C (ed.): *Dictionary of Practical Surgery, vol 2.* J. B. Lippincott Company: Philadelphia, PA, 1886.

1887

Beevor CE, Horsley V: A further minute analysis, by electrical stimulation, of the so-called motor region of the cortex cerebri in the monkey (*Macacus sinicus*). (Abstract.) *Proc R Soc Lond* 1887; 43: 86–88.

Beevor CE, Horsley V: A minute analysis (experimental) of the various movements produced by stimulating in the monkey different regions of the cortical centre for the upper limb, as defined by Professor Ferrier. *Philos Trans R Soc Lond, B* 1887; 178: 153–167.

Beevor CE, Horsley V: Recherches expérimentales sur l'écorce cérébrale des singes (Macacus sinicus). *C R Soc Biol (Paris)* 1887; 39: 647–652.

Horsley V: A note on the means of topographical diagnosis of focal disease affecting the so-called motor region of the cerebral cortex. *Am J Med Sci* 1887; 93: 342–369.

Horsley V: Notes on the pathology of inveterate neuralgia of the fifth nerve, illustrated by cases treated successfully by avulsion of the nerve close to the skull. *Br J Dent Sci* 1887; 30: 964–968, 1011–1015.

Horsley V: Notes on the pathology of inveterate neuralgia of the fifth nerve, illustrated by cases treated successfully by avulsion of the nerve close to the skull. *Trans Odontol Soc Gr Br* 1887; 19: 270–285.

Horsley V: Remarks on ten consecutive cases of operations upon the brain and cranial cavity to illustrate the details and safety of the method employed. (With a table.) *Br Med J* 1887; 1: 863–865.

Horsley V: Remarques sur dix cas d'opération pratiqués sur le crâne et le cerveau. *Prog Med (Paris)* 1887; 6 (2nd Series): 79–82.

Paget J, Brunton TL, Fleming G, Lister J, Quain R, Roscoe HE, Sanderson JB, Horsley V: Report of committee of enquiry into M. Pasteur's treatment of hydrophobia. *Vet J Ann Comp Pathol* 1887; 24: 82–93.

Horsley V: Witness testimony, June 28, 1887. pp. 3–31. In *Report from the Select Committee on Rabies in Dogs; Together with the Proceedings of the Committee, Minutes of Evidence and Appendix.* Henry Hansard and Son: London, 1887.

1888

Beevor CE, Horsley V: A further minute analysis by electric stimulation of the so-called motor region of the cortex cerebri in the monkey (*Macacus sinicus*). *Philos Trans R Soc Lond B* 1888; 179: 205–256.

Beevor CE, Horsley V: Note on some of the motor functions of certain cranial nerves (v, vii, ix, x, xi, xii), and of the three first cervical nerves, in the monkey (*Macacus sinicus*). *Proc R Soc Lond* 1888; 44: 269–277.

Beevor CE, Horsley V: Reports to the Scientific Grants Committee of the British Medical Association. Report on some of the motor functions of certain cranial nerves (v, vii, ix, x, xi, xii), and of the three first cervical nerves, in the monkey (*Macacus sinicus*). *Br Med J* 1888; 2: 220–222.

Bristowe JS, Horsley V: A case of paralytic rabies in man, with remarks. *Trans Clin Soc Lond* 1888; 22: 38–47.

Horsley V: Case of cerebral abscess successfully treated by operation. *Br Med J* 1888; 1: 636–637.

Horsley V: Case of cerebral abscess successfully treated by operation. *Proc Med Soc Lond* 1888; 11: 232–236.

Horsley V: A case of thrombosis of the longitudinal sinus, together with the anterior frontal vein, causing localised foci of haemorrhage, which produced remarkably localised cortical epilepsy. *Brain* 1888; 11: 102–106.

Cope AC, Horsley V: *Reports on the Outbreak of Rabies among Deer in Richmond Park during the Years 1886-7.* Eyre & Spottiswoode: London, 1888.

Horsley V: Ein Fall von Hirnabscess erfolgreich operirt. *Wien Med Bl* 1888; 11: 424–426.

Gotch F, Horsley V: Observations upon the electromotive changes in the mammalian spinal cord following electrical excitation of the cortex cerebri. Preliminary notice. *Proc R Soc Lond* 1888; 45: 18–26.

Gowers WR, Horsley V: Royal Medical & Chirurgical Society. A case of tumour of the spinal cord: removal: recovery. *Br Med J* 1888; 1: 1273–1274.

Gowers WR, Horsley V: A case of tumour of the spinal cord. Removal; recovery. *Med Chir Trans Lond* 1888; 71: 377–428.

Gowers WR, Horsley V: Case of tumour of the spinal cord; removal; recovery. (Abstract.) *Proc R Med Chir Soc Lond* 1888; 2: 406–409.

Gowers WR, Horsley V: Royal Medical & Chirurgical Society. Pemphigoid eruption, with changes in peripheral nerves – Tumour of spinal cord; removal and recovery. *Lancet* 1888; 131: 1194.

Horsley V: On hydrophobia and its "treatment:" Especially by the hot-air bath, commonly termed the Bouisson Remedy. *Br Med J* 1888; 1: 1207–1211.

Horsley V, Schäfer EA: A record of experiments upon the functions of the cerebral cortex. *Philos Trans R Soc Lond, B* 1888; 179: 1–45.

1889

Beevor CE, Horsley V: Recherches expérimentales sur l'écorce cérébrale des singes Macacus sinicus. *Trib Med (Paris)* 1889; 20: 248–250.

Horsley V: Die Functionen der motorischen Region der Hirnrinde. *Dtsch Med Wochenschr* 1889; 15: 777–779.

Horsley V: On rabies: Its treatment by M. Pasteur, and on the means of detecting it in suspected cases. *Br Med J* 1889; 1: 342–344.

Horsley V: On rabies: Its treatment by M. Pasteur; and on the means of detecting it in suspected cases. *Trans Epidemiol Soc Lond* 1889; 8: 70–79.

Semon F, Horsley V: On the central motor innervation of the larynx. A preliminary communication. *Br Med J* 1889; 2: 1383–1384.

Spencer WG, Horsley V: Reports to the Scientific Grants Committee of the British Medical Association. Report on the control of haemorrhage from the middle cerebral artery and its branches by compression of the common carotid. *Br Med J* 1889; 1: 457–460.

Wilson J, Cloncurry, Stirling P, Jones JB, Horsley V, Grant GM, Brown GT: Appendix D. Tuberculosis. Nature of the disease. pp. 16–24. In: *Journals of the House of Commons of the Dominion of Canada.* House of Commons: Canada, 1889.

Horsley V: Appendix D. Supplementary report on tuberculosis. p. 24. In: *Journals of the House of Commons of the Dominion of Canada.* House of Commons: Canada, 1889.

Horsley V: Mr. Victor Horsley on the Pasteur system. [Letter to the editor.] *Spectator* 1889; 63: 13.

Horsley V: Discussion on cerebral localization. *Trans Cong Am Phys Surg* 1889; 1: 340–350.

1890

Semon F, Horsley V: Ueber die centrale motorische Innervation des Kehlkopfs. Eine vorläufige Mittheilung. *Int Centralbl Laryngol Rhinol* 1890; 6: 389–392.

Beevor CE, Horsley V: An experimental investigation into the arrangement of the excitable fibres of the internal capsule of the Bonnet monkey (*Macacus sinicus*). *Philos Trans R Soc Lond, B* 1890; 181: 49–88.

Beevor CE, Horsley V: A record of the results obtained by electrical excitation of the so-called motor cortex and internal capsule in an Orang-Outang (*Simia satyrus*). *Philos Trans R Soc Lond, B* 1890; 181: 129–158.

Beevor CE, Horsley V: A record of the results obtained by electrical excitation of the so-called motor cortex and internal capsule in an Orang Outang (*Simia satyrus*). (Abstract.) *Proc R Soc Lond* 1890; 48: 159–160.

Horsley V: Further note on the possibility of curing myxoedema. *Br Med J* 1890; 2: 201–202.

Horsley V: M. Pasteur and hydrophobia. [Letter to the editor.] *Lancet* 1890; 136: 205.

Horsley V: Note on a possible means of arresting the progress of myxoedema, cachexia strumipriva, and allied diseases. *Br Med J* 1890; 1: 287–288.

Horsley V: Remarks on the surgery of the central nervous system. *Br Med J* 1890; 2: 1286–1292.

Semon F, Horsley V: A propos du centre cortical moteur du larynx. *Ann Oreille Larynx* 1890; 16: 387–388.

Semon F, Horsley V: On the central motor innervation of the larynx. *Br Med J* 1890; 1: 175–176.

Semon F, Horsley V: Des relations du larynx avec le système nerveux moteur. *Arch Laryngol Rhinol* 1890; 3: 213–229.

Semon F, Horsley V: Du centre cortical moteur laryngé et du trajet intra-cérébral des fibres qui en émanent. *Ann Oreille Larynx* 1890; 16: 305–310.

Semon F, Horsley V: Du centre cortical moteur laryngé et du trajet intra-cérébral des fibres qui en émanent. *Gaz Med Chir Toulouse* 1890; 22: 115–116, 124.

Semon F, Horsley V: Ein Schlusswort in der Controverse über die centrale motorische Innervation des Kehlkopfs. *Berl Klin Wochenschr* 1890; 27: 155–156.

Semon F, Horsley V: Erwiderung auf vorstehenden Aufsatz. Ueber die centrale motorische Innervation des Kehlkopfs. Eine vorläufige Mittheilung. *Berl Klin Wochenschr* 1890; 27: 82–85.

Semon F, Horsley V: An experimental investigation of the central motor innervation of the larynx. Part I. Excitation experiments. *Philos Trans R Soc Lond, B* 1890; 181: 187–211.

Semon F, Horsley V: An experimental investigation of the central motor innervation of the larynx. Part I. Excitation experiments. (Abstract.) *Proc R Soc Lond* 1890; 48: 341–342.

Semon F, Horsley V: On the relations of the larynx to the motor nervous system. *Med Press Circ* 1890; 101: 153–157.

Semon F, Horsley V: On the relations of the larynx to the motor nervous system. Ueber die Beziehungen des Kehlkopfs zum motorischen Nervensystem. *Dtsch Med Wochenschr* 1890; 16: 672–679.

Horsley V: Sur la chirurgie du système nerveux central. *Mercredi Med* 1890; August 27: 414–417.

Horsley V: Ueber die Chirurgie des Centralnervensystems. *Wien Med Presse* 1890; 31: 1453–1457, 1496–1500.

Horsley V: Ueber die Möglichkeit, das Fortschreiten des Myxödems und der Cachexia strumipriva zu verhindern. *Wien Med Bl* 1890; 13: 116–117.

Horsley V: Muzzling and hydrophobia. [Letter to the editor.] *Spectator* 1890; 64: 165.

1891

Horsley V: Address to the students of University College, London, Oct. 1, 1891. *Lancet* 1891; 138: 754–759.

Horsley V: On the analysis of voluntary movement. *Nineteen Cent* 1891; 29: 857–870.

Barlow T, Horsley V: The late Mr. John Marshall, F.R.S. [Letter to the editor.] *Br Med J* 1891; 1: 553.

Horsley V: On craniectomy in microcephaly, with an account of two cases in which the operation was performed. *Br Med J* 1891; 2: 579–581.

Horsley V: Die Function der Schilddrüse. Eine historisch-kritische Studie. In: *Internationale Beitrage zur Wissenschaftlichen Medicin. Festschrift, Rudolf Virchow gewidmt zur Vollendung seines 70 Lebensjahres.* vol. 1, pp. 369–409. Hirschwald: Berlin, 1891.

Gotch F, Horsley V: Croonian lecture. – On the mammalian nervous system; its functions and their localisation determined by an electrical method. (Abstract.) *Proc R Soc Lond* 1891; 49: 235–240.

Gotch F, Horsley V: Croonian lecture. – On the mammalian nervous system, its functions, and their localisation determined by an electrical method. *Philos Trans R Soc Lond, B* 1891; 182: 267–526.

Gotch F, Horsley V: Ueber den Gebrauch der Elektricität für die Localisirung der Erregungserscheinungen im Centralnervensystem. *Centralbl Physiol* 1891; 4: 649–651.

Spencer WG, Horsley V: On the changes produced in the circulation and respiration by increase of the intra-cranial pressure or tension. *Philos Trans R Soc Lond, B* 1891; 182: 201–254.

Horsley V: On the student and the practitioner. *Br Med J* 1891; 2: 736–741.

Horsley V: The student and the practitioner. *Med Press Circ* 1891; 103: 357–358.

Horsley V, Taylor J, Colman WS: Remarks on the various surgical procedures devised for the relief or cure of trigeminal neuralgia (tic douloureux). *Br Med J* 1891; 2: 1139–1143, 1191–1193, 1249–1252.

1892

Horsley V: An address on the origin and seat of epileptic disturbance. *Br Med J* 1892; 1: 693–696.

Horsley V: Antiseptic wax. [Letter to the editor.] *Br Med J* 1892; 1: 1165.

Beevor CE, Horsley V: On a case of traumatic abscess in the neighbourhood of the left angular gyrus, with right hemianopia (limited fields) and word-blindness, treated by operation. *Trans Ophthalmol Soc UK* 1892; 12: 204–219.

Horsley V: The function of the thyroid gland. [Letter to the editor.] *Br Med J* 1892; 1: 1113.

Horsley V: Introductory remarks delivered in the section of pathology. *Br Med J* 1892; 2: 248–249.

Horsley V: The morality of 'vivisection.' *Nineteenth Cent* 1892; 32: 804–811.

Horsley V: Remarks on the function of the thyroid gland: A critical and historical review. *Br Med J* 1892; 1: 215–219, 265–268.

Semon F, Horsley V: Ueber die Beziehungen des Kehlkopfes zum motorischen Nervensystem. *Verhandlungen des X. Internationalen Medicinischen Congresses, Berlin, 4–9 August 1890.* Vol. 4, pp. 132–144, 1892.

Horsley V: *The Structure and Functions of the Brain and Spinal Cord, Being the Fullerian Lectures for 1891.* Griffin: London, 1892.

Horsley V: The study of pathology. [Letter to the editor.] *Br Med J* 1892; 2: 435.

Horsley V: Traducing the profession. [Letter to the editor.] *Br Med J* 1892; 2: 1199.

Horsley V: The British Medical Association meeting at Nottingham. Pathology. *Lancet* 1892; 140: 275–276.

Horsley V: On the topographical relations of the cranium and surface of the cerebrum. pp. 306–355. In Cunningham DJ: *Contribution to the Surface Anatomy of the Cerebral Hemispheres.* Academy House: Dublin, 1892.

Horsley V: On some points of psychological interest in the cerebral localisation of function. *Int Cong Exp Psychol* 1892; Second Session: pp. 87–89, 109.

1893

Horsley V, Boyce RW: Reports to the Scientific Grants Committee of the British Medical Association. A preliminary report on oedema. *Br Med J* 1893; 1: 111–112.

Horsley V: A clinical lecture on paraplegia as a result of spinal caries (compression myelitis) and its treatment. *Clin J* 1893; 1: 321–328.

Horsley V: Discussion on the treatment of cerebral tumours. Remarks on the surgical treatment of cerebral tumours. *Br Med J* 1893; 2: 1365–1367, additional discussion 1369.

Barlow T, Horsley V: The memorial to the late Professor John Marshall. [Letter to the editor.] *Br Med J* 1893; 2: 762.

Horsley V: Introduction. pp. 1–41. In Wooldridge LC: *On the Chemistry of the Blood and Other Scientific Papers. Arranged by Horsley V, Starling E*. Kegan Paul, Trench, Trübner: London, 1893.

Horsley V: The discovery of the physiology of the nervous system. *Med Press Circ* 1893; 107: 317–319.

1894

Beevor CE, Horsley V: A further minute analysis by electric stimulation of the so-called motor region (facial area) of the cortex cerebri in the monkey (*Macacus sinicus*). *Philos Trans R Soc Lond, B* 1894; 185: 39–81.

Horsley V: The destructive effects of small projectiles. *Nature* 1894; 50: 104–108.

Horsley V: The destructive effects of projectiles. *Not Proc R Inst Gr Br* 1894; 14: 228–238.

Horsley V: Experimental degeneration of the pyramidal tract. [Letter to the editor.] *Lancet* 1894; 143: 370–371, 571.

Horsley V: L'effet destructif des projectiles de petit caliber. *Rev Sci* 1894; 1 (4th series): 746–752.

Horsley V: The Medical Defence Union. [Letter to the editor.] *Lancet* 1894; 143: 1341.

Horsley V: On the mode of death in cerebral compression, and its prevention. *Q Med J* 1894; 2: 305–309.

1895

Horsley V: Diagnosi differenziale dei tumori cerebrali. *Boll D Clin* 1895; 12: 315–319.

Horsley V: On the differential diagnosis of cerebral tumours, with some remarks on treatment. *Clin J* 1895; 5: 245–251.

Horsley V: Five cases of leontiasis ossium, in three of which the disease was removed by operation. *Practitioner* 1895; 55: 12–25.

Horsley V: Introductory address delivered at the opening of the winter session of the Sheffield School of Medicine. *Q Med J* 1895; 4: 1–18.

Horsley V: Midwives registration and the Midwives Bill. [Letter to the editor.] *Br Med J* 1895; 1: 1239–1240.

Horsley V: The Obstetrical Society of London and the midwives question. [Letter to the editor.] *Br Med J* 1895; 1: 1005, 1120.

Horsley V: Two cases of perforated gastric ulcer treated by operation. *Br Med J* 1895; 2: 78–79.

1896

Horsley V: An address on the physiology and pathology of the thyroid gland. *Br Med J* 1896; 2: 1623–1625.

Horsley V: The British Medical Association and the adoption of medical defence. *Med Mag* 1896; 5: 669–674.

Horsley V: The difficulty at Adelaide Hospital. [Letter to the editor.] *Br Med J* 1896; 1: 1354.

Horsley V: Direct representatives: Mr. Horsley and the Lancashire and Cheshire branch. [Letter to the editor.] *Br Med J* 1896; 2: 418, 534–535.

Horsley V: A discussion on the General Medical Council in relation to the medical profession. II. On certain undesirable powers possessed by the President of the General Medical Council. *Br Med J* 1896; 2: 499–502, correction 699.

Horsley V: The duties and function of the General Council of Medical Education and Registration. *Med Mag* 1896; 5: 109–122.

Horsley V: Election of direct representatives to the General Medical Council. Mode of voting at the election. [Letter to the editor.] *Br Med J* 1896; 2: 1679.

Horsley V: Election of direct representatives to the General Medical Council. [Letter to the editor.] *Lancet* 1896; 148: 1629–1630.

Horsley V: The General Medical Council: critics and candidates. [Letter to the editor.] *Lancet* 1896; 148: 491–492, 632–633, 907–908.

Horsley V: Abstracts of introductory addresses, etc., delivered at the London and provincial medical schools at the opening of the session, 1896–97. Yorkshire College, Leeds. Introductory address by Mr. Victor Horsley. *Lancet* 1896; 148: 932–933.

Horsley V: A lecture on traumatic neurasthenia. *Clin J* 1896; 7: 281–286.

Horsley V: The Medical Defence Union, Limited, and the London and Counties Medical Protection Society, Limited. [Letter to the editor.] *Lancet* 1896; 147: 735.

Horsley V: The question of medical defence. [Letter to the editor.] *Lancet* 1896; 147; 885.

Horsley V: Medical education and practice. *Br Med J* 1896; 2: 942–946.

Horsley V: The midwives registration bill. [Letter to the editor.] *Br Med J* 1896; 1: 1066.

Horsley V: The physiology and pathology of the thyroid gland. *Trans Med Soc Lond* 1896; 19: 290–300.

Horsley V: Poor assistant. [Letter to the editor.] *Lancet* 1896; 148: 1340.

Horsley V: The special meeting at Birmingham. [Letter to the editor.] *Br Med J* 1896; 2: 101.

1897

Horsley V: A clinical lecture on the diseases of the spinal cord requiring surgical treatment. *Clin J* 1897; 9: 177–183.

Horsley V: Das Sauerstoffbedürfniss des Organismus. *Munch Med Wochenschr* 1897; 44: 499–500.

Horsley V: The election of a direct representative on the General Medical Council. [Letter to the editor.] *Lancet* 1897; 150: 946.

Horsley V: Letter to the registered medical practitioners of England and Wales. *Lancet* 1897; 150: 1072.

Kramer SP, Horsley V: On the effects produced on the circulation and respiration by gun-shot injuries of the cerebral hemispheres. *Philos Trans R Soc Lond, B* 1897; 188: 223–256.

Horsley V: To the registered medical practitioners of England and Wales. Letters from candidates to the electors. *Br Med J* 1897; 2: 1210.

Löwenthal M, Horsley V: On the relations between the cerebellar and other centres (namely cerebral and spinal) with especial reference to the action of antagonistic muscles. (Preliminary account.) *Proc R Soc Lond* 1897; 61: 20–25.

Horsley V: Methylenblaufärbung der Blutkörperchen. *Munch Med Wochenschr* 1897; 44: 625.

Horsley V: Torticollis and its treatment. *Trans Hunt Soc* 1897; 79th Session, Part I: 1–12.

Horsley V: Direct representation on the General Medical Council. Mr. Victor Horsley's address to the registered medical practitioners of England and Wales. *Br Med J* 1897; 2: 835.

Horsley V: The vacancy in the General Medical Council. Mr. Victor Horsley's address. To the registered practitioners of England and Wales. *Lancet* 1897; 150: 808.

Horsley V: The General Medical Council election. Mr. Victor Horsley and Mr. Colin Campbell. *Br Med J* 1897; 2: 1021.

Horsley V: The General Medical Council election. Replies of other candidates to the "interrogatories." *Br Med J* 1897; 2: 1020.

Horsley V: Short note on sense organs in muscle and on the preservation of muscle spindles in conditions of extreme muscular atrophy, following section of the motor nerve. *Brain* 1897; 20: 375–376.

Horsley V: Torticollis. *Clin J* 1897; 10: 145–149.

Horsley V: Traumatic neurasthenia. *Trans Med Soc Lond* 1897; 20: 216–227.

Horsley V: Two clinical lectures on the treatment of trigeminal neuralgia. *Clin J* 1897; 11: 8–14, 17–23.

1898

Horsley V: An address on the Medical Acts of Parliament: As they are and as they ought to be. *Lancet* 1898; 151: 1–2.

Horsley V: An address on the Medical Acts of Parliament: As they are and as they ought to be. *J Br Dent Assoc* 1898; 19: 45–51.

Horsley V: Association intelligence. General Medical Council. Metropolitan Branch. *J Br Dent Assoc* 1898; 19: 79–82.

Horsley V: Abstract of an address on the work of the General Medical Council. *Lancet* 1898; 152: 1692–1695.

Horsley V: The business of the General Medical Council. [Letter to the editor.] *Br Med J* 1898; 1: 661.

Horsley V: A clinical lecture on penetrating wounds of the central nervous system. *Clin J* 1898; 12: 261–267.

Horsley V: A contribution towards the determination of the energy developed by a nerve centre. *Brain* 1898; 21: 547–579.

Horsley V: A discussion on the treatment of spinal caries. I. Treatment of early caries. *Br Med J* 1898; 2: 1127–1128.

Horsley V: The duties of the president of the General Medical Council. [Letter to the editor.] *Lancet* 1898; 151: 676.

Horsley V: Fifth report of Mr. Victor Horsley to the registered practitioners of England and Wales. *Br Med J* 1898; 2: 1761–1763.

Horsley V: Foreign practitioners and reciprocity. [Letter to the editor.] *Br Med J* 1898; 1: 1558, 1685.

Horsley V: General Medical Council. A fourth report by Mr. Victor Horsley to the registered practitioners of England and Wales. *Br Med J* 1898; 1: 1288–1289.

Horsley V: A fourth report to the registered practitioners of England and Wales. *Lancet* 1898; 151: 1349–1350.

Horsley V: The General Medical Council: The right of members to inspect the council's documents. [Letter to the editor.] *Lancet* 1898; 151: 1562.

Horsley V: Legislation as a remedy for medical grievances. [Letter to the editor.] *Br Med J* 1898; 1: 243, 340–341.

Horsley V: Legislation as a remedy for medical grievances. [Letter to the editor.] *Lancet* 1898; 151: 399–400.

Horsley V: Masseurs and medical electricians. [Letter to the editor.] *Br Med J* 1898; 2: 1846.

Horsley V: The midwives registration bill. [Letter to the editor.] *Br Med J* 1898; 1: 915.

Horsley V: Mr. Victor Horsley and the General Medical Council. A report to the registered practitioners of England and Wales. *Br Med J* 1898; 1: 225–226.

Horsley V: The penal powers of the General Medical Council: A report to the registered practitioners of England and Wales. *Lancet* 1898; 151: 253–254.

Horsley V: The Manchester Medico-Ethical Association. Address by Mr. Victor Horsley on the procedure of the General Medical Council and the reform of the Medical Acts. *Br Med J* 1898; 2: 1883–1887.

Horsley V: The General Medical Council. Second report to the registered practition [sic] of England and Wales. *Br Med J* 1898; 1: 720.

Horsley V: A second report to the registered practitioners of England and Wales. *Lancet* 1898; 151: 744–745.

Horsley V: The Society of Apothecaries and Mr. Victor Horsley. [Letter to the editor.] *Lancet* 1898; 151: 327–328.

Horsley V: General Council of Medical Education and Registration. Report by Mr. Victor Horsley to the registered practitioners of England and Wales. *Br Med J* 1898; 1: 1037–1038.

Horsley V: Third report to the registered practitioners of England and Wales. *Lancet* 1898; 151: 1075–1076.

Horsley V: The true interpretation to be placed on the Medical Acts. *Clin J* 1898; 11 (Suppl.): 1–6.

Horsley V: A report to the registered practitioners of England and Wales. *Clin J* 1898; 11 (Suppl.): [no page numbers].

Horsley V: Trephining in the neo-lithic period. *J Anthropol Inst Gr Br Ire* 1888; 17: 100–106.

1899

Beevor CE, Horsley V: On excitable fibres of the crus cerebri. *J Physiol* 1899; 23 (Suppl.): 10–11.

Horsley V: The amendment of the Medical Acts. [Letter to the editor.] *Br Med J* 1899; 1: 941, 999–1002, 1129.

Horsley V: The conference on medical politics at Newcastle-on-Tyne. *Lancet* 1899; 154: 1474–1477.

Horsley V: A deserving case. [Letter to the editor.] *Br Med J* 1899; 2: 315.

Horsley V: A deserving case. [Letter to the editor.] *Lancet* 1899; 154: 318.

Horsley V: Galen. *Middlesex Hosp J* 1899; 3: 37–52.

Horsley V: The General Medical Council and the Hunter case. [Letter to the editor.] *Br Med J* 1899; 1: 374–375.

Horsley V: The General Medical Council. Inspection of documents. [Letter to the editor.] *Br Med J* 1899; 1: 52–53.

Horsley V: "Hunter v. Clare." [Letter to the editor.] *Lancet* 1899; 154: 50.

Horsley V: Illegal certificates. [Letter to the editor.] *Br Med J* 1899; 2: 685, 879–880, 1138, 1223–1224, 1315, 1446–1447, 1587.

Horsley V: Illegal certificates of proficiency in medicine, surgery, or midwifery. [Letter to the editor.] *Lancet* 1899; 154: 511.

Horsley V: On injuries to peripheral nerves. *Practitioner* 1899; 63: 131–144.

Horsley V: The Medical Acts and the medical profession. [Letter to the editor.] *Br Med J* 1899; 1: 54.

Horsley V: The medico-political outlook. *Scalpel* 1899; 4: 395–399 [Not verified].

Horsley V: The Midwives Bill. [Letter to the editor.] *Br Med J* 1899; 2: 313.

Horsley V: The Midwives' Bill: Illegal certificates. [Letter to the editor.] *Br Med J* 1899; 2: 502.

Horsley V: The direct representatives' meeting at Newcastle. Mr. Victor Horsley's address. *Br Med J* 1899; 2: 1501–1504.

Horsley V: The proposed registration of midwives. *Lancet* 1899; 153: 1732–1734.

Horsley V: On the rational treatment of goitre. *Clin J* 1899; 13: 321–327.

Horsley V: Sixth report of Mr. Victor Horsley to the registered practitioners of England and Wales. *Br Med J* 1899; 2: 354–356.

Horsley V: Sixth report of Mr. Victor Horsley to the registered practitioners of England and Wales. *Lancet* 1899; 154: 425–427.

Horsley V: Diseases of the vertebral column, tumours, and compression palsies. In Albutt TC (ed.): *A System of Medicine*, vol. 6, pp. 854–871. Macmillan: New York, 1899, reprint 1903.

Horsley V: Roman defences of south-east Britain. *Not Proc R Inst Gr Br* 1899; 16: 35–44.

1900

Horsley V: An address on the surgical treatment of trigeminal neuralgia. *Practitioner* 1900; 65: 251–263.

Horsley V: A clinical demonstration of cases of compression paraplegia. *Clin J* 1900; 15: 257–262.

Jackson JH, Buzzard T, Carter RB, Bastian HC, Gowers WR, Ferrier D, Ormerod JA, Beevor CE, Tooth HH, Taylor J, Risien Russell JS, Turner WA, Batten FE, Semon F, Horsley V, Ballance CA, Gunn RM, Cumberbatch AE.: The medical staff and the management of the National Hospital for the Paralysed and Epileptic, Queen-Square. [Letter to the editor.] *Lancet* 1900; 156: 351–352, 463.

Horsley V: Conference on medical organisation at Manchester. The Medical Acts. *Lancet* 1900; 1: 1302–1303; reported also in Anon: Conference on medical organisation. *Br Med J* 1900; 1: 1123–1124.

Horsley V: Mr. Victor Horsley and the Medical Acts. [Letter to the editor.] *Lancet* 1900; 155: 1605.

Horsley V. The Midwives Bill. Objections to the Midwives Bill. *Br Med J* 1900; 1: 1035.

Horsley V: Traumatic neurasthenia. In Albutt TC (ed.): *A System of Medicine*, vol. 8, pp. 164–176. Macmillan: New York, 1900.

Horsley V: *The Effect of Alcohol upon the Human Brain. The Second Lees and Raper Memorial Lecture*. Lees and Raper Memorial Trustees: London, 1900.

1901

Horsley V: The General Medical Council election. The approaching election of direct representatives. The gallery of the council chamber. *Br Med J* 1901; 2: 1544, 1713.

Horsley V: The General Medical Council election, 1901. Meeting of candidates at Cheltenham. *Br Med J* 1901; 2: 374–375, additional discussion 377.

Horsley V: The coming election of direct representatives to the General Medical Council. Mr. Horsley's address. *Lancet* 1901; 158: 410–411, additional discussion 412.

Horsley V: Mr. Victor Horsley's report. [Letter to the editor.] *Br Med J* 1901; 1: 485.

Horsley V: Mr. Victor Horsley's report. [Letter to the editor.] *Lancet* 1901; 157: 579.

Horsley V: The General Medical Council election. The approaching election of direct representatives. England. A protest and a warning. [Letter to the editor.] *Br Med J* 1901; 2: 1610.

Horsley V: The General Medical Council election. The approaching election of direct representatives. England. The proposed conciliation board. [Letter to CHW Parkinson.] *Br Med J* 1901; 2: 1610.

Horsley V: Seventh report by Mr. Victor Horsley to the registered practitioners of England and Wales. *Br Med J* 1901; 1: 361–362.

Horsley V: Seventh report by Mr. Victor Horsley to the registered practitioners of England and Wales. *Lancet* 1901; 157: 425–426.

Thiele FH, Horsley V: A study of the degenerations observed in the central nervous system in a case of fracture dislocation of the spine. *Brain* 1901; 24: 519–531.

1902

Horsley V: The General Medical Council election. Address from Sir Victor Horsley. To the registered medical practitioners of England and Wales. *Med J* 1902; 2: 1091.

Beevor CE, Horsley V: On the pallio-tectal or cortico-mesencephalic system of fibres. *Brain* 1902; 25: 436–443.

Horsley V: The General Medical Council: Election of direct representative for England

and Wales. Sir Victor Horsley's address. To the registered medical practitioners of England and Wales. *Br Med J* 1902; 2: 811.

Horsley V: The election of a direct representative to the General Medical Council. Sir Victor Horsley's address. To the registered medical practitioners of England and Wales. *Lancet* 1902; 160: 761.

Horsley V: The recent election of a direct representative on the General Medical Council. To the registered practitioners of England and Wales. *Lancet* 1902; 160: 951.

Horsley V: The organization of a political bureau in the British Medical Association. *Br Med J* 1902; 2: 1051–1052, discussion 1053.

1903

Horsley V: An address on medical politics. *Br Med J* 1903; 2: 1573–1575.

Horsley V: An address on the purposes and maintenance of our universities. *Br Med J* 1903; 2: 953–956.

Horsley V: On the consolidation of the public and professional interests of medical men. *Br Med J* 1903; 1: 631–633.

Horsley V: Obituary, Samuel Woodcock, M.D. Brux., L.R.C.P. & S. Edin., J.P. *Br Med J* 1903; 2: 1619.

Horsley V: The Northern University triad. [Letter to the editor.] *Br Med J* 1903; 2: 1179, 1244.

Horsley V: The purposes and maintenance of our universities. *Birmingham Med Rev* 1903; 54: 615–630.

1904

Byles DB, Harcourt AV, Horsley V: Report of special chloroform committee of the British Medical Association. Third report of proceedings (1903–4). Appendix III. Estimation of chloroform dissolved in blood. Report of work done between December 1903, and July 1904. *Br Med J* 1904; 2: 169–171.

Horsley V: On tactile sensation. *Practitioner* 1904; 73: 581–596.

Horsley V: Witness testimony, March 16, 1904. pp. 384–387. In: *Report of the Inter-Departmental Committee on Physical Deterioration. Volume 1. – Report and Appendix*. His Majesty's Stationery Office: London, 1904.

1905

Horsley V: An address on haemorrhoids. *Clin J* 1905; 25: 273–278.

Horsley V: Discussion on vertigo, its pathology and treatment. Introductory address by Sir Victor Horsley. *Trans Otol Soc UK* 1905; 6: 72–79.

Horsley V: Alcohol and commercial efficiency. *Lancet* 1905; 165: 739–740.

Horsley V: *Alcohol and commercial efficiency*. National Temperance League: Great Britain, 1905 [Not verified].

Horsley V: *The Cerebellum: Its Relation to Spatial Orientation and to Locomotion*. John Bale, Sons, and Danielsson: London, 1905.

Clarke RH, Horsley V: On the intrinsic fibres of the cerebellum, its nuclei and its efferent tracts. *Brain* 1905; 28: 13–29.

Horsley V: The effect of alcohol upon the human brain. *Br J Inebr* 1905; 3: 69–91.

Horsley V: Obituary, Sir John Burdon-Sanderson, M.D., F.R.S. *Br Med J* 1905; 2: 1490.

Horsley V: On a trigeminal-aural reflex in the rabbit. *Brain* 1905; 28: 65–67.

Horsley V: Vertigo. *J Laryngol Rhinol Otol* 1905; 20: 403–409.

Horsley V: Witness testimony, May 18, 1905. pp. 61–73. In: *Report from the Select Committee on Registration of Nurses; Together with the Proceedings of the Committee, Minutes of Evidence, and Appendix*. His Majesty's Stationery Office: London, 1905.

Horsley V: Report on the procedure of the coroner for south-west London and the inaction of the government in relation thereto. *Br Med J* 1905; 2 (Suppl. 68): 146–148.

1906

Clarke RH, Horsley V: On a method of investigating the deep ganglia and tracts of the central nervous system (cerebellum). *Br Med J* 1906; 2: 1799–1800.

Horsley V: On Dr. Hughlings Jackson's views of the functions of the cerebellum as illustrated by recent research. *Brain* 1906; 29: 446–466.

Horsley V: The necessity of union in the profession. Address by Sir Victor Horsley. *Br Med J* 1906; 2: 1821–1824, additional discussion 1825.

Horsley V: Note on the taenia pontis. *Brain* 1906; 29: 28–34.

Russel CK, Horsley V: Note on apparent re-representation in the cerebral cortex of the type of sensory representation as it exists in the spinal cord. *Brain* 1906; 29: 137–152.

Slinger RT, Horsley V: Upon the orientation of points in space by the muscular, arthrodial, and tactile senses of the upper limbs in normal individuals and in blind persons. *Brain* 1906; 29: 1–27.

Horsley V: On the technique of operations on the central nervous system. *Br Med J* 1906; 2: 411–423.

Horsley V: On the technique of operations on the central nervous system. *Can Pract Rev* 1906; 31: 486–492.

Horsley V: Address in surgery on the technique of operations on the central nervous system. *Lancet* 1906; 168: 484–490.

Horsley V: On the technique of operations on the central nervous system. *Montreal Med J* 1906; 35: 601–629.

Broadbent WH, Tweedy J, Gould AP, Brunton L, Woodhead S, Barlow T, Eccles WM, Horsley V: The teaching of hygiene and temperance in elementary schools. Deputation to the President of the Board of Education. *Br Med J* 1906; 2: 1412.

Horsley V: *What Women Can Do to Promote Temperance. An Address Delivered at the Annual Meeting of the Women's Union (C.E.T.S.)*. Church of England Temperance Society: London, 1906.

Horsley V: On the technique of operations on the central nervous system. *St. Louis Med Rev* 1906; 54: 261–265.

Horsley V: Introduction. In Hoskyns-Abrahall W: *The Health Reader*, pp. xiii–xv. Cassell: London, 1906; 2nd edition 1907; 3rd edition 1909.

1907

Horsley V: The deputation to the President of the Board of Education. [Letter to the editor.] *Br Med J* 1907; 1: 1459.

Horsley V: Dr. Hughlings Jackson's views of the functions of the cerebellum, as illustrated by recent research. *Br Med J* 1907; 1: 803–808.

Horsley V: The early Notification of Births Bill. [Letter to the editor.] *Br Med J* 1907; 2: 414, 553.

Horsley V, Sturge MD: *Alcohol and the Human Body. An Introduction to the Study of the Subject.* Macmillan: London, 1907.

1908

Horsley V, Sturge MD: *Alcohol and the Human Body. An Introduction to the Study of the Subject, and a Contribution to National Health*, 2nd ed. Macmillan: London, 1908.

Horsley V: The antivivisection agitation. [Letter to the editor.] *Br Med J* 1908; 1: 1208.

Horsley V: Obituary, Charles Edward Beevor, M. D., F.R.C.P.Lond. *Br Med J* 1908; 2: 1785–1786.

Horsley V, Clarke RH: The structure and functions of the cerebellum examined by a new method. *Brain* 1908; 31: 45–124.

Horsley V: Inquests and operations. *Br Med J* 1908; 1: 1460–1461.

Horsley V: Note on the existence of Reissner's fibre in higher vertebrates. *Brain* 1908; 31: 147–159.

Horsley V: The Notification of Births Act. [Letter to the editor.] *Br Med J* 1908; 2: 772.

Horsley V: The operative treatment of optic neuritis. *Ophthalmoscope* 1908; 6: 658–663.

Horsley V: Presidential address on reasons for joining the British Medical Association. *Br Med J* 1908; 2: 65–67.

Horsley V: Witness testimony, November 13, 1907. pp. 118–149. In: *Royal Commission on Vivisection. Appendix to Fourth Report of the Commissioners. Minutes of Evidence, October to December, 1907*. His Majesty's Stationery Office: London, 1908.

Horsley V: Appendix A: Forms I. and II. pp. 308–310. In: *Royal Commission on Vivisection. Appendix to Fourth Report of the Commissioners. Minutes of Evidence, October to December, 1907*. His Majesty's Stationery Office: London, 1908.

1909

Horsley V: The Cavendish lecture, 1909: The cerebellum. *West Lond Med J* 1909; 14: 149–158.

Horsley V: A clinical lecture on chronic spinal meningitis: Its differential diagnosis and surgical treatment. *Br Med J* 1909; 1: 513–517.

Horsley V: Description of the brain of Mr. Charles Babbage, F.R.S. *Philos Trans R Soc Lond, B* 1909; 200: 117–131.

Horsley V: The Linacre lecture on the function of the so-called motor area of the brain. *Br Med J* 1909; 2: 121–132.

Horsley V: The kinaesthetic area of the brain. [Letter to the editor.] *Br Med J* 1909; 2: 577.

MacNalty AS, Horsley V: On the cervical spino-bulbar and spino-cerebellar tracts and on the question of topographical representation in the cerebellum. *Brain* 1909; 32: 237–255.

Ridge and 42 other doctors, including Horsley V: International medical temperance appeal, 1909. *Br Med J* 1909; 1: 1131–1132.

Anderson JF, Haslip GE, Horsley V, Ker HR, Shaw LE: Metropolitan counties branch. Central council election, 1909. *Br Med J* 1909; 1 (Suppl. 269): 386–387.

Horsley V, Sturge MD: *Alcohol and the Human Body. An Introduction to the Study of the Subject, and a Contribution to National Health*, 3rd ed. (special ed.) Macmillan: London, 1909.

1910

Horsley V: An address on surgical versus the expectant treatment of intracranial tumour. *Br Med J* 1910; 2: 1833–1835.

Horsley V: Die chirurgische Behandlung der intrakraniellen Geschwülste, im Gegensatz zu der abwartenden Therapie betrachtet. *Neurol Centralbl* 1910; 29: 1170–1178.

Horsley V: A lecture on the topographical diagnosis of tumours of the cerebral hemisphere. *Univ Coll Hosp Mag* 1910; 1: 9–17.

Horsley V: The localizing value of unequal papilloedema. [Letter to the editor.] *Br Med J* 1910; 1: 725.

May O, Horsley V: The mesencephalic root of the fifth nerve. *Brain* 1910; 33: 175–203.

Horsley V: A paper on "optic neuritis," "choked disc," or "papilloedema": Treatment, localizing value, and pathology. *Br Med J* 1910; 1: 553–558.

Horsley V: Prison doctors and the Home Office. [Letter to the editor.] *Br Med J* 1910; 1: 49–50, 173, 233, 352–353.

Sturge MD, Horsley V: Alcoholism and degeneration. [Letter to the editor.] *Br Med J* 1910; 2: 1656, 1817–1818, 1946–1947, 2048–2049.

1911

Butlin HT, Maclean EJ, Macdonald JA, Rayner E, Greer WJ, Pope FM, Horsley V: Committee on treatment of fractures. [Letter to the editor.] *Br Med J* 1911; 1: 843.

Horsley V, Finzi NS: The action of filtered radium rays when applied directly to the brain. *Br Med J* 1911; 2: 898–899.

Goodall EW, Horsley V, Keay JH, Rice-Oxley AJ, Shaw LE: The insurance commissionership. Letter published in the "Times" on December 7th. [Letter to the editor.] *Br Med J* 1911; 2: 1572.

Handelsmann, Horsley V: Preliminary note on experimental investigations on the pituitary body. *Br Med J* 1911; 2: 1150–1151.

Horsley V: Operative versus expectant treatment in diseases of the nervous system. *Dtsch Z Nervenheilkd* 1911: 41: 91–99.

Horsley V: The State Sickness Insurance Bill and the forthcoming representative meeting. [Letter to the editor.] *Br Med J* 1911; 2: 138–139.

Sturge MD, Horsley V: Alcoholism and degeneracy. [Letter to the editor.] *Br Med J* 1911; 1: 112, 333–336, 404.

Sturge MD, Horsley V: On some of the biological and statistical errors in the work on parental alcoholism by Miss Elderton and Professor Karl Pearson, F.R.S. *Br Med J* 1911; 1: 72–82.

Horsley V, Sturge MD: *Alcohol and the Human Body. An Introduction to the Study of the Subject, and a Contribution to National Health*, 4th ed. (Shilling ed.) Macmillan: London, 1911.

1912

Horsley V: Factors which conduce to success in the treatment of otogenic brain abscess. *Proc R Soc Med* 1912; 5: 45–51.

Horsley V: The profession and the politicians. [Letter to the editor.] *Br Med J* 1912; 1: 391.

Horsley V: The profession and politicians. [Letter to the editor.] *Br Med J* 1912; 1: 462.

Savill A, Moullin CM, Horsley V: Forcible feeding. [Letter to the editor.] *Br Med J* 1912; 2: 100–101, 151.

Savill A, Moullin CM, Horsley V: Preliminary report on the forcible feeding of suffrage prisoners. *Br Med J* 1912; 2: 505–508.

Savill A, Moullin CM, Horsley V: Preliminary report on the forcible feeding of suffrage prisoners. *Lancet* 1912; 180: 549–551.

Horsley V: *The Effects of Small Quantities of Alcohol, Tested by Doctors; Notes of a Lantern Lecture at the Friends' Meeting-House, Holloway, to the London Auxiliary of the Friends' Temperance Union*. Friends' Temperance Union: London, 1912 [Not verified].

Horsley V: Citizenship and Alcohol. pp. 125–134. In: *Fifty Doctors Against Alcohol. A Call to National Defence*. Brotherhood Publishing House: London, 1912.

1913

Horsley V: A constitutional point. [Letter to the editor.] *Br Med J* 1913; 1: 1299.

Horsley V: A constitutional point. [Letter to the editor.] *Br Med J* 1913; 2: 48–49.

Moullin CM, Horsley V: Case of Miss Lenton. Correspondence of the Home Office with the Royal College of Surgeons and Sir Victor Horsley with regard to the case of Lilian Lenton. I. Correspondence of the Home Office with the Royal College of Surgeons. Forcible feeding. *Lancet* 1913; 182: 191.

Savill A, Moullin CM, Horsley V: Case of Miss Lenton. Correspondence of the Home Office with the Royal College of Surgeons and Sir Victor Horsley with regard to the case of Lilian Lenton. I. Correspondence of the Home Office with the Royal College of Surgeons. The case of Miss Lenton. *Lancet* 1913; 181: 190–191.

Horsley V: Case of Miss Lenton. Correspondence of the Home Office with the Royal College of Surgeons and Sir Victor Horsley with regard to the case of Lilian Lenton. II. – Correspondence of the Home Office with Sir Victor Horsley. *Lancet* 1913; 182: 192–193.

Horsley V: Sir Victor Horsley and Mr. McKenna. [Letter to the editor.] *Lancet* 1913; 181: 1693.

Horsley V: Sir Victor Horsley and Mr. McKenna. [Letter to the editor.] *Lancet* 1913; 182: 41–42.

Horsley V: *The Effects of Small Quantities of Alcohol, Tested by Doctors; Notes of a Lantern Lecture at the Friends' Meeting-House, Holloway, to the London Auxiliary of the Friends' Temperance Union*, 2nd ed. Friends' Temperance Union: London, 1913.

Horsley V: Islington. pp. 25–27. In: *The National League for Physical Education & Improvement*. Eighth Annual Report: London, 1913.

1914

Horsley V: Antisepsis and asepsis in war. [Letter to the editor.] *Br Med J* 1914; 2: 861.

Horsley V: Care of the wounded. [Letter to the editor.] *Br Med J* 1914; 2: 813.

Horsley V: The cause of hernia in infants. [Letter to the editor.] *Br Med J* 1914; 2: 1120.

Horsley V: Discussion on the reform of the vital statistics of the nation; with special reference to death certification. *Br Med J* 1914; 2: 787–789.

Horsley V: British and German small arm ammunition. Memorandum communicated by the War Office respecting British and German service ammunition. Appendix I. Memorandum on the .303 (174 grains) Mark VII British service rifle bullet in reference to explosive effects. *Br Med J* 1914; 2: 896.

Horsley V: British and German small arm ammunition. Memorandum communicated by the War Office respecting British and German service ammunition. Appendix II. Note on the flat-nose revolver bullet, Mark IV, in reference to the provisions of the Hague Convention. *Br Med J* 1914; 2: 896.

Horsley V: Note on haemostasis by application of living tissue. *Br Med J* 1914; 2: 8.

Horsley V: Present-day lessons from the life work of Mitchell Banks. *Br Med J* 1914; 2: 657–661.

Horsley V: State registration of nurses. [Letter to the editor.] *Br Med J* 1914; 2: 315–316.

Horsley V: The treatment of wounds in the present war. [Letter to the editor.] *Br Med J* 1914; 2: 901, 949, 999.

Horsley V: The wounded in the war. [Letter to the editor.] *Lancet* 1914; 184: 1116.

Horsley V: Witness testimony, March 27, 1914. pp. 372–389. In: *Royal Commission on Venereal Disease. Appendix to First Report of the Commissioners. Minutes of Evidence: 7th November 1913 to 6th April 1914. Question 1 to Question 12,549*. His Majesty's Stationery Office: London, 1914.

1915

Horsley V, Sturge MD: *Alcohol and the Human Body. An Introduction to the Study of the Subject, and a Contribution to National Health*, 5th ed., enlarged. Macmillan: London, 1915 [a sixth edition was published in 1920, after Horsley's death].

Horsley V: An address on gunshot wounds of the head. *Lancet* 1915; 185: 359–362.

Horsley V: On the alleged responsibility of the medical profession for the reintroduction of the rum ration into the British Army. *Br Med J* 1915; 1: 203–206.

Horsley V: Discussion on gunshot wounds of the head. *Trans Med Soc Lond* 1915; 38: 112–128.

Horsley V: The prevention of tetanus. [Letter to the editor.] *Br Med J* 1915; 1: 576–577.

Horsley V: Remarks on gunshot wounds of the head. *Br Med J* 1915; 1: 321–323.

Horsley V: The rum ration. [Letter to the editor.] *Br Med J* 1915; 1: 359–360, 448–489, 529–530, 575, 621.

Horsley V: The treatment of wounds. [Letter to the editor.] *Br Med J* 1915; 1: 93.

Appendix 4: Sir Victor Horsley's Correspondence with *The Times* of London

Horsley wrote frequently to the editor of *The Times (London)* on medical or political issues and these were often controversial opinion pieces that provide insight to his beliefs and principles. The title of the correspondence, date of publication, and page number in the broadsheet are listed below in chronological order.

Surgery and vivisection. January 16, 1885, p. 7

"The Angel of Death." January 22, 1892, p. 15

Mr. Victor Horsley and Miss Cobbe. October 12, 1892, p. 12 and October 17, 1892, p. 7

Professor Horsley and Miss Cobbe. October 20, 1892, p. 14; October 21, 1892, p. 6; and October 25, 1892, p. 7

The vivisection controversy. October 28, 1892, p. 5

Re. Memorial to the late Professor John Marshall. September 22, 1893, p. 5 [with Barlow T]

"Reg. V. Priestley." June 1, 1896, p. 9

The General Medical Council. December 3, 1896, p. 7 [with Rateman AG]; December 3, 1896, p. 7; and October 8, 1897, p. 5

National Hospital for the Paralysed and Epileptic. July 28, 1900, p. 10

The National Hospital for the Paralysed and Epileptic. August 7, 1900, p. 6 and March 14, 1901, p. 11 [both with Jackson JH, Buzzard T, Carter RB, Bastian HC, Gowers WR, Ferrier D, Ormerod JA, Beevor CE, Tooth HH, Taylor J, Risien Russell JS, Turner WA, Batten FE, Semon F, Ballance CA, Gunn RM, and Cumberbatch AE]

Anti-vivisection methods. March 8, 1902, p. 12; March 12, 1902, p. 12; and March 20, 1902, p. 12

The Imperial Vaccination League. August 11, 1902, p. 19 [with Cantuar F, London AF, Northumberland, Kelvin, Westminster, Avebury, Broadbent WH, Chelmsford, Lawrence T, Blyth J, Montefiore CG, Acland CTD, Wood HT, M'vail JC, Tuke JB, Pollock F, Crichton-Browne J, Carter RB, Roffen E, Stepney CG, Forrest RW, Sinclair W, Gibson JM, Adler H, Allen T, Brook D, Church WS, Howse HG, and Hutchinson J]

The representation of the University of London. January 12, 1903, p. 8

Hospital for invalid gentlewomen. July 19, 1904, p. 10 [with Waldegrave, Lister, Tweedy J, Barlow T, Dyke T, Bennett W, Acland, Church W, Bowlby A, Critchett A, Godlee RJ, Griffith W, and Smith T]

The National Hospital for the Paralysed and Epileptic. December 6, 1904, p. 5 [with Dudley, Harrowby, Buzzard T, Gowers WR, and Power JD]

The teaching of hygiene and temperance. June 8, 1907, p. 19 and June 13, 1907, p. 15

A coroner on operations. June 6, 1908, p. 12 and June 12, 1908, p. 20

The Research Defence Society and Mr. Coleridge. December 30, 1908, p. 7 and January 5, 1909, p. 7

The vivisection dispute. January 8, 1909, p. 6.

Sir James Paget on total abstinence. January 23, 1909, p. 10

Brewers' challenge to teetotalers. February 22, 1909, p. 10; February 25, 1909, p. 10; and March 1, 1909, p. 4

The Nervous Diseases Research Fund. May 31, 1909, p. 4 [with Speyer E, Jackson JH, Buzzard T, Ferrier D, Gowers WR, and Power JD.]

The Artists' Rifles. June 4, 1909, p. 10 [with Brock T, Busk EH, Cope AS, Forbes-Robertson J, Poynter EJ, Thornycroft H, and Waterlow EA]

Forcible feeding. "Leigh v. Gladstone and others." December 11, 1909, p. 4

Forcible feeding. December 16, 1909, p. 12; December 18, 1909, p. 12; December 21, 1909, p. 10; and December 23, 1909, p. 8

The London University contest. November 26, 1910, p. 12

Sir Victor Horsley and the Galton Laboratory. January 13, 1911, p. 8

Alcohol and degeneracy. January 14, 1911, p. 10 [with Sturge MD.]; January 16, 1911, p. 7; January 19, 1911, p. 12 [with Sturge MD.]; January 28, 1911, p. 12 [with Sturge MD]

The great "betrayal." A reply to Dr. Smith. December 7, 1911, p. 10 [with Goodall EW, Keay JH, Rice-Oxley AJ, and Shaw LE]

The great betrayal. Policy of the doctors. December 11, 1911, p. 10 [with Goodall EW, Keay JH, Rice-Oxley AJ, and Shaw LE]

"The great betrayal." December 13, 1911, p. 7 and December 15, 1911, p. 12 [both with Goodall EW, Keay JH, Rice-Oxley AJ, and Shaw LE]

The Council's Position. The association and the profession. December 20, 1911, p. 10 [with Goodall EW, Keay JH, Rice-Oxley AJ, and Shaw LE]

The Insurance Act. The doctors' Guildhall meeting. Another adjournment. The British Medical Association. February 22, 1912, p. 7

Demands of the medical profession. Women on insurance committees. February 24, 1912, p. 9

Women on the insurance committee of the British Medical Association. February 27, 1912, p. 6

Sir Almroth Wright's letter. A protest by Sir. R. Douglas Powell. Reply by Sir Victor Horsley. April 1, 1912, p. 6

A defence of the Act. June 6, 1912, p. 7

Medicine and the Insurance Act. June 8, 1912, p. 6

Mr. McKenna and medical memorialists. July 11, 1912, p. 8 [with Savill A and Mansell Moullin C]

Horsley V: Tests of drunkenness. November 1, 1912, p. 15; Nov 8, 1912, p. 16; November 14, 1912, p. 4; November 19, 1912, p. 14; and November 23, 1912, p. 13

Sir Victor Horsley on the pledge. December 27, 1912, p. 6

Sir V. Horsley's Position. Reply to Mr. Turner. December 30, 1912, p. 8

The case of Miss Lenton. March 18, 1913, p. 6 [with Savill A and Mansell Moullin C]

The case of Lillian Lenton. July 15, 1913, p. 10 [with Mansell Moullin C]

Sir Victor Horsley and the Harborough division. November 17, 1913, p. 1

Registration of nurses. A reply to Lady Jersey. February 9, 1914, p. 11

Mothers of the race. April 13, 1914, p. 5

The Royal Commission on Venereal Diseases. April 22, 1914, p. 10

The care of our wounded. November 2, 1914, p. 9

Index

Acland, Sir Henry, 24
acquired immunodeficiency
    syndrome (AIDS), 154
activism. *See* Social activism
Adams, William, 57
aerophobia, 28
AIDS. *See* acquired
    immunodeficiency
    syndrome
Alabone, Edwin, 110–111
alcohol abuse, 143
    generational influences on, 143
    parental alcoholism and, 146
Alcohol and the Human Body
        (Sturge, M. and Horsley, V.),
        144, 145, 149
alcohol use
    in *British Medical Journal*, 147
    contemporary beliefs on, 143
    driving and, safety issues and,
        147–148
    generational influences on, 143
        parental alcoholism, 146
    health benefits from, 143
    Horsley opposition to, 143–149,
        173
    the Lancet manifesto, 144–145
    Pearson study on
        conflict with Horsley, 146–147
        criticism of, 146
        parental alcoholism as
            influence on, 146
    problems from, 143
    rum rationing, 148–149
        for British Expeditionary
            Force, 148
    at secondary schools, 145
    venereal diseases and, 153
alcoholism, parental, 146
Alexandra (Queen), 133–134
Allbutt, Thomas Clifford, 144
Althaus, Julius, 56
Alverstone, Lord, 131–132, 138
Amara War Cemetery, 164
ambidexterity, of Horsley, 92
American Neurological
        Association, 48, 93
Anderson, Elizabeth Garrett, 139
anesthetics, study of
    in animal experimentation, 130,
        131

dosing determinations, 61–62
    by Horsley, on himself, 15–16
    movement and, cerebral
        localization of, 41
    in neurosurgical techniques,
        63
Anglo-Persian Oil Company, 162
animal studies, experimentation
    and. *See also* comparative
    anatomy
anesthetic use in, 130, 131
British Medical Association
    support of, 134
    resolutions on, 129–130
Coalition for Medical Progress,
    135
with Horsley-Clarke stereotactic
    apparatus, 65, 67–68
International Medical Congress
    resolution on, 129–130
movement and, cerebral
    localization of, 40–41
for pituitary gland tumor surgery,
    78–79
for rabies, inoculation strategies,
    30–31
regulatory legislation of, 128
Annandale, Thomas, 77
anthrax, 23–24
Anthropological Institute, lecture
    at, 99–100
antibiotics, for venereal diseases,
    154
antiseptic approach
    infection risks and, 19–20
    at University College Hospital, 16
antivivisectionist movement, 18,
        172–173. *See also* animal
        studies
British Union for the Abolition of
    Vivisection, 134
Brown Animal Sanatory
    Institution as target of, 23
Brown Dog Affair, 124–125,
    131–133
    Bayliss and, 131–132
    lawsuit as result of, 131–132
    student protests as result of,
        133
Church of England and, 129
Cruelty to Animals Act and, 23

development and origins of, 128
Hadwen correspondence and,
    133–134
National Anti-Vivisection
    Society, 128, 131
in newspapers, 128–131
    Daily Mail, 134
    Daily News, 131
    New York Times, 130–131
    The Times, 128–129, 130, 132,
        134–135
*The Nine Circles of the Hell of the
    Innocent*, 128–131
opposition to Horsley, as
    candidate for Parliament,
    124–125
public rallies as part of, 128
Queen Victoria and, 128
Research Defence Society in
    opposition to, 135
Royal Commission of Enquiry
    into Vivisection, 128
Second Royal Commission on
    Vivisection, 134–135
Sherrington, C., and, 130
suffragists in, 128
University College as focus of,
    128
Victoria Street Society, 128
aphasia, 39
    Broca, Paul, on, 38–39
    Brown-Séquard, C. E., on, 39
    Wernicke, Carl, 39
arachnoiditis, spinal, 83
archaeological interests, of Horsley,
    100–101
Archibald, Edward, 70
Archway Hospital (London), 76
Armour, Donald, 70
Arnold, F. S., 129
Artists' Rifles, 156, 170
Asquith, H. H. (Prime Minister),
    112, 137, 138, 166
athetosis, surgical treatment of, 81
Austen, Jane, 1

Babbage, Charles, 49
Babtie, William, 160, 161,
    166
Baden-Powell, Robert, 1
Bailey, Percival, 91, 94

Balfour, Arthur, 113
Ballance, Charles, 15, 58, 70, 77, 130, 171
Barrington, Frederick, 67
Barry, Bishop Alfred, 129, 130
Bartholomow, Roberts, 48
Bastian, Charlton, 10
Baudelaire, Charles, 1
Bayliss, William, 131–132
Beatrice (Princess), 1–2
Beck, Adolf, 47–48
Beck, Marcus, 11–12, 19–20
Bedales School, 98, 170
Beevor, Charles, 8
  cerebral localization research, 34, 42–44
Bell, Charles, 5
Bell, Ernest, 132
Bellevue Hospital, New York City, 93
Bennett, James, 5–6
Bergmann, Ernst von, 73, 74–75
Bernard, Claude, 25, 96, 128
Berthold, Arnold Adolph, 25
Bingley, A. H., 162
Bloody Sunday, 19
Bloxham (Dr.), 107
Boer War, 119
Bond, Charles, 8, 15, 16
Bordeu, Théophile de, 25
Bouisson remedy, for rabies, 32
Boyce, Rubert, 18, 89
Bradley, David, 105–106
Brain, 12–13, 15, 40, 67
brain, of Horsley, preservation of, 170
The Brain as an Organ of Mind (Bastian), 10
brain development. *See* cerebral localization
brain studies, for cerebral localization of brain functions, 48–49
  by electrical stimulation, 48–49
brain tumors. *See* intracranial tumors
brain-mind relationship, 8–9
Bramwell, Eldred. *See* Horsley, Eldred
British Expeditionary Force, rum ration for, 148
British Institute of Preventive Medicine (Lister Institute), 33, 129
British Medical Association, 96, 108, 117–118, 173
  on animal experimentation, 134
    resolutions on, 129–130
  medical reforms as focus of, conflict over, 117–118
  National Insurance Bill and, 122, 123–124

nurses and, registration mechanisms for, 112
on venereal diseases, reform approach to, 152, 153
British Medical Journal, 8, 112, 118, 138, 148, 164–165
British Red Cross Society, 112–113, 158
British Temperance Society, 96
British Union for the Abolition of Vivisection, 134
Broadbent, Sir William, 144
Broca, Paul, 38–39
  aphasia, description of, 39
Brodie, Sir Benjamin, 4–5
Bronte, Charlotte, 1
Brotherhood Movement of Free Churches, 101, 159
Brown, Thomas, 22–24. *See also* Brown Animal Sanatory Institution
Brown Animal Sanatory Institution
  antivivisectionist movement and, as target of, 23
  Burdon Sanderson and, 22, 23–24
  clinical practices of, 22–23
    for vaccine development, 23–24
  closing of, 24
  establishment of, 22–24
  goals and purposes of, 22
  Horsley and, 24
    canine chorea and, 34
    cerebral localization and, 34
    rabies research by, 24, 27–34
    resignation of, 34
    thyroid gland research by, 24, 26–27
  Sharpey, W., and, 22
Brown Dog Affair, 124–125, 131–133
  Bayliss, W., and, 131–132
  lawsuit as result of, 131–132
  student protests as result of, 133
Brown-Séquard, Charles Édouard, 25–26, 27, 98, 128, 171
  on aphasic patients, 39
  on cerebral localization of brain functions, 49
Brunel, Isambard Kingdom, 4–5
Brunton, Sir Lauder, 28–30, 144
Buchanan, James, 1
Bucknall, Rupert, 20
Bucy, Paul, 81
Burdett-Coutts, Angela, 128
Buxton, Dudley, 8

Calcott, Augustus Wall, 1
Calcott, Elizabeth Hutchins. *See* Horsley, Elizabeth Hutchins
callosotomy, for epilepsy, 73
Cameron Prize, 95

canine chorea, 34
Carswell, Robert, 5–6
Carter, Brudenell, 110
Cat and Mouse Act. *See* Prisoners (Temporary Discharge for Ill-Health) Act
Caton, Richard, 47–48
Cecil, Lord Robert, 140
cerebral cortex, 38
  electrical activity of, 47–48
cerebral localization, of brain functions
  Beck, A., and, 47–48
  Beevor, C., and, 34, 42–44
  in brain studies, 48–49
    for electrical stimulation, 48–49
  Brown-Séquard, C. E., and, 39, 49
  Caton, R., and, 47–48
  in cerebral cortex, 38
    electrical activity of, 47–48
  Ferrier and, 48, 49
    Cruelty of Animals Act of 1876, 42
    Goltz and, confrontation between, 41–42
    motor cortex, 44
    for movement disturbances, 40–41
  Gotch, F., and, 46–48
  historical development of, 38
  Horsley involvement in, 42–49
    Croonian lectures and, 46–47
    Gotch and, 46–47
    Jackson, J. H., and, 39, 40–41, 48–49
  for language
    aphasia, 39
    Broca, P., and, 38–39
    Brown-Séquard, C. E., and, 39
    disturbances in, 38–39
    Wernicke, Carl, 39
  for motor cortex
    Horsley involvement in, 44–46
    laryngeal, 45–46
    perirolandic cortex, 44
    prerolandic cortex, 44–45
  for movement and its disturbances, 39–41
    anesthesia and, 41
    in animals, 40–41
    convulsive seizures, 40
    Ferrier, D., and, 40–41
  phrenologists and, 38
  Schäfer, E. *See* Sharpey-Schafer, Edward
  Semon and, 34, 42–44, 45
  Sharpey-Schafer, E. (previously Schäfer, E.) and, 34, 42, 44, 48
  Yeo, G., and, 41–42, 44
cervical dystonia (torticollis), 81

Chandler, Edward, 54
Chandler, Johanna, 54
Chandler, Louisa, 54
Charcot, Jean-Martin, 56, 57
Charlotte (Queen), 54
child welfare issues, 118–120
    during Boer War, 119
    under Children's Act of 1908,
        118–119, 144
    compulsory education
        requirements, 119–120
    in London, 119–120
    under Education Bill of 1902, 119
    medical inspections as part of,
        119–120
    nutrition requirements and
        standards, 119
    poverty as, 118–119
    social activism for, ix
Children's Act of 1908, UK,
    118–119, 144
Church of England,
    antivivisectionist movement
    and, 129
Churchill, Winston, 139
Clark, Andrew, 130
Clarke, Robert, 61, 64–68, 77–78.
    See also Horsley-Clarke
    stereotactic apparatus
Cleveland Clinic, 91, 96
Clinical Society of London, 26
Coalition for Medical Progress, 135
Cobbe, Frances Power, 128, 174
    The Nine Circles of the Hell of the
        Innocent and, involvement
        in, 128–131
Coleridge, Stephen, 128, 131, 134,
    135, 174
College of Nursing, 112–113
Collie (Dr.), 107
Colmore, Gertrude, 128
color-blindness, of Horsley, 5
Commission of Hydrophobia, 24
Companion of the Order of the
    Bath, 161
comparative anatomy, Horsley and,
    94–95
compulsory education
    requirements, 119–120
    in London, 119–120
Congress of American Physicians
    and Surgeons, 59
Conrad, Joseph, 1
"contract practice,", 120–121
convulsive seizures, 40
Cooper, Irving, 81
coroners, 113–114
    responsibilities of, 113
Cox, Alfred, 113
Cranbrook, Kent, Willesley country
    home, 2–5
    construction and design of, 2

as holiday home, 5
Cranbrook colony, 2–3
Cranbrook School, 3–4
    foundation of, 3–4
    foundationer students at, 4
cranial surgery procedure, of
    Horsley, 177–178
    bleeding during, control of, 178
    brain incision, 178
    closure, 178
    drainage, 178
    dura incision, 178
    hemostasis, 177–178
    operative exposure, 177
    staged procedures, 177
    suboccipital craniectomy, 177
craniectomy. See suboccipital
    craniectomy
Crichton-Browne, James, 40
Crile, George Washington, 91, 96,
    134–135
Critchley, Macdonald, 175
Croonian lectures, 46–47, 95
Crowden, Charles, 3–4
Cruelty to Animals Act, Great
    Britain (1876), 23, 42
The Cure of Consumption
    (Alabone), 110
Currie, Sir Donald, 10
Cushing, Harvey, 63, 70, 77, 157
    historical legacy of, 172
    Horsley and, 93–94, 172
    intracranial pressure studies by,
        74–75
Cushing's reflex/Cushing's law, 75

Dale, Henry, 131
Dandy, Walter, 77
Darwin, Charles, 5
Dawson, Margaret Damer, 128
Dax, Gustave, 39
Dax, Marc, 39
death, in Mesopotamia
    causes of, 163
    letters received after, 164–167
    during military service, ix, 156,
        163–164
decompressive surgery, for
    intracranial tumors, 76
Denholm (Dr.), 106–107
Despard, Charlotte, 128, 132
Dickens, Charles, 1, 106
Disraeli, Benjamin, 28–30
The Doctor (Fildes), 19
doctors. See physicians
Dolan, Thomas, 31–32
Dolbeau, Henri-Ferdinand, 63
domestic life, 96–99. See also family
    members; Horsley, Eldred
    children, 97–98
    home residence, 97–98
    marriage, 96–98

Paget, S., on, 97
Duff, Sir Beauchamp, 161, 166
Durante, Francesco, 52–53

education. See also compulsory
    education requirements;
    University College;
    University College Hospital;
    specific colleges and
    universities
Bedales School
    sons at, 98, 170
compulsory requirements,
    119–120
    in London, 119–120
Cranbrook School, 3–4
    foundation of, 3–4
    foundationer students at, 4
Edward VII (King), 11–12, 96
Egypt, during World War I,
    159–161
    family visits to, 160–161
    Gallipoli campaign and, 160–161
    in Mediterranean Expeditionary
        Force, 159–161
    in Royal Army Medical Corps
        (Territorials), 159
Elderton, Ethel, 146–147
electrical stimulation, 63–64
    for epileptic seizures, 72–73
Elements of Anatomy (Quain, J.),
    5–6
Elgar, Edward, 1
Ellis, G. Viner, 6
endocrine system, 6. See also thyroid
    gland
    internal secretions, concept of, 25
epileptic seizures
    electrical stimulation and, 72–73
    Jackson, J. H., and, 72
    localization of, 52
    neurosurgery for, 52–54, 71–73
        callosotomy, 73
        experimental work in, 72–73
        historical background on,
            71–72
        by Horsley, 52, 53–54, 61–62,
            64
        at National Hospital, 57, 61
expert medical witness, Horsley as,
    94

family members, 1–2, 4–5. See also
    specific people
    grandparents, 1
    parents, 1–2
    siblings, 2
Ferguson, Sir William, 57
Ferrier, David, 12–13, 41, 52, 56, 95,
    171
    on cerebral localization of brain
        functions, 48, 49

Goltz and, confrontation between, 41–42
for movement, 40–41
filariasis, 135
Fildes, Sir Luke, 19
Flaubert, Gustave, 1
Fleming, George, 28
Flexner, Abraham, 172
forcible feeding, of prisoners, 137–141
Ford, Isabella, 128
Forschungen und Erfahrungen (Research and Experience) (Semon), 94
Foster, Michael, 6
Foster Kennedy syndrome, 77
Fothergill Gold Medal, 95
foundationer students, at Cranbrook School, 4
Fox, Wilson, 10–11
France
cerebral localization of brain functions, historical development of, 38
Salpêtrière Hospital, 56
during World War I, 158–159
in Wimereux, hospitals in, 158–159
French, Sir John, 128, 141
Freud, Sigmund, 91
Freyberger, Ludwig, 113
Fritsch, Gustav Theodor, 40
The Functions of the Brain (Ferrier), 12–13, 41

Gallipoli campaign, 160–161
Galton, Francis, 5
Gaskell, W. H., 95
gender equality, social activism for, ix
General Medical Council, 10–11, 90–91, 96, 106, 108–111, 173
Alabone and, 110–111
Horsley and, election to, 109–111
Horsley election to, 109–111
Medical Act of 1858 and, 108–109
Medical Act of 1886 and, 108–109
Medical Register, 108, 109–110
midwives registration and, 111–112
purpose of, 108
registration mechanisms, for midwives, 111–112
General Nursing Council for England and Wales, 113
George, David Lloyd, 122, 123–124, 137, 148, 158. *See also* National Insurance Bill
George III (King), 54
George IV (King), 95
George V (King), 11–12, 19, 96

Germany, cerebral localization of brain functions, historical development of, 38
Gilbey, Captain Walter, 57, 70, 82
Gladstone, Herbert, 133, 138
Gladstone, William, 133
Glasgow Pathological and Clinical Society, 52–53
Godlee, Rickman, 11–12, 27, 52, 56, 117, 140, 174
row with Horsley, about cleansing war wounds, 158
Goltz, Friedrich, 41–42
gonorrhea, 151
Gordon Highlanders, 156
Gotch, Francis, 2, 6–7, 8, 46–48, 72, 95, 97
Gotch, Oliver Henry, 98
Gowers, William, 8, 11–12, 56, 58, 59, 77, 95, 145
The Grammar of Science (Pearson), 146
Grant Medical College, 161
Great Britain. *See also* London; *specific topics*
cerebral localization of brain functions, historical development of, 38
Cruelty to Animals Act, 23, 42
rabies in, 28–34, 172–173
animal control strategies, 32
eradication of, 33–34
outbreak in deer at Richmond Park, 31
quarantine regulations in, 33
Green, Joseph, 32
Greenfield, William, 24, 28
Grünbaum. *See* Leyton, Albert S. F.
Guillain-Barré syndrome, 32
Gulbenkian, Calouste, 170
Gull, Sir William, 26
gunshot wounds to head, research on, 156–157
clinical aspects of, 157
intracranial pressure intervention, 157
physics of, 156–157
at Royal Institution, 156

Haden, Charles Thomas, 1
Haden, Francis Seymour, 1, 4
Haden, Rosamund. *See* Horsley, Rosamund
Haden, William, correspondence with, 133–134
Hageby, Louise Lind af, 124–125, 128, 131, 132, 133
Handbook for the Physiological Laboratory, 23–24
Handelsmann, Dr., 78–79
Harcourt, Sir William, 105–106
Hardinge, Lord, 166

Harley, Vaughan, 18, 90
Hartley, Frank, 84
Heath, Christopher, 11–12, 18–19
hemostasis, during intracranial surgery, 63, 177–178
Henry VIII (King), 3–4, 24, 96
Herren, R. Y., 73
Hill, Berkeley, 11
Hine, J. E., 8
historical legacy, of Horsley, 171–175
Hitzig, Eduard, 40
Horsley, Eldred (née Bramwell) (wife), 17, 96–98, 135, 170
after death of Horsley (husband), 171
in Egypt, 160–161
suffragist movement and, 137
Horsley, Elizabeth Hutchins (née Calcott) (grandmother), 1
Horsley, Emma Mary (sister), 2
Horsley, Fanny Marian (sister), 2, 15
Horsley, Gerald Callcott (brother), 2, 4, 89
Horsley, Hugh John (brother), 2
Horsley, John Callcott (father), 1, 4
as celebrated painter, 1
of Princess Beatrice, 1–2
Horsley, Mary Elizabeth, 4–5
Horsley, Oswald (son), 98, 170
Horsley, Pamela Comfrey (née Robinson) (daughter), 98, 160–161, 170
Horsley, Rosamund (née Haden) (mother), 1–2
Horsley, Rosamund Brunel (sister), 2, 7–8, 98
marriage of, 2, 97
works of, 2
Horsley, Siward (son), 97–98, 170
Horsley, Victor. *See also specific topics*
last will of, 170
Horsley, Walter Charles (brother), 2
Horsley, William (grandfather), 1
Horsley-Clarke stereotactic apparatus, 61, 64–68, 77–78, 82
animal studies with, 65, 67–68
patents for, 67
prototypes for, 67
Hospital for Diseases of the Nervous System, 56
hospital ships, during World War I, 160, 164–165, 166
House, William, 77
Humphry, George, 130
hunger strikes, by suffragists, 138
in *British Medical Journal*, 138
forcible feeding as response to, 138, 139

hunger strikes (cont.)
government response to, 139,
140–141
Leigh v. Gladstone, 138
under Prisoners (Temporary
Discharge for Ill-Health)
Act, 140–141
Huxley, Thomas, 5, 33, 130
hydrophobia, 28. *See also* rabies
Society for the Prevention of
Hydrophobia, 33
hypothyroidism, 27

Imperial College of Science and
Technology, 5
Indian Medical Service, 160–161
Infamous Conduct (Alabone), 111
*Instincts of the Herd in Peace and
War* (Trotter), 19
"insuline," discovery of, 6
insurance reforms. *See* National
Insurance Bill
International Medical Congress, 59,
129–130
intracranial aneurysms, 82
intracranial pressure, experimental
studies of, 73–74
clinical aspects of, 75
Cushing and, 74–75
experimental approaches to,
73–74
intracranial tumors, neurosurgery
for, 75–77
decompressive surgery, 76
hemispherectomy, 76
lobectomy, 76
papilledema and, localizing value
of, 76–77
Ireland, home rule for, 125
Isaacs, Rufus, 131–132

Jackson, J. Hughlings, 39, 40–41,
48–49, 52, 56–57, 64, 77, 95,
171
Jenner, Sir William, 12, 58, 106
Jodrell, T. J. Phillips, 6
Jones, Ernest, 91, 92
Joyce, Thomas, 5

Keen, William, 48, 64, 70, 82
Kennedy, Robert Foster, 77,
92–93
Keogh, Sir Alfred, 160
Keynes, John Maynard, 146
Kingsford, Anna, 128
Kitchener, Lord, 157
Klein, Edward Emanuel, 42, 95
Kocher, Emil Theodor, 26, 74–75,
93, 171, 172
Kramer, S. P., 157
Krause, Feodor, 48, 64, 83, 84
Kronecker, Hugo, 74

Lancet, 55–56, 89, 106, 144–145, 152
Landry's paralysis. *See* Guillain-
Barré syndrome
language, cerebral localization of
aphasia and, 39
Broca and, 38–39
Brown-Séquard and, 39
language disturbances, 38–39
Lankester, Ray, 33
Lannelongue, Marie, 96
Lannelongue, Odilon, 96
Lannelongue Prize, 96, 143
laryngeal motor cortex, 45–46
Leigh, Marie, 138
Leigh v. Gladstone, 138
Leighton, Sir Frederic, 16
Lenton, Lilian, 140
Leyton, Albert S. F. (Grünbaum),
44–45, 89–90
Liberal Party, 124–125
Linacre, Thomas, 96
Lister, Joseph, 5, 10–11, 28, 33, 56,
95. *See also* antiseptic
approach
Lister Institute. *See* British Institute
of Preventive Medicine
Liszt, Franz, 1
Liverpool School of Tropical
Medicine, 18
Lobb, Harry, 55–56
lobectomy, 76
London, England. *See also* National
Hospital
Archway Hospital, 76
compulsory education
requirements in, 119–120
neurological hospitals in, 54–57
Hospital for Diseases of the
Nervous System, 56
London Galvanic Hospital,
55–56
London Infirmary for Epilepsy
and Paralysis, 56
National Hospital for the
Paralysed and Epileptic, 10,
49
West End Hospital for Diseases
of the Nervous System,
Paralysis, and Epilepsy, 56
London Galvanic Hospital, 55–56
London Infirmary for Epilepsy and
Paralysis, 56
Long, Walter, 33
Louis XV (King), 25
Löwenthal, Max, 64–65
Lukis, Sir Pardey, 161, 163

Macewen, William, 52–53, 96, 172,
178
spinal surgery by, 58, 84
MacNeece, James, 166
Magendie, François, 25, 26, 63

Magnus, Sir Philip, 5, 124–125
Magnus, Vilhelm, 70
malpractice protection, ix. *See also*
Medical Defence Union
Manson, Sir Patrick, 135
Maple, Sir John Blundell, 10
Maria, Lady Callcott (Horsley,
R. B.), 2
Marshall, Alfred, 146
Marshall, John, 10–11, 19–20, 34, 95
Martel, Thierry de, 70
Martin, Sidney, 18
Martin-Leake, Colonel, 95
McCann, Isabel, 92
McCarrison, Robert, 160–161
McKenna, Reginald, 139, 140
McMillan, Margaret, 119–120
McMillan, Rachel, 119–120
Medical Act, UK (1858), 106,
108–109
Medical Act, UK (1886), 108–109
Medical Defence Union, 90–91, 96,
105–108, 173
malpractice insurance and, 106
Medical Act of 1858 and, 106
membership levels in, 108
mixed reception to, 106
medical practices, development of
for antiseptic approach, 5
institutional reform of, ix
for nursing, 5
qualifications for nurses, ix
standardization of disease
certification, ix
treatment strategies for sexually
transmitted diseases, ix
Medical Protection Society, 108
Medical Register, 108, 109–110
Medical Reports, of West Riding
Lunatic Asylum, 40, 41
Medical Society of London, 95
medicine, as career. *See also* medical
practices; registration
mechanisms; University
College; *specific topics*
early interest in, by Horsley, 5
Mediterranean Expeditionary
Force, 159–161
Mellus, E. Lindon, 89
memorials, for Horsley, 171
*Mendelssohn and his friends in
Kensington* (Horsley, R. B.), 2
Mercier, Charles, 139, 148
Mesopotamia
Anglo-Persian Oil Company, 162
death of Horsley in
causes of, 163
letters received after, 164–167
during military service, ix, 156,
163–164
Horsley in, 161–163
Meyers (friend), 94

Middlesex Hospital Medical
Society, 100
Midwifery Council, 113
midwives, registration mechanisms
for, 111–112
by General Medical Council,
111–112
Midwifery Council, 113
Midwives Act, UK (1902), 111
military service
death during, in Mesopotamia, ix,
156, 163–164
of Foster Kennedy, 93
Mitchell, Silas Weir, 38
Money, Angel, 8
morality, venereal diseases and, 151
The Morning Post, 152
Morris, Sir Malcolm, 152
Mosso, Angelo, 74, 172
motor cortex, studies of
Horsley involvement in, 44–46
laryngeal, 45–46
perirolandic cortex, 44
prerolandic cortex, 44–45
Mott, Frederick, 8, 16
Moullin, Charles Mansell, 139, 140
movement disorders, neurosurgery
for, 81–82
athetosis, 81
cervical dystonia, 81
with Horsley-Clarke stereotactic
apparatus, 82
Parkinson's disease, 81
movement disturbances, cerebral
localization and, 39–41
anesthesia and, 41
in animals, 40–41
convulsive seizures, 40
Ferrier and, 40–41
Moxon, Frank, 141
Muirhead, Gertrude, 113–114
Murray, George Redmayne, 27
myxedema, 26. See also thyroid
gland

National Anti-Vivisection Society,
128, 131
National Hospital (at Queen
Square), 18, 54–55, 56–57.
See also neurosurgery;
individual physicians
Gowers at, 56, 59. See also
Gowers, William
Horsley at
admitting privileges for, 58–59
appointment to, 18, 56
spinal surgery by, 57–58
surgeries for epileptic seizures,
57, 61–62, 64
Jackson at, 56–57, 64. See also
Jackson, J. Hughlings

Kennedy at, 92–93. See also
Kennedy, Robert Foster
origins of, 54–55
peripheral nerve injury surgery
at, 85
staffing at, 56–57
National Hospital for the Paralysed
and Epileptic, 10, 49
National Insurance Bill, UK, ix, 117,
120–124, 158, 173–174
British Medical Association and,
122, 123–124
"contract practice" and, 120–121
physicians' public response to,
122–123
Royal Commission on the Poor
Laws and, 122
Naunyn, Bernhard, 74–75, 172
Neosalvarsan, 151
nervi nervorum, 17
neuralgia. See trigeminal neuralgia
neurological hospitals, in London.
See London
Neurological Institute, New York
City, 93
Neurological Society of London, 96,
170
neurosurgery
Cushing and
historical legacy of, 172
intracranial pressure and,
74–75
for epilepsy, 71–73
callosotomy, 73
experimental and clinical work
on, 72–73
historical background on,
71–72
Horsley's techniques for, 62–68
anesthesia use, 63
electrical stimulation, 63–64
hemostasis and, 63
historical legacy of, 85–86,
91–94
Horsley-Clarke stereotactic
apparatus, 61, 64–68, 82
for intracranial aneurysms, 82
for intracranial pressure, 73–74
clinical studies of, 75
Cushing and, 74–75
experimental approaches to,
73–74
for intracranial tumors, 75–77
decompressive surgery, 76
hemispherectomy, 76
lobectomy, 76
papilledema and, localizing
value of, 76–77
for movement disorders, 81–82
athetosis, 81
cervical dystonia, 81

with Horsley-Clarke
stereotactic apparatus, 82
Parkinson's disease, 81
for peripheral nerve injuries,
84–85
at National Hospital, 85
for pineal tumors, 80–81
for pituitary tumors, 78–80
animal studies for, 78–79
experimental work by Horsley,
78–80
in human subjects, 79–80
non-functioning tumors, 78
for posterior fossa tumors, 77–78
stereotactic surgery, 77–78
Scandinavian school, 70
for spinal surgery, 57–58, 82–83
arachnoiditis and, 83
tuberculosis disease, 82–83
for trigeminal neuralgia, 83–84
New York City. See Bellevue
Hospital; Neurological
Institute
New York Times, inspection of
Horsley laboratory and,
130–131
Nightingale, Florence, 5
St. John's Nursing Services, 54
The Nine Circles of the Hell of the
Innocent (Rhodes), 128–131
Nobel Prize, Horsley nominated for,
172
Norman, Priscilla, 158–159
Norman, Sir Henry, 158–159
North London or University College
Hospital Report of the
Surgical Register, 17–18
nurses, nursing and
British Red Cross Society,
112–113
Order of St. John of Jerusalem
and, 112–113
registration mechanisms for,
112–113
British Medical Association
and, 112
General Nursing Council for
England and Wales, 113
training for, 18
College of Nursing, 112–113
Royal College of Nursing, 113
nutrition and health care for
children, 119

Oliver, George, 6
On Failure of Brain Power (Althaus),
56
Oppenheim, Hermann, 80
The Origin of the Species (Darwin), 5
Osler, Sir William, 24, 58, 93–94,
123, 172

Paget, Sir James, 28, 33, 95, 1
    30
Paget, Stephen, 97
Pankhurst, Christabel, 137
Pankhurst, Emmeline, 137, 141
papilledema, localizing value of,
    76–77
Parkinson's disease, 81
Parliament, candidate for, 124–125
    antivivisectionist opposition,
        124–125
    in Liberal Party, 124–125
    symbolism of candidacy, 125
Pasteur, Louis, 95, 128
    rabies work of, 28–33, 134
Pathological Society of London, 152
La Patologia Chirurgica dell'Ipofisi
    (Surgical Pathology of the
    Hypophysis) (Verga), 79
Pattison, Granville Sharp, 5–6
Paul, Frank Thomas, 79
Pearson, Karl, 90, 143, 146, 173, 174
    alcohol use study
        conflicts with Horsley, 146–147
        criticism of, 146
        parental alcoholism as
            influence on, 146
Pease, Jack (Lord Gainford), 120
Penfield, Wilder, 48, 64, 96
peripheral nerve injuries,
    neurosurgery for, 84–85
perirolandic cortex, 44
Petit, François Pourfour du, 38
Philomathic Society, 8–9
phrenologists, 38
physicians
    educational standards for,
        establishment of, 106. See
        also General Medical
        Council; Medical Act, UK
        (1858); Medical Act, UK
        (1886)
    reaction to National Insurance
        Bill, 122–123
    Society for the Study of Inebriety,
        144
Pietri, Dorando, 133–134
pineal tumors, 80–81
pituitary tumors, 78–80
    animal studies and, 78–79
    experimental work by Horsley,
        78–80
    neurosurgery for, by Horsley,
        79–80
    non-functioning tumors, 78
pleuropneumonia, 23–24
politics. See Parliament; social
    activism
Pollard, Bilton, 8, 96
posterior fossa tumors, 77–78
poverty
    as child welfare issue, 118–119

Royal Commission on the Poor
    Laws, 122
prerolandic cortex, 44–45
The Pride of the Village (Horsley, J.), 1
Prison Act of 1898, UK, 137–138
Prisoners (Temporary Discharge for
    Ill-Health) Act, UK (1913),
    140–141
Public Health (Venereal Diseases)
    Regulations of 1916, UK,
    153–154
publications, of Horsley
    professional (scientific), 182–197
    in The Times of London, 198–199

Quain, Jones, 5–6
Quain, Richard, 5–6, 28–30
Queen Square, London. See also
    National Hospital (at Queen
    Square)
    National Hospital in, 18, 54–55,
        56–57
    St. John's Nursing Services, 54

rabies
    causes of, 27–29
    diagnosis of, 28
    in Great Britain, 28–34, 172–173
        animal control strategies, 32
        eradication of, 33–34
        muzzling and, 32
        outbreak in deer in Richmond
            Park, 31
        quarantine regulations in, 33
    Guillain-Barré syndrome and, 32
    mortality rates for, 27–28
    Pasteur's work on, 28–33, 134
    research on
        animal inoculations as part of,
            30–31
        by Horsley, at Brown Animal
            Sanatory Institution, 24,
            27–34
    symptoms of, 28
    treatment strategies for, 32–33
        Bouisson remedy, 32
Radcliffe, Charles, 98
Recollections of a Royal Academician
    (Skerrett), 1–2
registration mechanisms, 111–113
    for midwives, 111–112
        by General Medical Council,
            111–112
        Midwifery Council, 113
        under Midwives Act, 111
    for nurses, 112–113
        British Medical Association,
            112
        General Nursing Council for
            England and Wales, 113
Rent Day at Haddon Hall (Horsley,
    J.), 1

Research Defence Society, 135
Reverdin, Auguste, 26
Reverdin, Jacques-Louis, 26
Reynolds, Sir Russell, 11–12
Rhodes, G. M., 128–131
Rideal, Charles F., 106
Ridsdale, E. A., 162
Ringer, Sidney, 10–11, 19
Robinson, Edward Stanley Gotch,
    170
Robinson, Pamela Comfrey. See
    Horsley, Pamela Comfrey
Roman Empire, surgery during, 100
Romanes, George John, 95, 152
Roscoe, Sir Henry, 28–30, 33
Ross, Ronald, 1
Roy, Charles Smart, 24, 33
Royal Army Medical Corps
    (Territorials), 159
Royal College of Nursing, 113
Royal College of Surgeons of
    England, 10–11, 17, 91,
    110–111, 117, 140, 158
    Godlee, R., and, 117
    Horsley becomes a fellow of, 17
    lack of representation of
        members, 117
Royal Commission of Enquiry into
    Vivisection, UK, 128
Royal Commission on the Poor
    Laws, 122
Royal Society of London, 41, 58, 95,
    179
Royal Society of Medicine, 26, 77,
    80–81
Royal Society of Painter-Etchers
    and Engravers, 1
Royal Society of Printmakers, 1
Ruffer, M. Armand, 129
Rule 243A, UK (1910), 139
rum rations, 148–149
    for British Expeditionary Force,
        148
Runciman, Walter, 119–120
Russell, James Risien, 91

Sachs, Ernest, 67, 70, 81, 91
St. John's Nursing Services, 54
Salpêtrière Hospital, 56
Salvarsan, 151, 154
Sanderson, John Burdon, 6–7, 8, 9,
    17–18, 42, 46
    Brown Animal Sanatory
        Institution and, 22, 23–24
Sargent, Percy, 70
Savill, Agnes, 139, 140
Scandinavian school, of
    neurosurgery, 70
Schäfer, E. See Sharpey-Schafer,
    Edward
Schäfer, Edward. See Sharpey-
    Schafer, Edward

Schartau, Leisa K., 131, 132
Schiff, Moritz, 26, 171
scientific awards and honors, of
    Horsley, 95–96, 179–181
  Cameron Prize, 95
  Croonian lecture, 46–47, 95
  Fellowship of Royal Society, 95
  Fothergill Gold Medal, 95
  Lannelongue Prize, 96, 143
  Nobel Prize nominations, 172
  society memberships, 96
  Second Royal Commission on
    Vivisection, UK, 134–135
Semon, Felix, 26
  cerebral localization research, 34,
    42–44, 45
  relations with Horsley, 94
Semple, David, 160
sex education, venereal disease
    prevention for children, 153
Shaftesbury, Lord, 128
The Shambles of Science (Hageby
    and Schartau), 131, 132
Sharpey, William, 5–6
  Brown Animal Sanatory
    Institution and, 22
Sharpey-Schafer, Edward, 6–7,
    17–18, 26, 56, 95, 171
  cerebral localization research, 42,
    44, 48
  conflict with Horsley, 90
Shaw, Richard Norman, 2–3
Sherrington, Charles, 1, 34, 44–45,
    48, 64–65, 93, 174
  during antivivisectionist conflict,
    130
  conflict with Horsley, 89–90
Silk, John, 8
Skerrett, Marianne, 1–2
Smith, F. J., 123
social activism, ix, 173, 174. See also
    specific activities and
    organizations
  in suffragist movement, violence
    as part of, 137
  Lenton, L., and, 140
Society for the Prevention of
    Hydrophobia, 33
Spencer, Walter, 74
Spiller, W. G., 83
spinal arachnoiditis. See
    arachnoiditis
spinal surgery
  arachnoiditis and, 83
  by Horsley, at National Hospital,
    57–58, 82–83
  by Macewen, 58, 84
  tuberculous disease, 82–83
spinal tuberculosis, 82–83
spontaneous generation of life, 10
Squire, P. W., 63, 177–178
Stanley, Arthur, 112–113

Starling, Ernest, 131, 132, 134,
    135
stereotactic surgery, 77–78. See also
    Horsley-Clarke stereotactic
    apparatus
Stevenson, Robert Louis, 54
Sturge, Mary, 144, 145, 146–147,
    149
suboccipital craniectomy, 177
suffragette, as derogatory term, 128
suffragist movement, women's
    rights and
  activist violence as part of, 137
  Lenton, L., and, 140
  Horsley, Eldred, and, influence of,
    137
  organizations in, 137
  Sir Almroth Wright's letter in
    The Times, 139
  Women's Social and Political
    Union and, 137
suffragists
  in antivivisectionist movement,
    128
  hunger strikes by, 138
    in British Medical Journal, 138
    forcible feeding as response to,
      138, 139
    government response to, 139,
      140–141
    Leigh v. Gladstone, 138
    Prisoners (Temporary
      Discharge for Ill-Health) Act
      and, 140–141
  imprisonment of, 137–138
    under Rule 243A, 139
    under Prison Act of 1898,
      137–138
Surgical Pathology of the
    Hypophysis. See La Patologia
    Chirurgica dell'Ipofisi
surgical registrar
  Horsley as, 14–18, 152
  resignation from, 18
  responsibilities of, 17–18
Swayne, Martin, 163
Swedenborg, Emanuel, 38
Swetmore, Eliza, 105–106
Swift, James, 67
Swift, Sarah, 112–113
Sydenham of Combe (Lord), 152
syphilis, 151, 152. See also venereal
    diseases
  earliest appearances of, 151
  symptoms and long-term
    implications of, 151
  treatment of, 151, 152

Taft, William Howard, 1
Tait, Robert Lawson, 106–107, 130
temperance movement, 173. See also
    alcohol abuse; alcohol use

British Medical Association and,
    144
British Medical Temperance
    Association, 144
International Association of
    Abstaining Physicians, 144
medical advocates in, 144
National Temperance League,
    144
Society for the Study of Inebriety,
    144
Territorials. See Royal Army
    Medical Corps
Thackeray, William Makepeace, 1
Thane, George Dancer, 6–7
Third London General Hospital, 158
Thompson, Joseph John, 95
Thompson, Seth, 4
thyroid gland
  hypothyroidism and, treatment
    of, 27
  research on
    early influences on, 26
    history of, 24–27
    by Horsley, at Brown Animal
      Sanatory Institution, 24,
      26–27
    myxedema and, 26
The Times, 91, 114, 123, 138, 158,
    166
  antivivisectionist movement in,
    128–129, 130, 132, 134–135
  suffragist movement in, 139
torticollis. See cervical dystonia
Treatise on Medical Electricity
    (Althaus), 56
trephining, during Neolithic period,
    99–100
Treves, Sir Frederick, 19
trigeminal neuralgia, 83–84
Trinity College. See University of
    Dublin
Trollope, Anthony, 1
Trotter, Wilfred, 19, 20, 70
Troutbeck, John, 113–114, 173, 174
Truman, Harry, 19
Tubby, Alfred, 160
tuberculosis, spinal, 82–83
tumors. See specific tumors
Turner, George Grey, 164
Turner, Sydney, 33
Tyndall, John, 95

The Unexpurgated Case Against
    Woman Suffrage (Wright,
    A.), 139
United Kingdom (UK). See also
    Great Britain; specific topics
  Children's Act of 1908, 118–119,
    144
  General Nursing Council for
    England and Wales, 113

United Kingdom (UK) (cont.)
Medical Act of 1858, 106, 108–109
Medical Act of 1886, 108–109
Midwives Act, 111
National Insurance Bill, ix, 117,
120–124, 158, 173–174
British Medical Association
and, 122, 123–124
"contract practice" and,
120–121
physicians' public response to,
122–123
Royal Commission on the Poor
Laws and, 122
Prison Act of 1898, 137–138
Prisoners (Temporary Discharge
for Ill-Health) Act, 140–141
Public Health (Venereal Diseases)
Regulations of 1916, 153–154
Royal Commission of Enquiry
into Vivisection, 128
Royal Commission on the Poor
Laws, 122
Rule 243A, 139
Second Royal Commission on
Vivisection, 134–135
Venereal Diseases Act of 1917,
153–154
United States (US)
American Neurological
Association, 48, 93
cerebral localization of brain
functions, historical
development of, 38
Congress of American Physicians
and Surgeons, 59
University College, London, 5–9
antivivisectionist movement and,
128
appointments at, 16, 18, 19
establishment as medical school,
5–6
professors and, 5–6
fellow students, 8
Philomathic Society, 8–9
scientific approach at, 8
University College Hospital
administrative appointments
at, 19
antiseptic approach, 16
clinical appointments at, 15, 17–19
clinical training at, 10–13
establishment of, 10

teaching staff at, 10–13
Horsley as vice dean, 19
University of Dublin (Trinity
College), 22, 24
University of London, 5, 10, 19. See
also Brown Animal Sanatory;
University College, London

Van Wagenen, W. P., 73
venereal diseases, 151–152
alcohol use and, 153
gonorrhea, 151
morality and, 151
under Public Health (Venereal
Diseases) Regulations of
1916, 153–154
reform in approach to, agitation
for, 152
British Medical Association
and, 152, 153
through royal commission of
inquiry, 152–154
sex education of children as
element of, 153
syphilis, 151
earliest appearances of,
151
symptoms and long-term
implications of, 151
treatment for, 151, 153, 154
Venereal Diseases Act of 1917, UK,
153–154
Verdi, Giuseppe, 1
Verga, Giovanni, 79
Victoria (Queen), 1–2, 11–12,
156
antivivisectionist movement and,
involvement in, 128
Fox, W., as physician-
extraordinary to, 10–11
Victoria Street Society, 128
Vincent, Clovis, 70
Vincent, Sir William, 162
von Marxow, Fleischl, 47–48

Walshe, Sir Francis, 160,
161
Walter, Elvira, 2
Walton, Lawson, 132
Waterhouse, Paul, 10
Webb, Beatrice, 122
Webster, Thomas, 2–3
Wernicke, Carl, 39

West End Hospital for Diseases
of the Nervous System,
Paralysis, and Epilepsy, 56
Westminster Gazette, 124
Whitaker, Smith, 122–123
Whitehead, James, 32–33
Whitelegge, Benjamin Arthur,
2, 15
Wilks, Samuel, 130
will, of Horsley, Victor, 170
Williams, Dawson, 8, 118
Willis, Thomas, 38
Wilson, S. A. Kinnier, 67
Wimereux, France, hospitals in,
158–159
Wire, David (Alderman), 54
Women's Social and Political
Union, 137
Wood, Ethel, 98
Woodward, Anna Louisa, 132
World Medical Association, 173
World War I
Amara War Cemetery, 164
Artists' Rifles, 156
British Red Cross Society,
158
in Egypt, 159–161
family visits to Horsley,
160–161
in Mediterranean
Expeditionary Force,
159–161
in Royal Army Medical Corps
(Territorials), 159
in France, 158–159
in Wimereux, hospitals in,
158–159
in Gallipoli campaign, 160–161
Gordon Highlanders, 156
hospital ships during, 160,
166
as "insane folly,", 156
medical services during, criticism
of, 157–158
Godlee, R., and, 158
in Mesopotamia, 161–163
death of Horsley in, 156,
163–164
Wright, Sir Almroth, 139,
160

Yeo, Alfred William, 125
Yeo, Gerald, 41–42, 44

Printed in the United States
by Baker & Taylor Publisher Services